Martin Fleishman, MD, PhD

The Casebook of a Residential Care Psychiatrist

Psychopharmacosocioeconomics and the Treatment of Schizophrenia in Residential Care Facilities

Pre-publication
REVIEWS,
COMMENTARIES,
EVALUATIONS . . .

"**D**r. Fleishman's casebook is actually a unique literary work—a textbook, a how-to manual, a professional autobiography, and a plan for legislative/regulatory reform, all rolled into one. This book is a wealth of thoughts, reflections, and entertainment. From a technical standpoint, Dr. Fleishman provides very detailed treatment guidelines well-honed by thirty-five years of compassionate solo practice. The wisdom gained over time infuses his prose, which ranges from serious and direct to smile-inducing one-liners and laugh-out-loud comedic ramblings. I strongly encourage every resident to read and enjoy Dr. Fleishman's deeply thoughtful and uniquely entertaining casebook."

Daniel Ben Bleman, MD
Director of Psychiatry Residency Training,
UMDNJ–New Jersey Medical School

"**D**r. Fleishman presents a unique and relevant perspective on the dehospitalization process that affected many severely ill psychiatric patients during the last half-century. In addition, he offers an excellent description of the role of residential care in today's psychiatric practice in the United States. This book must be read by all psychiatric practitioners. It offers a clear and comprehensive view of the current mental health care system in the United States."

Pedro Ruiz, MD
Vice President,
American Psychiatric Association;
Past President,
American College of Psychiatrists;
Professor and Vice Chair,
Department of Psychiatry
and Behavioral Sciences,
The University of Texas
Medical School at Houston

More pre-publication
REVIEWS, COMMENTARIES, EVALUATIONS . . .

"This is a book of clinical wisdom and gems as well as musings, opinions, and arguments. Dr. Fleishman's self-revealing, irreverent humor and his original way of seeing situations and treating patients make reading this book a delight as well as a profound learning experience. Above all, this book is a strong plea for more psychiatrists to leave their offices and help treat the thousands of needy and fascinating patients who reside in residential care facilities. This is a much-needed book that sheds light on a formerly ignored subject."

Lawrence B. Lurie, MD, DFAPA
Chair, APA Committee on Managed Care;
Clinical Professor of Psychiatry,
University of California, San Francisco

"Dr. Fleishman presents the reader with an unusual blend of puckish humor, hard-earned wisdom, and compassionate understanding when describing the care of psychiatric patients in the residential setting. This book provides an abundance of helpful vignettes, pragmatic advice, and even 'Ten Commandments' for psychiatrists working in residential settings. Unifying all this is the author's zealous effort to understand our patients as fully constituted individuals."

Ronald Pies, MD
Clinical Professor of Psychiatry,
Tufts University School of Medicine

"No one will ever write a more lucid, comprehensive, clinically compelling text on how to provide psychiatric treatment in a residential care facility. Yet Fleishman has also created a masterful memoir of American psychiatry as he has practiced the craft over the last half-century. His fascinating clinical vignettes of dialogues with patients diagnosed with schizophrenia should be standard reading for every psychiatrist. And Fleishman imparts all of his wisdom in a book filled with grace, compassion, and the best sense of humor in American psychiatry."

Richard M. Berlin, MD
Associate Professor of Psychiatry,
University of Massachusetts
Medical School

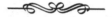

"This is a must-read for residents, teachers, community psychiatrists, and all those who have forgotten what our field is really about."

Stephen M. Goldfinger, MD
Professor and Interim Chair,
Department of Psychiatry,
State University of New York
Downstate Medical Center

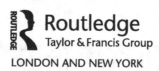
Routledge
Taylor & Francis Group

LONDON AND NEW YORK

The Casebook of a Residential Care Psychiatrist

Psychopharmacosocioeconomics and the Treatment of Schizophrenia in Residential Care Facilities

The Casebook of a Residential Care Psychiatrist

Psychopharmacosocioeconomics and the Treatment of Schizophrenia in Residential Care Facilities

Martin Fleishman, MD, PhD

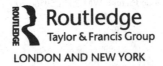

Routledge
Taylor & Francis Group

LONDON AND NEW YORK

First published 2005 by The Haworth Press, Inc.

2 Park Square, Milton Park, Abingdon, Oxfordshire OX14 4RN
605 Third Avenue, New York, NY 10017

Routledge is an imprint of the Taylor & Francis Group, an informa business

First issued in paperback 2020

PUBLISHER'S NOTE
Identities and circumstances of individuals discussed in this book have been changed to protect confidentiality.

Cover design by Jennifer M. Gaska.

Library of Congress Cataloging-in-Publication Data

Fleishman, Martin.
    The casebook of a residential care psychiatrist : psychopharmacosocioeconomics and the treatment of schizophrenia in residential care facilities / Martin Fleishman.
       p. ; cm.
    Includes bibliographical references and index.
    ISBN 0-7890-2372-5 (hard : alk. paper) — ISBN 0-7890-2373-3 (soft : alk. paper)
       1. Mentally ill—Institutional care—United States. 2. Mentally ill—Long-term care—United States. 3. Mental health facilities—United States. 4. Mental health personnel—United States. 5. Psychiatry—Practice—United States. 6. Psychoses—Treatment.
    [DNLM: 1. Schizophrenia—drug therapy. 2. Patient Care Team. 3. Psychiatry—methods. 4. Residential Facilities. 5. Socioeconomic Factors. WM 203 F5956c 2004] I. Title.
    RC443.F56 2004
    362.2'1'0973—dc22

                                   2004002767

ISBN 978-0-7890-2373-5 (pbk)

This book is dedicated to my father,
who taught me how to interact with people;
to my mother, who taught me ambition;
to my daughter, Raina, who taught me fatherhood;
and to my wife, Susan, who insisted that I eat
during the months it took me to complete the manuscript—
otherwise I might not have (eaten, that is).

ABOUT THE AUTHOR

Martin Fleishman, MD, PhD, has fifty years of experience in treating schizophrenia, originally as a clinical psychologist and later as a psychiatrist. At seventy-seven years of age, he still works full time, treating on average 250 patients a month. His work is focused on the provision of on-site treatment for the mentally ill residents of residential care facilities. He has written articles on the role of psychiatrists in board-and-care homes and on how Medicare should reimburse for treatment provided in these homes. Dr. Fleishman is working at the state level and with the American Psychiatric Association's Managed Care Committee to expand the definition of "medical necessity" for psychiatric patients to include information derived from the patient's family, legal representatives, and other professionals and nonprofessionals involved in a caretaking capacity to encourage psychiatrists to treat patients outside their offices and hospitals. The APA selected Dr. Fleishman to receive the 2001 Arnold L. Van Ameringen Award in Psychiatric Rehabilitation.

CONTENTS

PART VII: APPENDIXES

Foreword

In 1955 the peak of public asylum psychiatry in the United States was reached with more than half a million patients residing in state and county mental hospitals throughout the country. The length of stay averaged nearly a year, and many individuals spent their entire lifetime residing in such facilities. One out of two hospital beds in this country was occupied by a psychiatric patient. Described by the muckraking journalist Albert Deutsch as "the Shame of the States," many exposés and scandals related to this warehousing of the chronically mentally ill. In 1955 the world began to change as dramatic new medication technologies combined with economic opportunity and social policy changes and moved these patients from institutional to community settings, changing the prospects for care for many individuals with severe and persistent mental illness.

In 1955 chlorpromazine was introduced to the United States from France, which initiated the psychopharmacologic revolution that transformed hospitals and allowed for acute stabilization and discharge from inpatient care. These antipsychotic medications have improved over the past forty-five years and are often combined with other psychiatric and nonpsychiatric medications. Psychopharmacology is now a breakthrough and complex technology for psychiatry in the twenty-first century. But the story of de-institutionalization isn't just about medication; it's also about changing economic and social policy perspectives on where the mentally ill should reside and how they should be treated. It was in 1955 that Title II of the Social Security Act passed (the Social Security Disability Income Program), which initiated the federalization of long-term care throughout the United States. Title II of the Social Security Act eventually led to other Social Security titles such as Medicare, Medicaid, and the Social Security Income Program, which moved the financial support of long-term care from state to federal coffers as long as patients were residing in community settings. "Follow the money" and one can see why so many patients flowed out of institutions into community-based care. Reinforcing the psychopharmacological and economic imperatives was a growing ideology of community mental health that underscored the potential psychiatric morbidity of long-term institutional care and the advantages of treating individuals nearer to home and in general medical settings.

So, by 2004, fewer than 60,000 individuals reside in state and county facilities, whereas if not for the changes initiated in the mid-1950s there would be more than 2 million individuals in these hospitals today. Since the medications help but do not cure schizophrenia and other psychotic disorders patients are "better, but not well." Where do we find these patients today? Much has been written about the public health disaster of homelessness and incarceration of the mentally ill; some of the largest psychiatric facilities today are the Los Angeles County Jail and Rikers Island in New York. A substantial number of individuals now reside in a variety of residential facilities in the community, which although once were hoped to be transitional are now more or less permanent facilities for individuals suffering from the devastating illness of schizophrenia that strikes young people and creates lifelong disability. These residential facilities exist in every community across the country. Psychiatrists and other clinicians who care for these patients and are deeply committed to their quality of life need to provide care to the patients in these settings.

It is shocking but not surprising to find that many of these individuals are neglected and abused in residential care. The April 2002 exposé in *The New York Times* on the sad and disgraceful warehousing of chronically ill individuals in residential facilities reported on what is a growing national scandal similar to Deutsch's exposés of state hospitals in the 1940s.

Only a few psychiatrists have immersed themselves in treating patients in residential facilities and none more deeply and compassionately than Martin Fleishman. Here is a master clinician who understands the extraordinary complexities of modern psychopharmacology and interactions with multiple nonpsychiatric medications along with issues of psychosocial treatment and support and the legal and economic issues that require a broad agenda of reform. This book is much more than a manual of how to provide quality care on site in residential programs; it is also a road map to change in federal and state policies that would allow for a more effective and efficient approach in caring for individuals with serious and persistent mental illness.

Steven S. Sharfstein, MD
President and Chief Executive Officer,
Sheppard Pratt Health System
Clinical Professor of Psychiatry,
University of Maryland
President-Elect,
American Psychiatric Association

Preface

This book addresses the problems involved in the on-site treatment of mentally ill patients residing in residential care facilities. Such facilities are also known as board-and-care homes, adult residential facilities, adult foster homes, adult homes, community care homes, supervisory care homes, sheltered care facilities, continuing care facilities, transitional living facilities, group homes, domiciliary care homes, personal care homes, family care homes, and rest homes. In all probability there are other synonyms. Generally speaking, these facilities provide room and board, supervised medication, and assistance with the activities of daily living to chronic mental patients or individuals who are developmentally disabled. Because of the multiplicity of names, it is very difficult to accumulate statistical data regarding the number of people living in these homes, but I estimate the number to be in excess of 157,000 (as explained in Chapter 2).

I wrote this book knowing that many psychiatrists would not be interested in the problems involved in providing home visiting services to mentally ill occupants of residential care facilities. However, many other psychiatrists would be interested, as would other professionals involved in the provision of on-site services. This would include other nonpsychiatric physicians involved in long-term care, as well as psychologists, social workers, case managers, home visiting nurses, and pharmacists.

In Chapter 7 I describe the roles of these professionals and how they should interact with home visiting psychiatrists—and, conversely, how psychiatrists should relate to other involved professionals. I emphasize that these services are best accomplished through a team approach, and I stress the importance of regularly scheduled visits by the team, which should include a home visiting social worker and pharmacist. The inclusion of the pharmacist may seem surprising to some, but today the average psychiatric patient is usually on a multiplicity of medications, only some of which are for the treatment of psychiatric illnesses, the reasons for which are explained in Chapter 1.

I also wrote this book because there appears to be a relative lack of information about what psychiatrists should do when they make visits to residential care facilities. Previous textbooks in community psychiatry have described the role of psychiatrists in psychiatric hospitals, inpatient psychiatric units of general hospitals, alternative acute treatment settings, community mental health centers, rehabilitation programs, substance abuse clinics, psychosocial rehabilitation clubhouses, and shelters for the homeless. Psychiatrists in the community appear to be working almost everywhere—everywhere except in residential care facilities where the patients are living. When I searched the Entry-Pubmed online search engine using the phrase "the role of the psychiatrist in board and care homes," I received only two results, both of which were written by me (see Introduction).

Obviously this book was written from the perspective of a psychiatrist. However, most of the book will also be of interest to any professional mental health worker involved in the provision of on-site services to residential care facilities. This is especially true for social workers and other physicians involved in the provision of long-term care, including geriatric long-term care.

It will also be of interest to knowledgeable laypeople who have an interest in the problems of the mentally ill. Most of the book is written in nontechnical language. Chapter 17 focuses on the technique of administration of intramuscular (IM) medications and understandably may not be of general interest, although parts of the chapter are amusing—even though the subject is a how-to-do-it treatise on injection techniques. Chapters 14 and 15 discuss progress note problems and may not be of general interest. Chapter 12 focuses on legal issues.

Any physician who makes on-site visits to any kind of long-term care facility and who is concerned with Medicare coding problems— and there are many of them—will be interested in this book because I make specific recommendations as to how these visits should be conducted with regard to frequency, duration, and the types of Medicare procedure codes to utilize. I also have some specific recommendations about how the cost of treatment can be controlled, so the book should be of interest to anyone involved in the economics of health care (see Chapters 21-25).

In addition, this book addresses the legal implications regarding the interpretation of the guidelines for "medical necessity," particularly as it relates to the provision of services to custodial facilities. As such, the book will have some interest to forensic psychiatrists and those psychiatrists under pressure for providing services that were deemed "not medically necessary." (The penalty under the Health Insurance Portability and Accountability Act [HIPAA] for rendering unnecessary medical services can be severe.)

Sometimes the residential care facility is mistaken for a nursing home, but the two are quite different. The purpose of a residential care facility is to provide nonmedical personal care with the exception of the supervision of medication. Nursing homes, on the other hand, provide essential nursing care at a level somewhat less than that given in hospitals. Because they do not qualify for such nursing care, many geriatric patients remain in residential care facilities. In fact, the psychopharmacological principles described for the treatment of geriatric (and other) occupants of residential care facilities can be directly applied to the treatment of geriatric patients in nursing homes. Thus, anyone involved in geriatric care will also be interested. (As a rule, prior publications have focused on the treatment of geriatric patients only in nursing homes—otherwise designated as long-term facilities.)

It is my hope that publication of this book may contribute to a change in Medicare policy to allow greater psychiatric oversight for the residents of these facilities. Residential care facilities and all its synonyms are governed by the same Medicare policies that pertain to rest homes and domiciliaries. These facilities are described in the book titled *CPT 2004 Physicians' Current Procedural Terminology** published annually by the American Medical Association (AMA) as facilities that provide room, board, and other personal assistance services, generally on a long-term basis, but the services do not include a medical component.[1] According to Medicare policies, home visits to such facilities are not required with any specific degree of frequency—as opposed to nursing homes, in which monthly visits by physicians are mandated under the regulations of the Omnibus Budget Reconciliation Act (OBRA). Legislative neglect in this area has led, not surprisingly, to medical neglect, as is cited in Chapter 15.

I should write a few words about the title. My original title was *The Treatment of Schizophrenia in the Residential Care Facility.* This describes much of what the book is about, but the title is rather textbooky and ignores the strong autobiographical and sometimes admit-

---

*CPT © 2004 American Medical Association. All Rights Reserved.

tedly opinionated component that underlies much of what I have written. The next title I considered was *The Casebook of a Residential Care Psychiatrist*. The problem with this was that no such word as *casebook* was listed in my edition of *The New International Webster's Comprehensive Dictionary of the English Language*. I have the 1996 "Deluxe Encyclopedic Edition." *Book* is defined and *case* is defined and *bookcase* is defined, but not *casebook*. Perhaps the dictionary is not comprehensive enough, although it has more than 1,900 pages.

So "casebook" was abandoned—almost, until I found a definition of casebook—"a book in which the physician enters a record of his cases"—as it appeared in my copy of *Dorland's Illustrated Medical (Sexist) Dictionary* (Twenty-fifth Edition). (*Sexist* is my own addition to the title, and I shall explain later in the text about the personal idiosyncrasies which led me to construct such a proposed amendment.) However, in fairness to Mr. Dorland, or possibly Dr. Dorland, it should be explained that my copy was published in 1974, and times have changed, as I repeatedly acknowledge in the text. So I returned to the casebook and I have decided to use that in the title because the book is partly autobiographical—nostalgically so, admittedly so, and unapologetically so. It is what it is—a casebook of cases, and one of the cases is my case, and how I handled my case by doing things My Way.

Since a lot of My Way involves the techniques relating to the on-site treatment of schizophrenia, I decided to include the phrase *The Treatment of Schizophrenia in the Residential Care Facility* in the subtitle because much of the book has a how-to-do-it-manual quality, which the subtitle amply describes. However, in a sense the subtitle is somewhat unnecessarily restrictive because the techniques I describe are not necessarily limited to the treatment of schizophrenia. Many of the procedures described can also be applied to other patients with other kinds of mental illness.

Also, in addition to the long-festering administrative and economic issues in the treatment of the chronically mentally ill just described, the book addresses a new problem that has arisen as a result of the high cost of the newer so-called atypical antipsychotic drugs. The new generation of antipsychotic drugs has created a new type of addiction not amenable to treatment by conventional programs. This occurs in best-case scenarios in patients who have improved enough in response to these medications to resume a working career. However they have become psychopharmacosocioeconomic addicts—"psychopharmaco" because they are dependent on the new generation antipsychotic medications for emotional stability, "economic" because once they have improved enough to live independently they are unable to afford the drugs that induced the improvement, and "socio" because as a result of these factors they are locked into a social class that is dependent on government subsidies. Under such circumstances best-case scenarios have become worst-case scenarios. I know of no good way to estimate the number of patients who are, or will be, in this position, but the likelihood is that the high cost of these medications will prevent these patients' conversion from tax-revenue recipients to employable tax-revenue generators for the rest of their lives.

This last example is but one small but significant way in which psychiatric drugs have changed the world. Chapter 21 lists twenty-seven other changes induced by these medications, and this list is presumed not to be exhaustive. I first created the word *psychopharmacosocioeconomics* in an article titled "Issues in Psychopharmacosocioeconomics," which first appeared in an Economic Grand Rounds Column of *Psychiatric Services* in 2002.[2] Since the word has what might be called broadband applicability, I have decided to retain it in the subtitle because it is the only single word that describes the broad range of topics discussed in the book.

Thus, the title of the book remains *The Casebook of a Residential Care Psychiatrist* because of the autobiographical structure of the book with its occasional digressive ramblings, with the subtitle, *Psychopharmacosocioeconomics and the Treatment of Schizophrenia in Residential Care Facilities.*

Acknowledgments

I must first acknowledge Richard A. Shadoan, MD, who was the first to convince me that the admiration I had for my own work was actually shared by others—although the use of the plural here may be unwarranted. (Nevertheless, one must never underestimate the impact of flattery when administered to those who are in the formative years of their dotage, as happens to be true in my case.) Also a special thanks to Steven S. Sharfstein, MD, currently President-Elect of the American Psychiatric Association, who encouraged my early interest in psychopharmacosocioeconomics, and to Connie Gartner, editor of Psychiatric Services who persuaded me to include the word in the subtitle after a chance encounter during the meeting of the American Psychiatric Association in San Francisco in 2003.

Additional acknowledgments go to Ed Nasrah and Steve Protzel, pharmacists who have been of inestimable value to me in psychiatric and nonpsychiatric pharmacotherapy as part of the home visiting team; Gary Levenson-Palmer, Chief of the Administrative Support Bureau, Community Care Licensing Division, California Department of Social Service, for valuable information regarding statistics of residential care facilities in California; to Robyn Eisenbraun, my whiz kid computer consultant at Kinko's; to Maryann Zaremska and Nancy Phelps, medical librarians at St. Francis Memorial Hospital who helped me trace cold-case references that would have been otherwise untraceable; to my sharp-eyed photocopier at PIPs, John Kung, who prevented part of my manuscript from being printed upside down; and to Christine Potvin, editor of *Psychiatric Times* who had the courage to publish my first comedic efforts describing the predicament of Dr. Ecks, a fictional psychiatrist who was imprisoned at Terminal Island for upcoding Medicare bills (entirely non-autobiographical). The psychiatrist, Dr. Ecks, returns for a cameo appearance in this book.

Also special thanks to the staff at The Haworth Press including Jillian Mason, Jennifer Durgan, Amy Rentner, and Dawn Krisko. Also a very special thanks to Senior Production Editor Peg Marr, who prevented me from crossing my eyes, dotting my teas, and committing other kinds of orthographic malfeasances. She has demonstrated an extraordinary tolerance for my intrusive comedic digressions while patiently redirecting me to the land of the coherent. Last, but certainly not least, my enduring gratitude to Terry S. Trepper, PhD, my understanding editor who encouraged me in this pursuit by virtue of e-mail therapy and common sense, and who convinced me that it was important to maintain my sense of humor (which periodically insinuates itself in the text even when the going gets serious) despite the adversities inflicted by grammar, punctuation, and formalities of attribution.

Introduction

As a result of the depopulation of state hospitals in the 1960s, hundreds of thousands of patients were released into the community. In a relatively short period of time, a new system of residential community care emerged for people who would have otherwise had to spend a major part of the rest of their lives in an institution. Many of these patients were transferred to transitional residential facilities where they received support and assistance with the goal of returning them to independent living. This system included halfway houses, three-quarter way houses, cooperative apartments, crisis lodge facilities, specialized hotels, and residential care facilities.

As stated in the preface, residential care facilities are also known as board-and-care homes, adult residential facilities, adult foster homes, adult homes, community care homes, supervisory care homes, sheltered care facilities, continuing care facilities, transitional living facilities, group homes, domiciliary care homes, personal care homes, family care homes, and rest homes. Possibly there are other synonyms. Generally speaking these facilities provide room and board, supervised medication, and assistance with the activities of daily living to chronic mental patients or individuals who are developmentally disabled. In some instances an occupant of a residential care facility may not have a history of mental illness or developmental disability but this is rather rare. In this book I will be using the term *residential care facilities* preferentially to describe these facilities, and I will focus on the special problems involved in the provision of psychiatric on-site services to the occupants of these facilities.

Although there was a great deal of initial optimism that returning chronically hospitalized mental patients to community settings would facilitate rehabilitation, it also became apparent over time that many of these patients—mostly chronic schizophrenics—were unable to achieve their hoped-for independence because of the persistence of illness and the irretrievable loss of job skills. Consequently a great number of these residences that were originally conceived of as transitional became the permanent residences of many of their occupants.

The existence of this population created new systems of care and new problems for psychiatrists who were long accustomed to treating people in their offices, in clinics, or in hospitals. Psychiatrists were now faced with the option of treating these patients where mentally ill people congregate, as in psychiatric offices, clinics, or hospitals, or where mentally ill people live, as in the aforementioned residential care facilities.

This book addresses the problems that psychiatrists encounter when they attempt to treat schizophrenic patients in their places of residence. In that sense this text represents a break in tradition because the treatment of such patients has hitherto been principally restricted to offices, clinics, and hospitals. Residential care facilities represent one of the chief sources of placement for patients being discharged from long-term facilities and community hospitals.[1]

In fact, it is estimated that one-third of chronic psychotic patients in California now live in these facilities.[2] Similar figures probably exist for other states. Despite this, very little recent literature has been written about this population and how it should be treated: should follow-up be done on the premises or in office or clinic settings, and with what degree of frequency? Typically psychiatrists visit these homes once or twice a month and order medications for most of the residents to be dispensed by the staff at prescribed times. A classical study done before the advent of atypical antipsychotics reported that the average residential care patient was visited by a psychiatrist 1.72 times per month and received an average dose of 760 mg of chlorpromazine or chlorpromazine equivalents.[3]

The aforementioned study was done in 1979, but times change rapidly, especially in psychiatric time. The nature of residential care psychiatry has undergone a rapid evolution in the past ten years. In a series of articles I described the characteristics of residential care psychiatry as well as recent changes that have added to the complexity of the medication management of patients in these homes.[4] Among these changes are the development of new drugs, many of which have the capacity to accelerate or inhibit the metabolism of other drugs; the emergence of atypical antipsychotics (sometimes called "newer generation antipsychotics," or "second generation antipsychotics") now regarded by many as the first line treatment for schizophrenia; the increasing necessity to follow drug treatment with laboratory tests, some of which are legally mandated;

the increased frequency of newly emergent FDA warnings for rare side effects; and the emergence of more sophisticated treatment algorithms in which polypharmacy is presented as a viable alternative when patients do not respond to single drugs.[5]

Adding to this complexity is the tendency to release more disturbed patients from community hospitals, state hospitals, and other long-term facilities because of the increased costs associated with institutionalization. For many of these patients stabilization is dependent on complicated pharmacological regimens which may include but not be limited to typical antipsychotics, atypical antipsychotics, antidepressants, anticonvulsants, minor tranquilizers, beta-blockers, anti-Parkinsonian agents, lithium, and stool softeners. Sometimes these combinations are little more than hastily contrived pastiches in which a little bit of this and a pinch of that have been pasted onto a preexisting menu of antisomethings, following which the patient is released into the community-ocean wherein the dangers of drowning replace the perils of hospital decertification. More often, these combinations are carefully conceived and represent the best possible option to preserve psychiatric stability. The medication management of psychiatric patients is more complicated than ever before and more effective than ever before, in terms of facilitating the release of severely disturbed patients from long-term facilities.

Because of these factors, the treatment of psychiatric outpatients in residential care facilities has become very complicated and very expensive. As an example of this consider the monthly costs incurred by an insured patient on a combination of an atypical antipsychotic, a mood stabilizer, and an antidepressant—a not unusual combination. An atypical antipsychotic such as olanzepine (brand name Zyprexa) at an average dose of 12 mg per day would cost $309 per month. An antidepressant such as paroxetine at an average dose of 30 mg per day would cost about $102 per month. Valproic acid at an average dose of 2,000 mg per day would cost about $200 per month.[6] This combination of psychiatric medications would cost more than $600 per month. Of course, these are not out-of-pocket expenses to a consumer—they are the prices that an insurance company would pay for the medication. Out-of-pocket expenses to an uninsured consumer would be much higher because the consumer does not enjoy the reduced advantages of bulk purchasing.

However, this is only the cost incurred from psychiatric medications. Psychiatric patients, as with nonpsychiatric patients, are not inured to the diseases of aging, and psychiatric patients are now living longer because they receive better care. However, they are living longer with the diseases of aging, such as arthritis, osteoporosis, heart disease, hypertension, hypercholesterolemia, and especially diabetes, to name a few—diseases which also require treatment with medication. It has long been acknowledged that diabetes was more common among psychiatric patients[7] even before the use of some of the newer antipsychotic agents that are alleged to predispose some patients to diabetes by converting impaired glucose tolerance to frank diabetes.[8] Diabetes is the leading cause of renal failure, blindness, and nontraumatic amputations, and its treatment is estimated to amount to about 15 percent of all health care expenditures in the United States.[9]

Unfortunately, these increases in expenses are coming at a time when there is an increasing necessity to reduce these expenses because of the expanding costs of health care. Additional economic pressures are created by the growth of entitlements, the need to balance the federal budget, and the perceived threat of Medicare insolvency within the next decade. The presence of high-cost treatment has added to the impetus to control costs on the part of managed care providers, third-party payers, and government agencies. Consequently, all health care providers are coming under increasing scrutiny by local and federal agencies to justify their role.

The legislative mechanism for such oversight is now in place in the form of the Health Insurance Portability and Accountability Act of 1996, otherwise known as the Kennedy-Kassebaum Act, or HIPAA. This act requires that the secretary of Health and Human Services set up a health care fraud program to coordinate the efforts of federal, state, and local law enforcement agencies with the authority to investigate the delivery of health care to all health plans—both public and private. The implications of this legislation will be discussed in the chapter addressing the legal problems (Chapter 12) associated with the delivery of services to residential care facilities.

The impetus for the enactment of these punitive laws is the widespread existence of health care fraud by physicians, other health care providers, health maintenance organizations, laboratories, and even prestigious university hospitals. The extent of fraud is staggering; it is believed by some to be as high as 10 percent of the approximately

$1 trillion that Americans spend every year on medical treatment.[10] The fact is that Medicare was basically an honor system which did not work because the rules were broken by too many dishonorable people. In short, somebody had to do something.

The upshot of all this is that psychiatric services to occupants of residential care facilities are medically complicated and of great economic importance to third-party payers, including Medicare. That means it is of great significance to taxpayers and to the nation. It therefore is of vital importance to determine the most effective way that services can be delivered to this population. At the same time psychiatric practitioners who provide on-site services to this population will come under increasing suspicion by Medicare auditors because they will be targeted as practicing their profession in an atypical way. This is true because on-site services to the residential care population generally involves the provision of services to multiple patients at the same site. This is very different from office psychiatry where services are provided on a one-to-one basis. Because of this the service of the on-site psychiatrist is generally conceived of as statistically different from the office psychiatrist. It is this very fact of atypicality which triggers computer-generated audits that can result in severe financial penalties and even in incarceration. While service to the patient is the primary consideration of health care providers, they must also have a clear understanding of the problems involved in treating multiple patients at the same site including problems created by the concepts of medical necessity, visitation frequency, and progress note documentation. Moreover, such providers and the psychiatric profession in general, as well as third-party payers, should be made aware of the treatment advantages afforded by on-site visits.

It is rather strange that the value of on-site visits to residential care facilities has been questioned. It is generally acknowledged that the population of residential care facilities is largely composed of those who, in darker days, would have had to spend the rest of their lives in mental hospitals. The value of a doctor on a mental hospital staff treating a mentally ill patient in a hospital—on site, as it were—has never been questioned, so why should such on-site services be regarded as substandard when rendered to mentally ill residents of residential care facilities? This is a profoundly important question, yet the practice and issue of on-site services to residential care facilities has remained a neglected area in psychiatry, as will be documented in Chapter 1.

THE GOALS OF THIS BOOK

In writing this book I originally had four goals in mind, all of them somewhat grandiose. Briefly put, these goals are (1) to provide a set of guidelines for on-site residential care services, (2) to change the American Psychiatric Association's definition of "medical necessity," (3) to suggest an alternative way in which Medicare could assess penalties to make them more equitable, and finally (4) to suggest certain changes in the Medicare policies regarding the appropriateness of on-site services rendered to residential care facilities.

Two additional goals—(5) suggesting legislative changes and (6) recommending university-approved psychiatric rotations in residential care facilities—were not in the original plan of the book. These latter goals slowly emerged only as I was in the process of writing the book. It was only after I had read what I had written that I developed the courage to make certain additional recommendations. The article in *The New York Times* (Chapter 15) detailing abuses and neglect in the residential care system also contributed to my decision to make these recommendations.

It is my hope that as a result of this book, more psychiatrists will be motivated to focus on the care of chronically ill psychiatric patients in long-term facilities through the provision of on-site visits. To my knowledge this is a neglected aspect of psychiatry, and room exists for a subspecialization in this area. The provision of on-site services to the chronically ill in nonhospital settings is not at all unprecedented in other specialties since some internists and geriatricians specialize in the long-term care of the chronically ill. In fact, a periodical titled *Annals of Long-Term Care* is devoted to the care of patients in long-term facilities. However, to my knowledge, no university residency training program in psychiatry includes monitored experiences in a residential care facility. In addition, aside from influencing psychiatrists about the utility of on-site services, I hope to convince third-party payers that this is an economically efficient way to render psychiatric care.

Why Should Psychiatrists Visit Residential Care Facilities?

The concept of a psychiatrist making home visits has been described in the literature as generally occurring in response to crisis situations. Generally when such visits are made the psychiatrist is part of a home visiting team and the visits are conducted in response to emergencies as reported by neighbors, clergy, relatives, landlords, the police, or social service organizations.

This type of approach is crisis oriented and serves a distinct purpose in terms of preventing exacerbations and hospitalizations. In contrast this book focuses on the value of maintenance and routine nonemergency visitations as a way of preventing emergencies. Although emergency situations can be minimized by such routine home visits, they cannot be prevented entirely. When such emergencies occur, I generally will refer to the kind of home visiting mobile crisis team that Sullivan and Cohen describe in their chapter titled "The Home Visit and the Chronically Mentally Ill" in *Psychiatry Takes to the Streets*.[11] Their article emphasizes the utility of the team approach.

The focus of this book is somewhat more specialized in that it concentrates on the role of the psychiatrist and not on the team as such—although the value of the team concept is acknowledged and discussed with some of my own personal convictions as to who should be on the team. Also this book has a narrower focus in that it concentrates on the problems that a psychiatrist will encounter when rendering services to a particular kind of home, this being the residential care facility. Outreach services to family homes or apartments or hotels present other problems and are described in other books. In contrast, this book addresses the problems involved in the provision of on-site services to residential care facilities.

The Problem of Defining Chronic Mental Illness

There remains the additional problem of defining chronic mental illness. This is easier said than done since no one is happy with the term. Fortunately for me, others have done a credible job here. Goldman notes that this population includes persons who are currently in hospitals or nursing homes, those who are discharged, and those who have no prior hospital or psychiatric experience so that they cannot simply be described as deinstitutionalized patients or chronic schizophrenics.[12] He refers to Bachrach's definition which describes chronically mentally ill patients as "those individuals who are, have been, or might have been, but for the deinstitutionalization movement, on the rolls of long-term mental institutions, especially state hospitals."[13] This definition is a good example of how definitions may be changed by social policies. Goldman defines the chronic state as "an illness of long duration, which may include periods of apparent wellness interrupted by flare-ups of acute symptoms and secondary disabilities."[14]

The Problem of Anecdotal Observations

The contents of this book reflect my own experiences in servicing residential care facilities over a thirty-year period. I hope what I have to say will be helpful to other psychiatrists engaged in such work. Some of what I have to say may be controversial or even wrong, but if it stimulates discussion on this hitherto ignored area of psychiatry, so much the better. Besides, no one in psychiatry is right 100 percent of the time. The psychiatric writer must learn to treat criticisms as welcome guests. Otherwise he or she is destined to dwell indefinitely among his or her enemies. I suspect that after I express some of my opinions in this book, my circle of welcome guests will expand appreciably.

To the extent that this book recapitulates many of my own anecdotal experiences in residential care psychiatry, it is part diary. To the extent that I offer my own opinions about how residential care should be conducted, it is partly a how-to-do-it manual. The manual-type information and its related guidelines evolved principally from my personal experiences rather than the experiences of others as described in the literature because of the scarcity of how-to-do-it literature on the subject.

It is safe to say that residential care psychiatry has never enjoyed a prestigious place in American psychiatry. There are many reasons for this, possibly involving a feeling of hopelessness regarding the treatment of the seriously mentally ill, possibly involving the reluctance of psychiatrists to leave their offices, or possibly because chronic schizophrenics were (and are) regarded as nonproductive citizens who could rarely pay for professional services. Whatever the reason, this professional apathy continues to exist, and psychiatrists engaged in this area are frequently regarded as practicing an inferior brand of psychiatry. As previously implied, psychiatric residency programs involving a residential care facility rotation are few and far between, and at the present time I would be hard put to cite even one such program. Moreover, the literature on the techniques of psychiatric on-site evaluations is virtually nonexistent.

The role of psychiatrists practicing in residential care facilities has also received short shrift in the literature. In a recent compendium addressing community psychiatry titled *Practicing Psychiatry in the Community*[15]—described by some as the most comprehensive book on community psychiatry in the past twenty years—residential care psychiatry received somewhat less than short shrift. In fact, it received no shrift at all, short or otherwise—not in the table of contents or the text or the index. The role of the psychiatrists was described in psychiatric hospitals, inpatient psychiatric units of general hospitals, alternative acute treatment settings, community mental health centers, rehabilitation programs, substance abuse clinics, psychosocial rehabilitation clubhouses, and shelters for the homeless. Psychiatrists in the community appear to be working almost everywhere—everywhere but in the residential care facilities where the patients are living. I cannot fault the editors for this omission since the concept of on-site psychiatric services to patients at their place of residence appears by some to be so outlandish as to be totally overlooked.

Other excellent and otherwise comprehensive books on the treatment of schizophrenia lack references to residential care facilities. If, for instance, one attempts to look up *residential care* in the index of *Schizophrenia—A New Guide for Clinicians,*[16] the references are limited to *residential care, acute* or *residential care, late phase.* Pursuit of the "acute" reference leads to a description of acute residential care. Acute residential care facilities are described as "respite care" or "crisis centers" providing "24-hour nursing or other mental health staff, and supervision by a psychiatrist." Pursuit of the "late phase" index reference leads to a description of nursing homes for geriatric schizophrenic patients. It is interesting that the concept of residential care is limited to acute problems, as may be manifested by the young schizophrenic, or to "late phase" problems, as may be manifested by the aging schizophrenic. No reference identifies a residential care facility as a domicile for those patients in their middle years who are not undergoing a crisis. Such patients do not seem to have a national identity.

Since no national identity exists for this population, practically no professional interest is expressed in this group by articles in the literature. Thus no abstracts address the problems of patients in residential care facilities—or any of its aforementioned congeners—in *The Year-book of Psychiatry and Applied Mental Health.*[17] *The Yearbook of Psychiatry and Applied Mental Health* is a literature survey service providing abstracts of significant articles in psychiatry including articles in child and adolescent psychiatry, psychotherapy, alcohol- and substance-related disorders, psychiatry and the law, community psychiatry, clinical psychiatry, biological psychiatry, and psychopharmacology. One cannot blame the editors for this omission since it is impossible to present abstracts of articles that have not been written.

The Problem of the Conceptual Desert

The upshot of all this—the lack of reliable statistics and the inability to agree on a common name for the domiciles for the chronically mentally ill—has led to a conceptual desert regarding how such patients should best be treated in their places of residence, or whether in fact they should be treated at all in their places of residence. Only a minimal literature at best addresses the advisability or describes the techniques of providing maintenance on-site care as a way of avoiding crises for the nongeriatric psychiatric patient. To the extent that such literature exists, it does not focus on the role of the psychiatrist in these facilities. When I accessed the Entry-Pubmed search engine with the subject "the role of the psychiatrist in board and care homes," only two results appeared. I will provide the search engine results from September 5, 2002.

1.
TITLE: The changing role of the psychiatrist in board-and-care homes.
AUTHORS: Fleishman M
SOURCE: Psychiatr Serv. 1997 Apr;48(4):510-3.
CIT. IDS:PMID: 9090735

2.
TITLE: The role of the psychiatrist in board-and-care homes.
AUTHORS: Fleishman M
SOURCE: Hosp Community Psychiatry. 1989 Apr;40(4):415-8. No abstract available.
CIT. IDS:PMID: 271475

I wrote these two articles to describe the functions of a psychiatrist in a residential care facility. Obviously, not many people are addressing this issue. Because of this, the references at the end of each chapter of this book are sparse, and some of them are old. I had to go back to 1979 to find the most recent reference addressing the problem of frequency of visits to residential care facilities.[18]

In the course of treating the chronically ill residents of long-term facilities, internists who specialize in this area provide routine on-site nonemergency-dictated services. This has been found to be medically preferable and economically more efficient than waiting until the patient's condition deteriorates and then administering treatment either in emergency rooms or hospitals.

Why does this tradition not exist in psychiatry? Possibly the answer is that one customarily thinks that a real difference exists between medically ill residents of long-term care facilities and psychiatrically impaired residents insofar as the medically ill residents are confined to the facility whereas the psychiatrically impaired are ambulatory and therefore able to come to psychiatrist's offices. These differences, however, are more apparent than real. Many chronically ill psychiatric patients, while technically ambulatory, choose not to exercise their ambulatory status. Some of them are too intimidated to utilize public transportation, either because of irrational reasons or because they have no experience in doing this. Also others either deny illness or, while not denying illness, deny the need for treatment.

The question may arise as to whether a patient who denies illness should be treated at all. This question has two answers: First, the denial of illness may emanate from the pathologically impaired judgment that is the product of illness. Second, the denial for treatment may lead to a hospitalization—which is more expensive for the patient if he or she is able to pay for this, or more expensive for the community if the patient is unable to pay. The second alternative is more likely to occur. Aside from the problem of economic expense, it is generally accepted that periodic exacerbations of a psychiatric illness usually worsen during the long-term course of the illness. Conceivably, Medicare auditors may question the "medical necessity" of treating patients who deny illness, and quite possibly our customary definitions of medical necessity might have to be amended. This goal of the book will be pursued in Chapter 12.

After the previous disappointing Internet search results, I tried substituting the subject heading from "the role of the psychiatrist in board-and-care homes" to "the role of the psychiatrist in adult residential facilities." This produced zero results. I then changed the search engine query to "the role of the psychiatrist in residential care facilities." The results were somewhat better. Five results addressed the issues presented by children or the developmentally disabled, but none of them described the role of the psychiatrist in the treatment of the adult mentally ill in these facilities.

1.
TITLE: Diagnosis, guardianship, and residential care of the mentally ill in medieval and early modern England.
AUTHORS: Neugebauer R
SOURCE: Am J Psychiatry. 1989 Dec;146(12):1580-4.
CIT. IDS:PMID: 2686477

2.
TITLE: Children's rights on entering therapeutic institutions.
AUTHORS: Miller D, Burt RA
SOURCE: Am J Psychiatry. 1977 Feb;134(2):153-6.
CIT. IDS:PMID: 835735

3.
TITLE: The role of the certified social worker in England's social services.
AUTHORS: Johnston JA
SOURCE: Hosp Community Psychiatry. 1976 Dec;27(12): 872-5.
CIT. IDS:PMID: 186379

4.
TITLE: The responsibilities and role of the doctor concerned with the care of the mentally handicapped.
AUTHORS: Godber G
SOURCE: Br J Psychiatry. 1973 Dec;123(577):617-20. No abstract available.
CIT. IDS:PMID: 4797864

5.

TITLE: The role of the residential treatment center in the treatment of children and adolescents with emotional problems.
AUTHORS: Quackenbush JF
SOURCE: South Med J. 1971 Jun;64(6):671-5. No abstract available.
CIT. IDS:PMID: 5089140

The advantage of this kind of attribution is that it saves me the tedium of typing a lengthy bibliography with its irritating rules involving commas and colons. I believe I have already implied that I am not writing a standard medical text. Unfortunately, as emphasized above, not much evidence-based information exists regarding the efficacy of on-site treatment at residential care facilities so that one is heavily reliant on anecdotes to illustrate issues. Still, my suggestions are based on many years of providing services to the occupants of residential care facilities, so they are presumed to have some validity. To put it somewhat more candidly, they are presumed by me to have some validity. The dearth of literature carries disadvantages as well as advantages. The disadvantage of being a self-proclaimed authority on an aspect of psychiatry that is so arcane as to be unaddressed by others is that one cannot attribute to others opinions or policies which may be inherently controversial. The buck, in this instance, stops with me.

PART I:
THE PLACES

Chapter 1

What Is a Residential Care Facility?

Given the widespread lack of interest in residential care facilities, it is not surprising that many but infrequently asked questions arise. Following is a list of such questions (IAQs).

INFREQUENTLY ASKED QUESTIONS

Q. What is a residential care facility?

A. A residential care facility is a privately owned facility that functions to provide unlocked shelter, three meals a day, and supervision of medication to psychiatric patients.

Q. What is a residential care psychiatrist?

A. A residential care psychiatrist is a psychiatrist who makes routine on-site visits to residential care facilities for the purpose of treating the residents of this facility. In California residential care facilities are statistically divided into two categories, residential care facilities for the elderly (RCFEs) and adult residential facilities (ARFs).

Q. How do adult residential facilities (ARFs) differ from residential care facilities (RCFs)?

A. The adult residential facility is another name for the residential care facility. Residential care facilities also have other names in other states. Residential care facilities are also known as board-and-care homes, adult residential facilities, adult foster homes, adult homes, community care homes, supervisory care homes, sheltered care facilities, continuing care facilities, transitional living facilities, group homes, domiciliary care homes, personal care homes, family care homes, and rest homes. Although California officially uses the term *adult residential facilities* (ARFs) to describe residential care facilities for the nonelderly, I don't like the term because of its inherent vagueness insofar as it is possible to use the term to describe the situation of people living in retirement homes or hotels. Also ARFs inevitably invoke the inappropriate image of the balloons that come out of the head of barking dogs in comic strips. The reasons for the California preference for this term is a long story and is described in Appendix A.

Q. How do residential care facilities differ from nursing homes?

A. Residential care facilities differ from nursing homes in that the purpose of a residential care facility is to provide nonmedical personal care with the exception of the supervision of medication. Nursing homes, on the other hand, provide essential nursing care at a certain level. A licensed practical nurse must be available twenty-four hours per day. In addition, a registered nurse must be available for eight hours per day.

Q. Are nursing homes the same as skilled nursing facilities?

A. Not exactly. Not all nursing homes are qualified as skilled nursing facilities although most are. Skilled nursing facilities are specialized nursing facilities that can provide a level of care almost equivalent to that of hospitals.

Q. Are residential care facilities the same as residential treatment facilities?

A. No, they are not.

Q. What is the difference?

A. In residential care facilities, the treatment, with the exception of the visiting psychiatrist (if one exists) and the administration of medication, is done off the premises. Residential treatment facilities, on the other hand, provide treatment on the premises and are known as acute diversion units, halfway houses, three-quarter way houses, and possibly other fractional equivalents. Residential treatment facilities are richly endowed with mental heath professionals who live or work on site compared to residential care facilities where professional help is generally referred to an outside source. The principal exception to this is the on-site services rendered by a visiting residential care psychiatrist and visiting social worker.

Q. What about psychiatrists who treat residential care patients in their offices? Aren't they residential care psychiatrists?

A. Such psychiatrists are practicing standard office psychiatry in the treatment of patients who are residents of residential care facilities. This is fine except that it is not an efficient way to treat this population as a whole, although it may be the preferable treatment for an individual patient.

Q. Why is it not the most efficient way to treat this population as a whole?

A. There is no quick answer to that question. That is what this book is about.

Q. Is there a subspecialization called "residential care psychiatry"?

A. If there is such a specialization, sub or otherwise, I have not been able to find it via Internet searches. Also, I am not aware of any university psychiatric residency program that offers a rotation in residential care psychiatry or any of its synonyms. Therefore the answer is no, but in my opinion there should be such a specialization.

Q. Why?

A. Again, that is what this book is about.

Chapter 2

The Problem of the Problem

As stated in the Introduction and elsewhere, residential care facilities are known by different names in different states. Generally speaking, all these facilities provide room and board, supervised medication, and assistance with the activities of daily living to chronic mental patients or individuals who are developmentally disabled.

No clear information is available on how many mentally ill residents are serviced nationwide in residential care facilities. There is a dearth of literature on this subject and a surprising lack of reliable statistics. This presents a problem in that the diversity of names prevents adequate national statistical categorizations. Without reliable statistics, it is difficult to identify a constituency. This has contributed to the legislative neglect of this population when compared to the legislative mandates affecting nursing homes. Where no identifiable constituencies exist, there are no lobbies militating for legislative oversights. However, regardless of what they are called, all these facilities share the essential characteristic of being the domiciles of mentally ill patients in their adult years, some of whom may be considered borderline geriatric patients.

In a sense these facilities are long-term care facilities. For many people long-term care necessarily connotes a facility for the elderly, but in fact many chronic psychotic patients spend much of their young and middle years in facilities designed for the nongeriatric. Many chronic schizophrenic patients spend most of their lives in a residential care facility, and in that sense the long-term care provided by these facilities is probably longer in duration than the long-term care provided by facilities for geriatric patients.

Chronic psychotic patients get older and eventually qualify for placement in the geriatric long-term care facility. However, although much has been written about the treatment of geriatric patients—both psychiatric and nonpsychiatric—in long-term care facilities, very little has been written about the treatment of the nongeriatric psychiatric patients in the other types of long-term care facilities.

Because of the multiplicity of names, it is difficult to determine how many chronic psychotic patients are living in nongeriatric long-term care facilities on a nationwide basis. Perhaps the least ambiguous descriptive name to define the function of these residential care facilities is "long-term care facilities for the nongeriatric mentally ill," but this term is somewhat cumbersome and does not lend itself to easily articulated acronyms that trip off the tongue. Besides, some of the older patients in their middle years gradually become geriatric and if they are in reasonably good physical health, they tend to remain in the residential care facility rather than be transferred to a selectively geriatric facility. To make matters even more confusing, many nonpsychotic developmentally disabled residents also live in these facilities.

The problems of terminology are even more complicated than just suggested, and it is for this reason that I have previously referred the reader to Appendix A. However, because there is no agreement regarding terminology, I have decided to use the term *residential care facilities* because it appears to enjoy the widest usage in California.

Proposals to conduct national surveys have failed because of the high costs of data collection and the difficulty of reliably identifying residential care facilities. Improvement in the quality of information pertaining to residential care facilities is important because of the need to increase the number of residential care facilities while improving the quality of care received by the residents. This information is particularly important with respect to mentally ill residents because of the increasing tendency by psychiatric hospitals to make quick discharges to community facilities in response to the tendency of third-party payers to decertify payment. Because of this, it is easy to see how economic trends will cause residential care facilities to proliferate. The decennial census should be the primary source of national statistics on residential care facilities, but unfortunately the rules addressing the classification of living arrangements have created insurmountable barriers to accumulating meaningful information regarding the numbers of residential care facilities or the characteristics of their occupants.

THE PROBLEM OF DATA COLLECTION

One of the problems of data collection is that a continuum of facilities provides varying degrees of care and protective oversight to a variable number of residents. Some of these facilities are institutions, but it can be difficult from the statistical point of view to distinguish noninstitutional residential care facilities from institutions, especially since the number of residents alone is an insufficient basis for differentiation. The problem is compounded by the fact that states have different licensing laws and in some states the distinction between nursing homes and residential care facilities is not clearly delineated.

In 1987 a national survey of state licensing agencies was conducted by the National Association of Residential Care Facilities, which represents residential care facility owners and operators. The survey reported a total of 41,381 homes with 562,837 beds. Of this total, approximately 10,000 homes with about 264,000 beds were identified as primarily geriatric, with the rest servicing the developmentally disabled or the mentally ill.[1]

The association stated that its estimates were incomplete due to the wide variety of definitions included in licensing as well as the fact that some states were just beginning to license some homes. Confusion about the size of this population is not new. During congressional hearings in 1981, the Department of Health and Human Services estimated that boarding home population was between 500,000 and 1.5 million, but that it was unclear as to how many of these residents lived in homes that could be defined as board-and-care homes.[2] There was an insufficient breakdown of residents into separate geriatric, developmentally disabled, and mentally ill categories. Also it was acknowledged that the bottom line estimate of 500,000 was necessarily an undercount because of the lack of information on the number of unlicensed facilities. Some facilities were unlicensed because the state criteria excluded them from licensing requirements. Other homes were able to meet criteria but remained unlicensed due to lack of enforcement efforts. Thus, unfortunately, there is no nationwide information on the number of unlicensed homes. No clear nationwide information exists on the number of licensed homes.

However, in California the statistics are somewhat clearer in that we have statistics regarding licensed residential care facilities statewide, and a breakdown as to how these homes are divided among the aged, the mentally ill, and the developmentally disabled. In California in 2000, there were 4,639 licensed nongeriatric residential care facilities with a bed capacity of 37,985.[3] These facilities are categorized as residential care facilities by the Department of Social Services and are occupied by the mentally ill and the developmentally disabled. Of the RCF beds, 26,590 (70 percent) were occupied by residents diagnosed as developmentally disabled and 11,395 (30 percent) RCF beds were occupied by patients with mental illness.

In September 2000 in California the total number of nursing home patients (NH) was estimated at 107,084.[4] We already know that mentally ill residential care facility occupants totaled 11,395. We now have a RCF/NH ratio for California (11,395/107,084 or 10.6 percent). If we label the 10.6 percent as the California ratio, it is possible to use this ratio to estimate the nationwide population of mentally ill residential care facility occupants as follows: According to the HCFA Online Certification and Reporting statistics the national number of nursing home beds for this time period was calculated at 1,490,155.[5] We can now compute an estimate of the nationwide number of residential care facility beds by multiplying the nationwide nursing home beds by the California ratio of 10.6 percent. This produces an estimate of 157,956 as the number of residential care facility beds nationally.

It can be argued that such an extrapolation is unwarranted because California is not a typical state because it has a higher incidence of mental illness than the rest of the country. Although this inference may appear to be true by observing the pedestrian traffic at certain intersections in San Francisco, it is not true of the state as a whole. There may be no way to prove that California is typical of the rest of the country but the fact that California accounts for one-eighth of the national population makes it extremely unlikely that California-derived statistics would be seriously unrepresentative.

However, life is not that simple. It is probable that many more mentally ill patients occupy residential care facility beds than the 157,856 beds estimated from the California ratio,

First, the California statistics for the residential care facility population are based on licensed homes. The number of residents in unlicensed facilities is still unknown. Second, and even more important, many mentally ill residents, when they attain geriatric status at age sixty, are frequently transferred to residential care facilities for the elderly. These patients continue to be mentally ill, but they no longer occupy recognized mentally ill beds. From the statistical point of view they have literally disappeared.

This problem is increasing in importance because more schizophrenic patients are attaining geriatric status and are thus in danger of disappearing statistically. Schizophrenic patients are now living longer because many of them are being effectively treated for concurrent medical diseases such as arthritis, diabetes, heart disease, hypertension, hypercholesterolemia and the various forms of chronic obstructive pulmonary diseases—to name only a few. To make matters somewhat more complicated, many geriatric patients have no prior history of mental illness and develop psychopathology during their residency in the facilities for the elderly. When these factors are considered it is highly probable that many more than the 157,956 nationwide residential care facility beds exist for the mentally ill than indicated by simple extrapolative methods based on the California statistics.

This is not to say that 157,956 patients are residing in licensed residential care facilities nationwide. Some states may not have residential care facilities or their equivalents. Some states have substituted other facilities such as specialized hotels to subserve the functions that would otherwise have been delegated to residential care facilities. Yet this gives some indication of the scope of the population that is in need of the services of these facilities whether they exist or not.

In addition to this population, another population of geriatric schizophrenic patients are too disabled to reside in residential care facilities for the elderly and currently occupy beds in nursing homes. In many instances the nursing home has replaced the state hospital as the repository for the severely disabled geriatric schizophrenic patient. In fact, the statistics for nursing homes are much more accurate with respect to mental illness than are the statistics for the residential care facilities for the elderly. Thus, in 1999 it was estimated that the psychiatric (mostly schizophrenic) population of nursing homes comprised 14.5 percent— or 216,072—of the total nursing home population of 1,490,155.[6] If we add this to the number of psychotic patients living in residential care facilities or their equivalent (157,956), we get a total in excess of 370,000 mentally ill patients living in either nursing homes or residential care facilities. This is an estimate of the number of occupants, but does not give us information about the number of mentally ill patients who can benefit from placement in such facilities but are unable to utilize them because the number of facilities is inadequate. I am talking about the mentally ill homeless.

The mentally ill homeless can be defined as those individuals lacking fixed nighttime domiciles and experiencing clinically diagnosable psychiatric disorders. Many of these patients would have been the chronic residents of state hospitals—for better or worse—but are now left to the tides of fate and chance wherein they drift across the intersections of urban America with shopping carts full of pitiful belongings. It is estimated that more than 500,000 individuals in the United States are homeless, and that at least one-quarter of this population is mentally ill.[7]

In addition to this population, another population may have or would have benefitted from residential care facility placement but will not have the opportunity to do so because it is in prison. The estimates for the mentally ill prison population range between 200,000 and 300,000, with prisons holding three times more people than psychiatric hospitals.[8]

Chapter 3

The History

This chapter focuses on my early experiences as a psychiatrist working in residential care facilities in San Francisco. My original descriptions of my early experiences were first published in the November 1985 edition of *Psychiatric Annals,* and some (but not all) of this chapter includes a recapitulation of these experiences.[1]

In 1952, Delay and Deniker first published their observations on the use of chlorpromazine in France.[2] Heinz Lehmann took the drug to Canada and by 1953 the word of the new miracle drug had spread to the United States. By 1956, for the first time in 175 years, the number of patients in psychiatric hospitals began to decline.[3] Contributing to this accelerating depopulation was an unlikely confluence of events in which economic frugality, civil rights activism, and social psychiatry, as well as chemistry, all played their part. It would be difficult to devise a stranger cast of bedfellows. This was one of the few times that the political right and the political left joined forces to combat a common enemy—the state hospital system.

In 1955 the Federal Mental Health Study Act was passed, authorizing the formation of the Joint Commission on Mental Illness and Health. Recommendations included that immediate care be provided to mental patients living in the community; that treatment of major mental illnesses be recognized as the responsibility of mental health service systems; that large and remote state hospitals be replaced by smaller institutions; that community-based aftercare and rehabilitation services be greatly expanded; and that fully staffed mental health clinics be available to the whole population.

In 1957, the Short Doyle Act was passed in California creating financial inducements to counties for reducing their use of twenty-four-hour inpatient care.[4] In 1963, the Community Mental Health Centers Aid was passed, thereby creating, over a period of years, a network of outpatient facilities and agencies at the national level.

Also, the federal government assumed unprecedented responsibility for persons in the community disabled by mental illness, resulting in the establishment of more than 750 community mental health centers and resulting in the appropriation of more than $2.9 billion in federal money. Also, the act allocated federal funds for the states but not for patients who remained in state hospitals, the effect being to encourage discharges into the community.

Also in 1963, persons in California disabled by mental illness became eligible for financial support under the Categorical Aid to the Disabled as part of changes in California welfare regulations. This was formerly called ATD and is now called Supplemental Security Income (SSI) and is managed by the Social Security Administration.

In 1965 Medicare and its companion program Medicaid (which insures indigent recipients) were signed into law by President Lyndon Johnson as part of his Great Society program. (A brief history of Medicare is described in Appendix F.) One of the effects of the 1965 law was to establish standards of care for nursing homes which indirectly preceded state-established standards for residential care facilities. Subsequent judicial decisions have mandated an increase in the standards for adequate and appropriate treatment. Legislation was passed that guaranteed broader privileges to patients in mental hospitals, such as the right to be admitted voluntarily, to make a will, to manage their affairs, to communicate with friends and relatives, to seek legal counsel, and to marry.

The net effect of these changes was that warehousing in large institutions became expensive for the states, and community placement became relatively economical—or so it seemed. Thus it was that in this relatively short period, a new system of residential community care emerged for people who would have otherwise had to spend a major part of the rest of their lives in an institution. As previously stated in the Introduction, this system includes halfway houses, three-quarter way houses, cooperative apartments, crisis lodge facilities, specialized hotels, and residential care facilities with all their aforementioned names and pseudonyms. In addition, let it not be forgotten that many patients were able to return to their homes and families but many of these patients continued to be impaired so that their familial members were thrust into caretaking roles whether prepared for this or not.

Thus the unintended consequences of the deinstitutionalization movement were that patients were placed in a variety of environments in which responsibility for program development and implementation was scattered across multiple agencies and involved various levels of government. Thus payment for services to mental patients came principally from the federal government, while administration for the programs was left to the states and municipalities. Consequently, services to the mentally ill became a complex patchwork involving many agencies and many people with different professional backgrounds. A potential advantage of the residential care facility is that it can provide a geographical setting which can be a focus for the provision of various professional services. This is also true for agency, clinic, and hospital settings, the difference being that caretakers are more easily accessible at the home. Generally speaking, caretaker and caregiver input is solicited in initial interviews at agencies, community clinics, and hospitals but later this input tends to get lost in the shuffle with ongoing treatment. Ideally the professionals who provide services to the patients in the residential care facility setting should be in contact with one another, with the patient, and with the caretaker. My own preference is that various professional services should be simultaneously administered in team meetings with patients and caregivers by members of the Modern Psychiatric Team (capitalized for reasons described in Chapter 7) to the extent that such a convergence in space and time is possible.

RESIDENTIAL CARE FACILITIES IN SAN FRANCISCO

Although most residential care facilities in the San Francisco area are licensed for six residents, they range in census from one to fifty-five and encompass a wide variety of facilities ranging from small, family-type homes to small hotels. Typically, residents share their rooms and bathrooms with other ex-patients. They generally have shared access to a television. Residential care facility patients have the freedom to come and go as they please, although they are encouraged to participate in various programs—day treatment programs, social skills programs, partial hospitalization programs, and rehabilitation programs—as offered by a variety of agencies throughout the city. The patient population reflects the Caucasian, African-American, Hispanic, and Asian mix of San Francisco, although the majority of residents are Caucasian. Obviously, this is a multicultural mix, although I became immersed in this practice more than thirty years ago, before multiculturalism became a buzzword. The homes are scattered throughout San Francisco, but mostly in certain lower-class or lower-middle-class neighborhoods not well known to the tourist, such as the Western Addition, Mission, Ingleside, and Haight-Ashbury. I like to think of them in a proprietary way as Dr. Fleishman's neighborhoods.

Because of the trend toward deinstitutionalization, residential care facilities assumed an ever-increasing degree of importance as more and more patients were channeled into the community. To appreciate the magnitude of this migration, consider that the bed capacity of the California state hospital system has shrunk from 37,500 beds in 1959 to 5,000 beds in 1989, half of which were reserved for the judicially committed.[5] However, one of the problems that residential care facility patients (and administrators) had was that relatively few psychiatrists were prepared to meet the special problems of residential care facility occupants in innovative ways.

PERSONAL HISTORY

My first contact with the residential care facility system occurred in 1968 at the request of a social worker within the State Department of Mental Hygiene who asked me if I would follow the patients in a board-and-care home. Since I was young and impulsive at the time, and since I didn't like to alienate social workers, I agreed to do this without even knowing what a board-and-care home was. I certainly did not realize that this off-the-cuff agreement would dominate my professional career for the rest of my life. This is a classic example of how professional careers are determined by imprecise decisions in which all possible factors are scrupulously disregarded.

At that time, a large number of patients were living in residential care facilities and relatively few psychiatrists were working in this field. As a consequence, many of these patients were poorly followed. One option was to have the patient visit a psychiatrist (called the convalescent leave psychiatrist) who worked at the central office of the Bureau of Social Work (an agency within the California Department of Mental Hygiene). The patients were given appointments to see the convalescent leave psychiatrist who would then evaluate the patient and send the patient home after prescribing medications that were kept on the premises. At that time the choices were limited to Thorazine and Stelazine; sometimes these were prescribed singly and other times, in combination. If all went well, patients honored their appointments, and went home with their supplies of Thorazine or Stelazine, or both, in a brown paper bag. There were a lot of brown paper bags in those days.

However, frequently all did not go well. Many patients were too confused to keep their appointments and generally had to be accompanied by their administrators. Yet administrators frequently did not have the time to accompany the patients or found it impossible to do so because they were required to remain on the premises. Because of this, I decided that it would be more practical to visit the patients at home. Also, this afforded certain theoretical advantages in that I could see how patients behaved on their own turf, I could become acquainted with their roommates and fellow residents, and I could meet with and consult with the administrators and other caregivers, such as cooks and housekeepers. Also by making routine home visits I could evaluate patients during their noncrisis periods and get some appreciation of their baseline status. Many psychiatric patients will consent to psychiatric services only following a crisis. By intervening in a prodromal precrisis stage, the psychiatrist may be able to avert a crisis and avoid a hospitalization.

Within a matter of months I was seeing as many as 400 patients in about thirty residential care facilities. I would like to think all this occurred because I was a brilliant psychiatrist, but in fact very few other psychiatrists were willing to do this kind of work. I was working a ten-hour day and a six-day week and beginning to entertain grandiose delusions about how I was pioneering in the field of epidemiological psychiatry. At night I had a recurring dream of hearing music from *The Sorcerer's Apprentice* and would visualize residential care facilities proliferating exponentially instead of brooms. A second dream had me in the wooden shoes of the little Dutch boy, trying to plug the holes in the dike, except that the holes were getting farther and farther apart. I was definitely working too hard. Since that frantic time I have decreased my practice to more manageable levels, seeing less than 200 patients.

This latter dream, however, led to a creative idea. If I could arrange the holes so that they were closer, I could then do my job more effectively. Subsequently I splurged on a street map of San Francisco and placed purple dots on each residential care facility location. I could then plan my visits on the basis of the home's accessibility to freeways and their geographical proximity to one another. Although such a strategy is well known to postal carriers and UPS drivers, it occurred to a slow-witted psychiatrist only through the unconscious imagery associated with dreamwork. I still have that map, and when I present it with my lectures to residential care facility administrators and mental health professionals (and I sometimes do), it is received with remarkable reverence—as if it were an important historical document like the Declaration of Independence or the Magna Carta.

Prior to this experience I was a conventional office psychiatrist, but the sudden emergence of a large-volume practice, replete with emergencies, did not adapt well to the luxuries of the meditative one-on-one office life. What I mean by this is that I no longer had the time to actively engage in long periods of pipe-smoking reflective silences while pondering the implications of a patient's response. Consequently, I developed a system of techniques that allowed me to rapidly evaluate patients. This system became very useful and has served me well in the subsequent thirty years I have been involved in residential care facility psychiatry. I have described them in Chapter 8.

Because of the generalized reluctance of psychiatrists to become involved in this type of practice, my commitments to residential care facilities grew rapidly and I was invited into many new homes. My initial impressions were that I was sometimes greeted with warmth and appreciation, much as I might have been at an isolated Midwestern farmhouse on a wintry day—a feeling quite unfamiliar to me as a psychiatrist and not at all unpleasant; at other times I was met with reserve and suspicion, possibly because of the feeling that I could not really do very much to change the isolated and hallucinated pattern of the occupants. But respect is the handmaiden of success, and when I succeeded in the sense that I could facilitate the improvement of the patients, respect replaced suspicion.

As in all fields, certain administrators excelled in their work, bringing to it sensitivities and energies that were truly remarkable; others did not. As a class, they deserve considerable respect, because residential care facility work is a twenty-four-hour-a-day commitment which exists seven days a week. Although administrators are essentially private entrepreneurs who must make a profit to stay in the business of board and care, it is not an easy way to make money. In the long run, it can be truly exhausting and the rate of burnout among administrators is quite high.

The problems of the administrators have been compounded by the inflationary cycle in that state-approved deductions for residential care facility payments have not kept up with increases in the costs of energy, food, and mortgage money. The net effect of this is that new residential care facilities are not being generated and attrition is taking its toll. Thus the total number of residential care facility beds in San Francisco has shrunk from 1,200 in 1978 to approximately 600 in 2004.

THE PIONEERS

Much of the foregoing I wrote more than twenty years ago. Since that time I and a few other psychiatrists in San Francisco—Richard A. Shadoan, Mel Blaustein, and Paul Heim—were pursuing our on-site residential care facility duties, each of us convinced that what we were doing was important in the sense of facilitating patient improvement, decreasing the incidence of rehospitalizations, and, in addition, saving the state lots of money. Our concept of our services was not necessarily in agreement with the value that other psychiatrists placed on our services.

With these issues in mind and with the intent of stimulating interest in this hitherto (and subsequently) ignored area of psychiatry, Mel Blaustein edited a special edition of *Psychiatric Annals* in 1985 dedicated to residential care.[6] Following this he organized a symposium which was presented at the American Psychiatric Association meeting in Washington, DC, in 1986. It was his hope and the hope of the panelists—which included myself, Paul Heim (the former vice chairman of the psychiatric department at St. Francis Memorial Hospital) and Richard Shadoan (ex-president of the California Psychiatric Association, ex-member of the board of trustees to the American Psychiatric Association, and ex-a lot of other things)—that we could popularize these issues and possibly make an impact in the way psychiatric services were delivered to the chronically mentally ill. We young Lochinvars had come out of the West with stars in our eyes and hopes in our hearts. We were soon to be disabused of our stars and our hopes.

The first clue that something was amiss lay in the logistics of the meeting. The planning committee, possibly as a result of the perceived triviality of residential care, banished our symposium to a site as far away from the convention center as possible—to the farthest reaches of the District of Columbia still within the borders of the continental United States. Whether this unfortunate selection was unintentional or deliberate is of little import, although the geographical isolation of the symposium symbolized residential care psychiatry's essential estrangement from mainstream psychiatry.

As a result of this internal exile, the only people present were the panelists, the wives of the panelists, and myself, plus one colicky infant whose paternity was established only later in the program. The situation was not without its comedic aspects: Following each presentation, the wives clapped enthusiastically, and even this uninvited, one-year-old, remarkably accomplished baby could and did applaud on cue, while simultaneously shouting "Daddy, Daddy" in response to his ambitious mother's insistent prodding. The one-year-old was still too young to harbor the primordial murderous patricidal hatreds that preoccupy the minds of the Oedipal theorists, but at least the rest of us then knew who his father was. Given the opportunity, any one of us could have done the patricide.

However, since I was single at the time, no wife was applauding for me and no precocious infant egged me on. He didn't even manage one adventitious clap. I think as a result of his phenomenal precociousness that perceptive little future psychoanalyst sensed I was not eligible for the adulation which ordinarily accompanies consanguinity, much like an ineligible receiver downfield, as they say in football. Because of these factors, my presentation was greeted with a gimlet-eyed silence. I mean, if silence could really be deafening, I would now be wearing bilateral hearing aids. I was mortified by the stony nonresponsiveness of the merry wives of Washington. The situation was all the more galling because I was sandwiched between two layers of adored husbands whose presentations were greeted with wildly enthusiastic proprietary applause by their spouses who obviously had entered into a cabal involving a barter system in which equal units of acclaim would be exchanged—you applaud for mine and I will applaud for yours—that sort of thing. When I returned to San Francisco I decided to get married.

Unfortunately the panel suffered similar indignities at future psychiatric conventions in Chicago in 1987, in New Orleans in 1988, and in San Francisco in 1989, again playing to spectacularly unpacked houses and again organized by the indefatigable Dr. Blaustein, a man blessed by the gods with the same kind of "irrational exuberance" that Alan Greenspan correctly attributed to the stock market of the late 1990s. Three weeks after that accusation Alan got married, so God only knows what he was thinking about. To my knowledge, nobody has ever remarked on this strange concatenation.

The final performance of our road trip was at an annual meeting of the California Psychiatric Association at the Asilomar Conference Center in Pacific Grove—same cast, same subject, same intimate devoted audience of wives but now grown world-weary from the obligatory annual conventional convention migrations. The only difference was that the infant was now four years into his unruly tykehood and still regrettably unorphaned. In the course of his precocious maturation he had mastered the remarkable facility of being able to applaud with both upper extremities for people (other than myself) while using both lower extremities to simultaneously toddle.

To ensure our isolation, the planning committee—possibly acting on enduring instructions from the planning committee of the prior Washington, DC, convention—scheduled our symposium opposite a psychiatrist, Denny Zeitlan, who was also a jazz concert pianist. I had never seen so many dedicated California psychiatrists who were suddenly patrons of the arts—even some of my best friends, although I suspect their frenzied rush for the exits resulted more from a distaste of the symposium's board-and-care theme (which should have been rechristened the Bored-and-Don't Care Symposium) rather than from a true love of music. This time when I returned to San Francisco I immediately started taking piano lessons with the intent of enhancing the box-office appeal of the symposium by providing mood music as a background accompaniment to my colleagues' lectures on mood stabilizers.

Subsequently the rest of the panel underwent a collective reactive depression and, since none of them responded to SSRIs, we never presented this symposium again despite the entreaties of the unflinchingly ebullient Dr. Blaustein. Even he, in the course of time, eventually abandoned his career as an itinerant impresario and finally found a steady job—as chairman of the Psychiatry Department at St.

Francis Memorial Hospital in San Francisco, where his tenacious cheerfulness in the face of recurrent adversity proved to be of inestimable value given the current state of chaos in Hospitalland. Because of this he is frequently referred to as Chairman Mel, an appellation stemming from genuine affection and a well-deserved admiration of his prodigious talents as an administrator, so much so that he no longer craves the adulation of packed houses, much to the relief of his applause-weary wife. In a sense, St. Francis Memorial Hospital became the packed house, and not just on opening night. Thus ended one of the most forgettable odysseys in the annals of American psychiatry, and one that has been hitherto entirely undocumented, possibly justifiably so.

I like to think of this group as pioneers, but we weren't pioneers at all, despite the heading under which this paragraph appears. Basically we were little more than a team of failed traveling salesmen in the Arthur Miller style—a bunch of Willy Loman hucksters hawking little bits of wisdom plucked from the board-and-care-home tree of knowledge and trying to distribute this produce free of charge but with no takers. It would be an exaggeration to say our enthusiastic efforts were greeted with apathy—collective somnolence would be more accurate.

Eighteen years have now passed since that nonhistoric meeting of the American Psychiatric Association in Washington, DC, in 1986, and as I look back upon the intervening events—given the philosophical maturity that accrues with mellowed retrospection—I remain convinced that these lamentable events are someone's fault and that somehow I should get even with him or her. Board-and-care psychiatry, as it was known then, still remains a stigmatized field, which partially explains its etymological evolution from "board and care" to "residential care." Thus, board-and-care homes are now referred to as "residential care facilities," and I have deferred to this designation. In San Francisco the city has found it necessary to hire a psychiatrist on the civil service payroll to make home visits because private practice psychiatrists refuse to do so. Perhaps that is the wave of the future.

Contributing in no small way to the reluctance of private practice psychiatrists to enter residential care facility work is the attitude of Medicare, which insists that a progress note be submitted for each residential care encounter (unlike office visits) before compensation may be made. Personally speaking, I still do it—that is to say I make my facility visits (formerly home visits) and in a grandiose way I still like to think of myself as an urban country doctor trudging through the San Francisco snows to do important business despite the hazards involved in generating aberrant computer profiles and the accompanying dangers of incurring Medicare audits.

Chapter 4

The Facility

Much of the material in this chapter is drawn from my own experiences working in residential care facilities and was originally described by me in one of the early articles that I wrote for *Psychiatric Annals* titled "Board-and-Care Homes, 1984: Return of the House Call." [1]

What can I say about the typical residential care facility except that there is no such entity? They are as different as families are different. The smaller homes tend to be more familial in the sense that a greater degree of personal involvement occurs between the administrator and the resident. Dependence, affection, and obligations vary as they might in families, with each parent interpreting his or her role somewhat differently.

Larger homes more nearly resemble residence clubs. Ties between administrator and resident are necessarily diluted. In a small home, the administrator may dine with the residents, whereas in a larger home this would not be true. While some patients prefer the intimacy and familial support that might be obtained in smaller homes, many others prefer the greater degree of anonymity and independence of the larger homes.

THE EVOLUTION OF RESIDENTIAL CARE FACILITIES

It is important to realize that there is no ideal home, only an ideal option—this being one in which a variety of homes are available to prospective patients who have a variety of needs. The variety of homes arises because individual personalities are not molded on the same template. Administrators endow their homes with their own habits, their own personalities, their own prejudices, and their own ideas about the kinds of patients they admit. Sometimes they are pressured to accept patients whom they might otherwise not admit.

The standardization factor enters the picture, as it should, via licensing regulations about the provision of food, shelter, and staffing patterns. Residential care facilities are categorized into homes for the developmentally disabled, homes for the mentally ill (with a stipulated age range between eighteen and sixty-five), and homes for geriatric patients. Each type of home has its own problems, as might be expected, and in the course of evolution many homes have become subcategorized with respect to their populations. Thus within the broad category of the developmentally disabled, several levels of care are offered, depending on the needs of the patient. The levels are defined by licensing. Therefore, some homes are approved for the moderately developmentally disabled (able to perform activities of daily living, educable, trainable), and others are licensed for the more severely impaired disabled (needs assistance with dressing, bathing, etc.).

Evolutionary subcategorization also characterizes the development of homes for the mentally ill so that one frequently finds homes specializing in the needs of the young chronic versus the middle chronic. Chronically ill young people tend to present more frequent problems insofar as they are characterized by increased lability, impulsivity, and intrusiveness, as well as a greater potential for violence and self-destructiveness. More and more placements now occur within this category, and residential care facility resources are now being pushed to their limits with respect to the referral of young mentally ill patients with violent and impulse-ridden histories. This is true because of the destruction of the state hospital system, the exorbitant costs of hospitalization at the community level, and the tendency of third-party payers and managed care organizations to discharge mental patients after only short periods of stay. Despite this, most residential care facilities are successful in the sense of preventing rehospitalizations and preventing violence. It is only the violent failures that make the headlines. Successful placements are not particularly newsworthy.

CASE HISTORIES

Here are extracts from the admission summaries of two violent patients as described by me a long time ago in a previous article who did not make the headlines and made successful adjustments to two different kinds of homes.

The first patient made a successful adjustment to a large residential home, the second to a smaller more familial home.

Case No. 1

This thirty-year-old single Hispanic male was admitted for the eighth time to this hospital on August 4, 1980, with a diagnosis of schizophrenia, paranoid type. This patient has a history of previous hospitalization dating back as far as 1974 with the diagnosis of schizophrenia, paranoid type. He also has a history of many antisocial behaviors and incarcerations since 1965, ranging from assault, theft, and shoplifting, to burglary. The patient was admitted this time with charges of assault. In June 1980, this patient struck a Chinese woman on the face with his fists without provocation, and after the woman fell down he started kicking her and jumping on her. On admission the patient claimed that this woman was messing up his mind. On admission he was noted to be alert, oriented, guarded, suspicious, and he denied any delusions. However, his behavior on the ward indicated auditory hallucinations with gross delusions. He was talking or mumbling to himself and thought there were invisible people on the ward. At one time he became hostile to the ward doctor and threatened to kill him. The patient was unable to go to trial because the judge and the court psychiatrists found him unable to cooperate with the defense and unable to comprehend the nature of the trial. He was then transferred to the Aspen ward to get the patient settled down and stabilize him so he would be ready for the trial. While at the Aspen ward, he continued to be hostile, suspicious, and withdrawn. He continued to have auditory hallucinations, complained that people were making plots against him and that people were still messing up his mind. He had been involved in a couple of fights with other male patients and from the reports it is noted he was always the aggressor. Part of his delusions included his distorted perception of women, who he thinks are simple. In the psychological testing done in October 1976, he considered himself "the right arm of God to punish these sinful women." He has unresolved conflicts with women, including guilt from his distorted perception of sex as well as masturbation. In the last several months of his stay at Aspen ward, he was fairly cooperative to ward routines but hadn't really gotten involved actively in any treatment programs. He refused to take an industrial assignment. He continues to be withdrawn and remains a loner. He is at times receptive to individual interviews. Just prior to this visit to jail for another court evaluation, he was starting to interact more with his peers.

Case No. 2

This thirty-year-old, single Chinese male was admitted as a transfer. He is under a conservatorship. He was admitted to the hospital on February 17,1972. He had a history of multiple hospital admissions since 1965; periods of violent behavior, including threatening and choking relatives. He attacked a sixteen-year-old white girl and was charged with battery. She was in a bookstore where he punched her down to the floor and lacerated her. He was in state hospitals from September 1965 to April 1971. Delusional, hallucinated, exhibits inappropriate high-pitched laughter. Sticks hands and feet into the air. Past history of violence in his home. Threatened family with knives and beat brothers. Never regularly employed.

Middle-aged chronic schizophrenics include a wide range of impaired behavior: The well-stabilized middle-aged chronic schizophrenic patient is set in his or her habits, predictable, with no recent hospitalizations and a minimum of medication changes needed to control the course of illness. On the other hand, the severely impaired middle-aged schizophrenics are poorly controlled with medications and are frequently described as "dilapidated." Sometimes the condition is aggravated by an admixture of alcohol, drugs, and incipient senescence. Occasionally there is a history of lobotomy. He or she may be episodically incontinent, may or may not choose to wear underwear, or conversely may wear multiple layers or outer clothing even on hot days. He or she frequently chain smokes to the point of retrieving butts from ashtrays and panhandling, and may frequently have multiple suprasternal holes in blouses or shirts where live ashes came to rest and made their mark.

Within these groups, administrators have preferences, and it is not always for the least worrisome as is exemplified by the cases just cited. The preferences and capabilities of residential care administrators become well known to placement workers and referrals are made accordingly.

SPECIALIZED REFERRAL PATTERNS

Specialized referral patterns can produce interesting reactions. Homes characterized by excessive loading of patients who are non-social middle-aged chronics leads to a clustering of patients around ashtrays and televisions, but with a degree of lack of comprehension that is amazing and apparent only with questioning. I remember one day entering a room in which eight men were gathered around a television set watching a football game apparently in rapt attention. *That's great,* I thought. "What's the score?" I asked. Nobody knew. "Who's playing?" Nobody knew that one either.

To the untrained eye, it would appear that some residential care facilities facilitate withdrawal and regression by tolerating such unwitting convocations. This critical appraisal tends to underestimate the extent to which nonsocialization may be a profound characterological allegiance not readily subject to change.

Granted that it is better for patients to go to activities, groups, trips, therapy sessions, etc., some patients will resist this with all the zeal of the professional revolutionary. It is easy to underestimate the commitment to avolition. This can be thoroughly exhausting and demoralizing to other types of professionals who have a vested interest in making therapeutic progress. In the real world sooner or later the isolates tend to cluster around their ashtrays and televisions, and the mental health professionals busy themselves with the more receptive and appreciative clients. The important point is to not allow the isolates to get too isolated. Make minimal contact within their tolerances so that they do not become too derailed or regressed. Generally, I can do this via monthly or twice-monthly brief encounters. After a time, I am acknowledged, eventually recognized, and sometimes even greeted.

PART II: THE PEOPLE

Chapter 5

Who Should Do It?

When I discuss residential care psychiatry and who should do it, I do so on the basis of my own experiences working in large homes containing ten or more residents. In small homes with just a few residents, it is possible to practice residential care psychiatry as one does in office settings—primarily in one-on-one situations in the luxury of a private room with the additional luxury of an allotted interval of time dedicated to an individual patient. This is one way to practice residential care psychiatry, but it is basically office psychiatry practiced in a residential care facility setting. My experiences in residential care facility psychiatry have been principally in large homes where the physical limitations were such as to discourage private sessions and where the time pressures were such that dedications of prolonged periods of time to selected patients were not practicable. Thus my comments about residential care psychiatry should be understood in that context. When I describe residential care facilities, I am focusing on large homes with many patients, most of whom have serious and severe mental illness of long duration and where the time demands were such so as to not allow the twenty-five-minute hour, much less the fifty-minute hour.

Most of the long-term residents of residential care facilities carry the diagnosis of schizophrenia—either as an undifferentiated reaction or one of its variants. The treatment of schizophrenia includes advantages and disadvantages. One of the advantages is that when schizophrenic patients get worse, either by virtue of increasing hallucinations, delusions, depression, or disorganization, usually something can be done about it, either through medication changes or some other kind of personal intervention. Frequently schizophrenic patients will improve rapidly in response to changes in medication or dosages.

By and large, such rapid improvements are generally associated with the treatment of the so-called positive symptoms of schizophrenia such as hallucinations and delusions. However, the negative expressions of the illness—such as flat affect, lack of motivation, and lack of interests—are much more resistant to treatment. In that sense the treatment of most of the residents of residential care facilities is ameliorative rather than curative. Sometimes negative symptomatology is a side effect of conventional antipsychotic medication, but many times it is an expression of core illness that does not respond to any known treatment. Residential care psychiatrists must adjust their therapeutic objectives on the basis of what can be accomplished rather than what they can hope for. Failure to do so will result in therapeutic demoralization and physicians leaving the field. Sometimes it is better to allow our therapeutic appetites to be satisfied by crumbs from the table rather than the feast which lies upon it. Sometimes crumbs are better than nothing.

Thus one of the qualifications of the successful residential care facility psychiatrist is the ability to survive professional starvation in the sense of being able to live on such crumbs. It is not our fault that we cannot cure schizophrenia. Despite all that I have said or will say about psychopharmacology, it has its limitations. It cannot make up for years of lost learning, lost job experiences, and whatever genetic vulnerabilities may exist. Rehabilitation of schizophrenic patients requires more than psychopharmacology. It requires the hard work of other disciplines and other orientations, including social work planning, psychosocial training, and cognitive therapies. But psychopharmacology can prepare the brain to assimilate new material. There can be no learning without the capacity to learn.

I am understating the gratifications that can occur in the long term, such as preventing relapse and participating in the rehabilitative process by working with other professionals—a process which I describe more fully in Chapter 7. Unique long-term gratifications can also occur as a consequence of working with residential care facility patients over a period of many years because for many patients their stays in residential care facilities may last for the rest of their lives. In the course of time the residential care facility psychiatrist will get to know the patient better than will any other professional. That works both ways in that the psychiatrist can become a significant other in the patient's life, especially in those who have lost contact with their families. Unfortunately this includes a large percentage of patients; the telephone calls I get from concerned family members are few and far between.

As a rule residential care psychiatry does not involve the treatment of psychoneurotic patients wherein sickness may interfere with productivity but does not prevent it. Psychoneurotics are usually not so severely impaired that they must live in a protective living facility. Generally speaking, psychoneurotics can continue with their work or schooling given the appropriate treatment by a patient and caring psychiatrist. It was my inability to provide such patient care that led me away from the treatment of psychoneurotics. Each of us in psychiatry must decide where our strengths lie and adjust our practices accordingly. Very few of us can be effective psychiatric general practitioners in the sense of handling anything that comes along. I exempted myself from seeing a certain kind of patient who was repetitive and offered resistances that I did not have the talent to overcome. Patience has never been one of my great virtues and at times I have felt the very unprofessional urge to tell some of my obsessive patients to snap out of it. I suspect other psychiatrists have had similar thoughts but would not acknowledge such heretical ruminations unless subject to some kind of an ethics inquisition.

If I am ever "a person of interest" in an auto-da-fé or placed on the rack, I know that after several hours of torture I would eventually break down and admit that I have sometimes conveyed my sense of impatience to patients by subtle clues such as not-so-furtive glances at my watch or drumming my fingers on the desktop in the middle of a sad story that should elicit a sympathetic ear rather than digital akathisia. One does not have to take remedial reading courses in body language to understand the import of such movements. If a tribunal decreed that this is sufficient to justify expulsion from the land of psychiatry and that I should forever be enjoined from the treatment of psychoneurosis, I would not necessarily argue the point. However I would not particularly like to see this as a framed disclaimer adjoining my other walled honorific plaques proclaiming competence in my profession. Perhaps one of the qualifications of a residential care facility psychiatrist is the inability to perform gainful work in other areas.

PSYCHOTHERAPEUTIC CONSIDERATIONS

It is safe to say that most psychiatrists who practice psychotherapy in an office—either their own office or in a semipublic setting such as a hospital or a clinic—would not want to work in the residential care facility settings I have just described. To do such work successfully requires a short but focused attention span, a quick wit, the ability to be folksy and colloquial when indicated, the ability to interact at a collegial level with nonprofessionals, and an optimistic trust in the effects of psychopharmacology. This is not to say that psychotherapy has no place. In fact, good psychopharmacology is dependent on personal interactions. The psychiatrist must be able to communicate with patients about their current cognitive or behavioral states, aside from the usual professional homage to hallucinations, delusions, and depression, the psychiatrist should be aware of changes in behavioral functioning relating to appetite, sleep, continence, bathing, bowel habits, dressing, and other aspects of personal hygiene. These are generally described by the acronym ADL, standing for activities of daily living.

ADLs are but one aspect of communal life. The residential care facility psychiatrist should also know about the patient's interaction with other residents of the facility. Is the patient appropriate in his or her interactions with other residents? Does the patient take advantage of others, or is the patient someone that others take advantage of? Does the patient have a history of stealing? Does the patient have a pattern of annoying others or disrupting others in minor ways, such as turning the televison set off while others are watching it or switching to another channel without consulting others? Does the patient monopolize the phone? Does the patient bring strangers into the home? People living together can intrude on the respective spaces of others in many ways, and the more the psychiatrist knows about such idiosyncrasies, the better he or she will be able to cope with the multiplicity of problems that can arise from such intrusions.

Also changes in interactive patterns may be the first signs of a resurgence of illness.

The first clue to an impending exacerbation may be subtle, as in the sudden absence of socially appropriate smiling. Similarly the first clue to an improved status may be superficially trivial but nevertheless significant, as when a disorganized schizophrenic patient told me that he was now able to brush his teeth. I responded to this information quite seriously with the comment that this was a notable achievement, because it indicated that he was now becoming more interested in self-care and more interested in assuming responsibility for his life. As it turned out, this was the signal event in what subsequently became a dramatic improvement. At that point I was acting more like a psychotherapist than a pharmacotherapist, but the fact is that frequently a psychopharmacological diet requires a psychotherapeutic garnish for optimal results.

When pinned to the wall I will reluctantly admit that on occasion I have committed psychotherapy, but with this patient psychotherapy would not have been effective without the necessary and preliminary improvement effected by pharmacotherapy. Before one crosses home plate one must traverse the bases. To put it another way, psychopharmacology is to psychotherapy as passport photos are to portraiture. We may need both, but without a passport photo one does not get a passport. When one is working with the chronically mentally ill, one hopes to enable them to obtain a passport to productivity.

Good psychopharmacology is not simply discussing drug side effects and measuring serum levels but is dependent on behavioral observations that involve the whole person over a twenty-four-hour cycle. If psychiatrists spend two hours of their day in a residential care facility, that means they are not there for twenty-two hours. Time is a zero-sum game. That means psychiatrists are strongly dependent on the information they receive from caregivers regarding the behavior of the patient when the psychiatrist is not on site. This is one of the reasons why psychiatrist should act in such a way as to be approachable by the house staff including cooks and housekeepers.

Also the psychiatrist should be alert to the nuances of language as it is used by the less well educated. On one occasion an alert administrator informed me that a patient was acting "funny." Now "funny" is in itself a funny word which frequently does not mean funny, as is exemplified by this sentence. I am generally not interested in funny unless I am writing a book, which I do about once every seventy-five years. But funny can have different meanings for different people, and it is a word that can be used to describe a wide range of pathological behavior. So I asked him what he meant by "funny," and he said, "You know, funny," so I said, "What do you mean by, 'you know, funny'?" So he said, "Like something funny," so I said, "Show me what you mean by something funny." The end result of this scintillating colloquy was that "funny" was used to describe a patient who was increasingly dysarthric and tremulous—and on lithium.

A quick trip to the nearest emergency room showed a serum lithium within the toxic range. The patient was subsequently hospitalized and made an uneventful recovery, but the story might have been quite different if the patient's toxic state had been allowed to continue in which case "funny" would not have been so funny. This ease of communication must also exist when the psychiatrist is not on the premises, so if the psychiatrist is someone who craves telephonic inaccessibility—as many of us do—it is probably not a wise choice to enter residential care work. This example also illustrates the importance of visitation frequency since if visits are not made with any reasonable degree of frequency, such events might not be discovered in a timely manner. I shall describe this case in greater detail in the chapter addressing frequency issues (Chapter 9).

THE ADVANTAGES OF A SENSE OF HUMOR

It is advisable, if at all possible, that residential care psychiatrists should have a sense of humor or sense of humors—whichever is correct. Actually, they are both correct. I know that the use of the plural version is an affront to the sensitivities of some, but there is more here than meets the bilious eyes of irate grammarians. When I use the term *sense of humors* I am referring to the medieval humors of blood, phlegm, yellow bile, and black bile, and which, according to Galen, are supposed to give rise to the sanguine, choleric, phlegmatic, and choleric temperaments respectively. But it was Hippocrates who originally postulated that an imbalance among the humors resulted in pain and disease. According to Hippocrates, good health was achieved when the four humors were in balance. Physicians—and even psychiatrists—should know this because we did take his oath before we were allowed to practice medicine. Besides, it is precisely this kind of knowledge that creates the impression of Renaissance-man omniscience, should the subject ever arise during one of the interviews with the chronic schizophrenic patient. In other words, it is simply good PR.

However, the sense of humor—in the singular sense—is even more important.

By sense of humor, in this sense, I am referring to the capacity to perceive, appreciate, or express that which is funny, incongruous, amusing, or ludicrous. It is a quality not shared by any of our phylogenetic relatives despite the reputed preponderance of DNA commonalities. We may share life, death, sleep, appetite, and aggression with our mammalian relatives. We do not share humor. Since only humans demonstrate it, that in itself implies a higher level of functioning notwithstanding the claims of animal activists who might consider this statement as indicative of speciesism. However, I will grant that humor is not evenly distributed among all the members of this species.

At the outset it should be clearly stated that humor is not essential in the performance of one's duties in residential care psychiatry. However, it is facilitative and can be used to defuse situations that might be destructive, as I shall describe shortly. Actually I don't know how one obtains a sense of humor even though this is a how-to-do-it-type book. I know that for me developing a playful sense of humor was particularly difficult as a result of spending many of my formative years in a quasi-psychoanalytic environment. I vividly recall being advised to never touch a patient. I believe we spent about two years practicing not touching patients, which I did while simultaneously trying to develop my emotional maturity. I remember those years with unusual clarity if only for the reason that they were so forgettable. Anyway, the first time a patient offered to shake my hand I blew it entirely. I became panicky and refused the offer in some socially clumsy way that I am still too embarrassed to describe, even to this day, but writing books demands honesty. I believe I said something like, "I am not allowed to touch you." The patient thought I was somewhat strange. In retrospect I believe what I should have done was to have assessed the situation calmly and said something like, "Professional ethics prevent any type of physical contact with you, however trivial that may seem." I think that may have resolved the situation.

Medical school gave me a different outlook regarding handshaking. I will now admit that I am now a vigorous handshaker, and when I do shake hands I have extraneous thoughts that are entirely unrelated to social rituals. Thus in the course of handshaking, I dutifully note the presence of flaccidity, coarse tremor, fine tremor, bradykinesia, sweaty palms, Dupuytren's contractures, palmer erythema, hypothenar atrophy, ulnar deviation, Heberden's nodes, tobacco-stained fingers, dirty fingernails, and even bitten-down fingernails. I admit to being a compulsive handwatcher. Later I also check the patient's hands.

By now the intelligent reader will have deducted that I am not averse to what is popularly known as "kidding around" with patients. At times, however, I try to make a serious point and it is obscured by my unrestrained levity. This is something I cannot control. If there is a bon mot lurking in that part of my brain in which comedic material accumulates, then it must be expressed or I get very nervous even if it leads to digressive ramblings—as is exemplified by this paragraph and to an extent, throughout this book. In fact, these comedic ruminations create the same kind of cognitive urgency that compel the coprophilic utterances of a patient in the final throes of Tourette's syndrome, a strange eponymic affliction possibly caused by some random cosmic ray hit producing the mutation of a single gene, as in cystic fibrosis or Mediterranean thalassemia. These thoughts demand expression or I get very nervous in an obsessive-compulsive way, experiencing much the same emotions as the checker who cannot check or the groomer who cannot groom—to say nothing of the discomfort experienced by the compulsive hand-washer with limited access to a faucet or the exquisite agony of the symmetry freak when encountering asymmetrical effronteries.

When the chips are down I can't really explain this humor thing. I will accept the explanation that it must be expressed because, like Everest, it is there. Occasionally these hypomanic cyclical excursions take me into uncharted waters, but, like Henry the Navigator, the fabled prince of Portugal, I always manage to find my way back. It is also historically true that Henry the Navigator never made any voyages himself. I hope that will not be true of me.

However, this book is not about me. This book is about me in relation to others. Having explained that, let me say that "kidding around" can be very useful. Sometimes the ability to kid around is the first sign of a patient's improvement. Seriously disturbed or preoccupied patients do not have the ability to kid around, and I do not attempt it with them, nor do I even think about it. The emotional tenor of an encounter with this type of patient does not lend itself to any kind of frivolity, so I do not do it. It's not as if this refusal to kid around is a contrived manipulation designed to test the patient; it's simply that I do not spontaneously invoke it and there is no cognitive effort involved in terms of thinking about whether it is appropriate or productive. Possibly this comes from a primordial self-protective instinct that subserves an evolutionary function in that it is used to assess who is friendly and who is not. Perhaps this is teleological over-reaching, but as I say I do this without thinking about whether it should be done, and I refrain from kidding around without thinking about whether it should not be done. However, if I had to make rules about humor, I would say that generally speaking it serves no useful purpose with patients who are depressed, paranoid, or seriously cognitively impaired.

Loss of a sense of humor has never been defined as a negative symptom or included in the deficit pattern of schizophrenia along with anhedonia, alogia, avolition, affective flattening, and social withdrawal, but perhaps it should be included as "ahumor" or an equivalent synonym with an "a-" prefix, connoting difficulty in responding to or recognizing humor.

Ahumor has never been officially designated as a symptom because it can exist as a character trait in people who are otherwise clinically normal. However, when humor does exist as a component of the premorbid personality, it frequently fluctuates with the course of an illness and in that sense it can be regarded as a symptom. As such it may be transitory or permanent. Ahumor can exist as a transitory symptom when one's underlying capacity to express or respond to humor is impaired by a cyclical depression, although it is not generally listed among the more typical depressive symptoms such as depressed mood, diminished interest in activities, changes in appetite, changes in sleep pattern, exaggerated feelings of guilt, excessive fatigue, impaired concentration, or suicidal thoughts.

The opposite of ahumor occurs in the manic state in which humor is expressed in the hyper form so that it is uncontrollable, poorly focused and inappropriate. In this case the expressed humor seems funny to self, but not to others. In a sense humor may be regarded as having a dimensional quality with ahumor at the low end and unfunny hyperhumor at the high end. Hyperhumor plays to an empty house in the sense that it is entertaining to the self but not to others. Hyperhumor, as might be displayed by someone laughing uproariously to himself or herself, immediately conveys the impression of profound irrationality even to the unsophisticated observer. One can think of hyperhumor as stuff which exists in a state of increased pressure, causing its inappropriate release, just as the overtalkativeness of mania is regarded as a product of increased pressure of speech. The analogy invites the phrase "increase pressure of humor" to describe hyperhumor.

In contrast, humor in the middle of the spectrum is other-directed. It is necessarily interactive and invites reciprocity if only by engendering a laugh or encouraging some other kind of friendly response. The only time midspectrum humor is not interactive is when it plays to a sitcom laugh track. This media machine-generated push-button gimmick is so ubiquitous that we have become inured to the fact that it is an essentially deceptive representation of interactive spontaneity, in that the viewing public is led to believe that it is hearing the responses of a live on-site audience. Nobody worries about this. Nobody even cares about this and there is no price to pay. Laugh track engineers are not going to be expelled from West Point for PR cheating even though this is clearly what it is. The manufacturers of synthesized hilarity may not be in violation of truth-in-advertising laws but they are clearly in violation of truth-in-presentation traditions. Humor may be the only quality that is unique to the human species now that primates can learn language through signing and have been observed using tools and making war.

In evaluating patient progress one must learn to recognize the early signs of the return of humor in the first faint glimmerings of an incipient smile as it evolves from the formerly slitlike fissure of a frozen face. This epiphenomena, more like a nudge than an awakening, may be the first sign of improvement, much as the dawn precedes the sunrise.

The following incident illustrates how midspectral humor (if I can call it that) can be applied to counteract a potentially unpleasant situation: I was asked to complete a conservatorship application form for a paranoid patient. He objected vigorously to the wording of the form and accused me of claiming that he could not handle his affairs. I countered with the statement that I didn't even know he had affairs. The patient was able to react to the humorous implications of my remark and the incident was defused.

When I encounter such resistances, I generally do not embark on plodding pedestrian psychoanalytic misadventures into the jungles of the unconscious in search of the holy grail of insight. At times I have asked myself whether such breezy responses originate from a superficial relationship with my patients, and that what I am doing is simply a form of post–Johnny Carson late-night talk-show hucksterism, a kind of stand-up comedian performing his functions while never leaving the sitting position. But it is more than that. Sometimes what appears to be superficial is only superficially superficial. First, this kind of response enables me to gracefully extricate myself from a situation that might otherwise be confrontational. In a sense this is self-serving, but sometimes it is acceptable for the self to be served. Second, it allows the patient a face-saving release from an aggressive posture so that another self is served besides my own self. Third, I am providing possible options for patients who might otherwise have knee-jerk aggressive responses to aggressive provocations. Finally, by so doing, I am preserving something of inestimable value—a friendly relationship with a patient who otherwise could not tolerate friendship. Although a good relationship with any patient is important, it is more important with this patient because he refuses to acknowledge that he is ill and refuses to see any other psychiatrist. In this instance, kidding around functions as a preservative for the relationship.

In a sense I have functioned as a role model to this kind of patient. I realize that I am talking as a psychotherapist now despite the fact that what I am doing is primarily psychiatric pharmacotherapy. However, in the process of years of such admittedly narrow interactions, the psychopharmacologist unwittingly assumes the mantle of the psychotherapist. If the patient picks up on this, the rewards can be great because humor can deflect aggression. Humor and aggression cannot coexist in the same mind-set. Humor can be aggressive, but only in a verbal sense and not in the physical sense. People are not incarcerated and lives are not destroyed by aggressive humor. It is the aggressive act that creates the problems. Victims held hostage by bank-robbers do not witness the criminals engaged in humorous interchanges as they go about their banking business.

Sometimes my quests to promote patient insights through humor take controversial routes, as indicated by the following colloquy during an initial interview:

ME: What medicines are you taking now?

PATIENT: I am taking Zyprexa, Xanax, Celexa, Loxitane, and amoxetine.

ME: Has it ever occurred to you that all the medicines you are taking are spelled with an x?

It is small wonder then that some of my attempts at insight are more inciteful (not a real word) than insightful (a real word) but actually this patient thought my initial questions were quite perceptive and this paved the way for a productive relationship. Eventually she described our intial interview as "refreshingly different." I don't know why I do things like that except that sometimes I think that the principal difference between the treater and the treatee is that the treater is in possession of the keys, if only in a symbolic sense because residential care facilities are unlocked by definition and by licensing laws. Symbolic or not, I find that sometimes I hold on to these keys with an uncommon degree of ferocity—which is not quite the word I am looking for, but which approximates the emotions elicited. Perhaps that—or something like that—is what underlies the origin of the phrase "losing one's grip." Be that as it may, my initial instincts were correct. The problem, however, was not that all the medicines she was taking were spelled with an x, but that she was taking too many medicines that were spelled with an x. She improved dramatically after two of the x-spelled medicines were ex'ed out.

Sometimes my humor is not appreciated, as in the following interchange.

PATIENT: Doctor, I am concerned about who will take care of me when you die. Have you made any arrangements for someone to take over your practice?

ME: When I die, my obligation to take care of you ends.

My little joke died and appears to have preceded my own death by many years, but I actually have made arrangements for such utterly impossible contingencies, though I did not choose to go into detail. Instead, I used the opportunity to discuss the fact that in life nobody has 100 percent guarantees about anything, including the time sequences with which people die, and it is possible to worry too much about such events. I once took care of a fifty-year-old very dependent schizophrenic patient who was living with his ninety-two-year-old mother, and he really was not concerned about his mother dying. However, the social worker was. She would telephone and ask me what arrangements I would make for Loren when his mother died. Shouldn't I get him into a program or shouldn't I encourage him to be more independent or shouldn't I try to place him in a residential care facility or shouldn't I do this or shouldn't I do that, until one day I asked her, "Shouldn't you stop calling me?" What happened next is that Loren died before his mother. That social worker no longer calls me. In fact, she doesn't even write. It's like I no longer exist.

Sometimes humor can be used to trespass upon territories that might otherwise be avoided, as illustrated in the following progress note written by me on March 5, 2001:

> A sixty-one-year-old chronic schizophrenic male, currently a resident of the Ritz-Carleton residential care facility [not the real name] whom I have been following since 1994. Good handshaker, good eye contact, but pt. somewhat malodorous. Smells as if he is incontinent of urine. Staff reports that he has to be reminded to shower and shave and change his underwear. He only does this twice a week.

I discussed this problem in the presence of the caretaker. What I said was this:

> Joe, do you remember all those ads on the radio that used to describe body odor as BO? Remember how they used to say, "Even your best friends won't tell you"? Well, we are better than your best friends—we tell you, Joe. Joe, you've got BO.

I presented it as a rhyming jingle. In this case, this gingerly approach to the indelicate, eased by humor's lubricant, had its advantages. The patient laughed, the administrator laughed. I laughed. Everyone had a fantastic time. Joe countered with, "I promise to be a good citizen and not smell of urine anymore." More hilarity—and all done without the assistance of a laugh track. In fact, I don't like laugh tracks, or did I already say that? As I said before, this approach is not prescriptive in the sense that it can be used on everybody. One has to know the territory in the sense of anticipating how the patient will respond to this technique. In many instances humor can be counterproductive. My response to the patient who told me about brushing his teeth was not humorous, and I believe a cavalier or dismissive response under those circumstances could have had a destructive effect.

I suppose one can think of humor as a new form of alternative medicine—laugh therapy—something like aroma thereapy but without the smells. The truth of the matter is that I generally prefer alternatives to alternative medicine—this being an acquired taste—a taste aquired only by dint of long years of nonattendance at the Harvard Medical School.

Humor can even be used with people who have severe communication problems—even with the total language barrier of people who were described in harsher days as "deaf and dumb," two ugly four-letter, one-syllable, mean-spirited, old-fashioned words which nevertheless convey the grim profundity of this impairment much more accurately than the insipid "hearing impaired." One such patient with that disability was living alone—in a sense—amid a population of the hearing unimpaired. At times I could feel his eyes on the back of my neck as I was busily engaged as a progress note scribe. At other times, from my central seat in the eye of the hurricane—a metaphor which I shall explain in a subsequent chapter—I could observe him, standing at the periphery of the crowd, always clean-shaven, always well-groomed with an alert face that was hungry for communication in the way that deprived children's hungers are expressed in their eyes when they flatten their noses against tantalizing storefront windows at Christmastime looking at brightly colored toys they wish they could have but know they never can. Only the deprivation endured by this man did not have the temporal limits of Christmas—it endures in perpetuity, day after day and year after year and minute after minute in stone silence. It was years until I found out that I could communicate with him by writing notes in large block capital letters which he was then able to read and to which he could respond in kind. Nothing in his chart indicated that he had this capability, and he could not tell me about it because he was unwillingly sworn to secrecy. Following this chance discovery I was able to establish a relationship with him and even engage in a little kidding around as is indicated in the following written colloquy. Here is the progress note that we co-authored on December 1, 2003.

(Me): OSCAR, HOW ARE YOU FEELING?
(Him): GOOD.
(Me): HOW ARE YOU SLEEPING?
(Him): GOOD.
(Me): ANYTHING NEW HAPPENING?
(Him): BURTHDAY.
(Me): WHEN?
(Him): JAN 9 2004.

(Me): HOW OLD?

(Him): 60.

(Me): WOW, OLD MAN!

He then cracks up in his own way. He convulses in silent laughter, and starts walking in a bent posture taking small Parkinsonian-like steps as old men do, and draws his hand over the lower part of his face as if fingering an old man's beard.

At one time in America's past the governor of North Carolina, John Motley Morehead, is reputed to have said to the governor of South Carolina, James H. Hammond, that it was a long time between drinks. For Oscar without-a-motley-last-name, it has been a long time between laughs. I think I made his day—maybe I even made his year. Sometimes I think if I were to die, that is to say—if I were to ever die, Oscar would cry a silent tear.

BEHAVIORAL THERAPY APPLICATIONS

Sometimes humor can be combined with behavioral therapy as indicated by the following incident. A young African-American patient who had a long-standing delusion that he was being pursued by Mexicans was getting into difficulty because every morning he would go into the backyard next to the NIMBY neighbors' backyards and shout that the Mexicans were after him. Not only was he disturbing the other residents but he was also disturbing the neighbors. Now the residents are usually not much of a problem because, being mentally ill themselves, they have an intuitive understanding and tolerance for the idiosyncrasies of their fellow residents, but neighbors are another story. Disturbing the neighbors is a serious offense in the residential care facility world because disturbing the neighbors can cause a NIMBY backlash that can result in the patient being expelled from the home, or under more dramatic circumstances, it can result in the home being expelled from the neighborhood.

Therefore it was imperative that I do something. I attempted various kinds of sophisticated psychopharmacological approaches all to no avail. I then asked the patient to show me what he did. He then started a little hip-hop routine and after a while he shouted, "The

Mexicans are after me; the Mexicans are after me." This resulted in the following therapeutic interchange:

ME: It's too loud. [I then simulated the hip-hop movements—to the best of the ability of a presumptuous seventy-five-year-old white man—and repeated the words, "The Mexicans are after me; the Mexicans are after me" in a softer cadence. I then told him to do it my way.]

PATIENT: The Mexicans are after me; the Mexicans are after me.

ME: Softer.

PATIENT: The Mexicans are after me; the Mexicans are after me.

ME [louder]: Softer.

PATIENT: The Mexicans are after me; the Mexicans are after me.

ME [even louder]: Softer!

PATIENT: The Mexicans are after me; the Mexicans are after me.

ME: I think you've got it. By George, you've got it.[1]

Now if the truth be told, he didn't get it in one session (but neither did Eliza Doolittle), and there had to be several rehearsals on subsequent visits, but eventually he did get it.

Did you notice how in the last dialogue I described myself as a "seventy-five-year-old white male" and then quickly left the subject as if embarrassed by this revelation? Actually getting old or older (a more pleasant word) has certain advantages in psychiatry. I have noticed that the longer I live, the longer is my relationship with patients, the greater is my degree of understanding. In psychiatry, increasing age does not necessarily impair one's professional skills. Retired surgeons luxuriating in Boca Raton should have it so good. It is said that wisdom comes with age. It doesn't quite work that way. Wisdom is not an automatic accompaniment of aging—like arthritis and flaccidity, but it does happen. The way it works is that when you get older, patients and colleagues seem to pay more attention to what you say. Therefore, you must be more careful about what you say, lest you may be branded as an old fool—and there is no fool like an old fool. So, the appearance of wisdom evolves partly as the result of what you say, partly as a result what you do not say, and partly as a result of the expectations that others have of you—and your reaction to their expectations.

I also described "the ability to be folksy and colloquial when indicated." I should also mention that sometimes the residential care facility psychiatrist should be somewhat autobiographical in contrast to
the SOP (standard office procedure) psychiatrist. The following incident illustrates the application of these elements:

The administrator recommended that I see a patient who was arrested on a minor charge and was refusing to keep a court appointment.

PATIENT: No way am I going to see the judge.

ME: When I was a kid [autobiographical mode] and if I had a bad attitude, they would take my bubble gum away [folksy mode] but if
you have a bad attitude as an adult they can put you in the slammer
[colloquial mode], and that's a lot worse than taking your bubble
gum away [reversion to folksy mode]. Nowadays there are dudes
[colloquial] doing hard time [colloquial] and the only reason for
this is that someone dinged them [colloquial] with a bad attitude
rap. Now there's such a thing as being street-smart [colloquial
again] and street-stupid [original mode]. Don't be street-stupid
[more original mode stuff]."

PATIENT: "Thanks, Doc. I really appreciate your advice."

Here is the progress note I entered for February 28, 2001:

> Pt. has court appointment for Mar 3 or 5, but he doesn't want to go be-
> cause he is afraid they will lock him up. I lectured pt. about the advis-
> ability of being cooperative. He then agreed he should be cooperative
> and have a good attitude and go to court.

This visit, coded as medication management, really happened and
possibly saved everyone, including the justice system, a moderate
amount of time and trouble. Two weeks later I entered the next progress note.

> Continues in good spirits. Pt. states that after his talk with me he kept
> his appointment with the judge. Now he has signed up for treatment
> with the Haight-Ashbury Free Clinic Drug Treatment Program. Contin-
> ues on Prolixin 10 mg twice a day, Cogentin 2 mg twice a day. No ap-
> parent adverse side effects. Staff reports no interim management
> problems.

GROUP PSYCHOTHERAPY CONSIDERATIONS

I haven't said much about conducting group psychotherapy in residential care facilities. I won't say this has no place, but it's not necessarily the best place to be for the psychopharmacological psychiatrist. I will say more about this issue in Chapter 7 when I discuss the "Medical Care Guidelines for Psychiatric Patients in Residential Care Homes" issued by the Northern California Psychiatric Society. For now I will restrict myself to a quotation from an article I wrote nineteen years ago.[2] I quote it now because what I said then is still true:

> The problem with ongoing group therapy or community meetings with the stabilized chronic patient is that it is likely to be ongoing year after year—with the same participants, and the script is likely to become repetitious. Sometimes signs of progress or of what the group therapist regards as progress, are not necessarily evident to others, and if the administrator feels she is participating in an essentially nonproductive, time-wasting enterprise, her relationship to the psychiatrist can be adversely affected. A psychiatrist insisting on involving a reluctant administrator in this endeavor can quickly find himself or herself persona non grata.

Chapter 6

The Job Description

Several years ago, a visiting social worker from the licensing department requested that I submit a letter to a residential care facility administrator describing the duties of psychiatrists who visited his home. I have always resented nosy people who ask me what I do in life, partially because there are times when I am not quite sure. Insecurity is the mother of resentment. However, on reflection, her request was quite reasonable because at the time nobody appeared to know what a residential care facility psychiatrist does or should do. This state of ignorance continues to the present time and is the principal reason why I am writing this book.

At the time there appeared to be an unwritten assumption that the skills necessary for a successful office practice are directly transferable to residential care facility settings, which, of course, was not true. The following letter was written in response to that request and was notable for two reasons: It established the framework for the formulation of an official job description, and it convinced me that I could write publishable material, since the letter was the basis for an article published in *Psychiatric Annals*.[1] Prior to this time the only written materials I had ever produced were unpublishable letters to the editor.

Dear Mr. Administrator:

This letter is being sent to you in response to the licensing worker's request that you obtain a letter from me explaining the functions of a residential care facility psychiatrist. [The original wording was board-and-care psychiatrist].

These functions are quite varied, and so I have classified them into four categories: evaluation, treatment, consultation, and miscellaneous. However, considerable overlap occurs among these categories.

1. *Evaluation:* Evaluation of patients may necessitate on-site operations such as observation of the patient and consultation with the administrator regarding the patient's symptomatology within the recent past. Thus a patient may seem relatively well during the period of time that the psychiatrist is at the house but may be confused or inappropriate during the night or preceding day. The psychiatrist might not be aware of this if he did not confer with the administrator, which is why this consultation is very important in evaluation.

Also, evaluation may involve off-site operations such as review of historical documents in the psychiatrist's office file. Such a review may additionally help to understand the reasons for the recurrence of symptoms.

2. *Treatment:* The treatment of patients is dependent upon the evaluation and may involve psychotherapy and/or pharmacological therapy. Pharmacological therapy may involve stopping, starting, increasing, or decreasing medications. It may involve the evaluation of drug-drug interactions, including drugs not specifically used for psychiatric purposes. It always involves an estimate of risk-benefit ratios. It may require periodic laboratory examinations. It may involve the administration of intramuscular drugs especially when previous therapy with oral medications has proved to be ineffective.

Treatment of patients may necessitate a psychiatric hospitalization during which time the house psychiatrist may treat the patient within the hospital and upon improvement may refer the patient back to the house, or may advise against this.

3. *Consultation:* Consultation with the administrator involves helping the administrator to understand and cope with behavioral patterns, and helping the administrator recognize the early signs of a psychosis of increasing severity, the hope being that accelerated therapy in the early phase of an illness can prevent a severe psychosis with a resultant hospitalization.

Consultation may involve a discussion of the side effects of medication. It may involve the admission of new residents, or the readmission of former residents in assessing the effect of their presence on the other residents of the house.

Consultation is not limited to the above, and may involve a discussion of other subjects as they pertain to the treatment of residents.

4. *Miscellaneous:* The following functions may be additionally categorized, but for purposes of brevity are summarized as miscellaneous. Hence the residential care facility psychiatrist may perform any of the following services, some of which are rendered on site, some of which are rendered off site:

   a. Confers with the house internist because of the possibility of drug-drug interactions
   b. Confers with the house internist because of the recognition of early signs of an impending physical illness

c. Requests a home visiting team to see a resident for purpose of obtaining a 5150 commitment when a resident with a severe psychiatric illness refuses the option of voluntary hospitalization

d. Checks bottles of medications in the house cabinet to see that they are in accord with physician's directions

e. Telephones the pharmacist to clarify directions on the medication bottle labels, or to order new medications

f. Confers with various mental health agency social workers re: specific patients

g. Communicates with the Medi-Cal consultant to order nonformulary drugs for patients on Medi-Cal (need for these drugs must be justified by documenting the inefficacy of formulary drugs that patient has used in the past)

h. Completes various and sundry forms including, but not limited to, applications for disability, renewal of disability, ability to handle funds, conservatorships, etc.

i. Writes to hospitals and other institutions to obtain previous case history information

j. Calls laboratories to order tests as indicated

k. Writes progress notes in house charts

l. Calls ambulance in possibility of medical emergency for transportation to an emergency room

m. Communicates with relatives as necessary

This list is not necessarily complete, nor should it necessarily be interpreted as what a residential care facility psychiatrist should do, but it is a rough description of what I do.

By way of implementing the above, I find it desirable to visit the house on a scheduled basis, although in the event of an emergency, or as the situation demands, I also make nonscheduled visits.

Sincerely yours,
Martin Fleishman, MD

Looking back upon this job description, with the objectivity that accrues with passing years, it becomes apparent to me that I gave psychotherapy rather short shrift. In fact, this was not true in the early years of my commitment to residential care facilities.

Thus, at that time, when my caseload was minimal, greater emphasis was placed on psychotherapy, both in a one-on-one setting and in group settings. In the course of time as my practice increased, and the amount of time per patient necessarily decreased, I spent a greater portion of my time in targeted psychopharmacology, crisis management, and hospitalization. Psychotherapy was left, for the most part, to social workers, rehabilitation therapists, or other mental health professionals. Also, as our experience with chronic schizophrenics in the community grew, it became increasingly apparent that the kind of psychotherapy which appeared to be most fruitful to those patients was psychosocially oriented with an emphasis on the here and now— a therapy with a pragmatic focus such as the problems involved in budgeting, personal cleanliness and hygiene, and the importance of observing social amenities. This is a therapeutic style for which psychiatrists are not necessarily the best suited. One has to acknowledge that the constraints of time sometimes lead to therapeutic minimalism. However, what may be construed as a minimalistic approach to chronicity actually contains hidden advantages.

Many schizophrenics cannot tolerate relationships—or if they can, only in an attenuated form. For these, a quick hello and a quick good-bye is sometimes a necessary prelude to more meaningful encounters. Only after several months of these rituals are they ready for more. Wise psychiatrists understand the rhythm of these social gradualists; if they do not push too far too soon, they may accomplish far more than any of their predecessors. I have had many negative-symptom, withdrawn, avoidant schizophrenics request to continue as office patients after having left the residential care home, and I believe this to be true partly because I was not pushy or intrusive.

I would make other changes if I had to rewrite the job description. Present-day psychiatry has become much more medically oriented and the psychiatrist now has a much greater involvement in decisions that require medical sophistication. This job description was written in the days before the advent of cytochrome P450, and at the time we didn't have to worry about such electrocardiographic niceties as the QTc interval and its worrisome prolongations.

As the residential care psychiatrist's patient care load grows he or she will necessarily be more involved with issues involving crisis management, psychopharmacology, hospitalization, and organization of community treatment facilities. As a result of this, psychiatrists in large residential care practices will spend a great deal of their office time on the telephone. They will be spending much time in patient care that is not face-to-face time. Such time is not legally compensable as it is in hospitals, where compensable time does not have to be face to face. This use of time is compensable in hospitals because it is understood by third-party payers that hospitalizations necessitate prodigious paperwork and interactive obligations with other professionals. These noninterpersonal interactions are paid for on the basis of floor time—this being the amount of time physicians spend on the floor, hopefully while standing; taking care of their patients. Residential care facilities do not have compensable floors.

While traditional psychotherapeutic approaches may be applicable in small residential care facility practices, psychiatrists in larger practices will find that they spend a greater percentage of their time in crisis management and psychopharmacology. Also they will be spending a great deal of their office time taking care of patients they are not seeing in the office. They will write to hospitals about patients seen at the residential care facilities, assimilate their case histories, and communicate with other professionals regarding various aspects of patient care. This may be part of the inevitable curse of bigness and may be regarded as either a curse or a blessing, depending on the psychiatrist's interests. Psychiatrists who prefer the more traditional one-on-one approaches should probably stay small.

Chapter 7

The Cast

The cast consists of the patient, the psychiatrist, the social worker, the pharmacist, the administrator, the case worker, and possibly later, the psychologist. I have left the psychiatrist out of this chapter since he or she is the focus of most of the other chapters.

We will start with the patient, since the patient is the most important part of the cast. Without the patients, there would be no cast.

THE PATIENT

There is no typical residential care facility patient. However, most of them share some characteristics, such as having had multiple psychiatric hospitalizations. Most of them also carry the diagnosis of one of the following schizophrenic diagnostic subcategories. The categories are reprinted with permission from the *Diagnostic and Statistical Manual of Mental Disorders,* Fourth Edition.[1]

A. **Characteristic symptoms:** Two (or more) of the following, each present for a significant portion of time during a 1-month period (or less if successfully treated):

1. delusions
2. hallucinations
3. disorganized speech (e.g., frequent derailment or incoherence)
4. grossly disorganized or catatonic behavior
5. negative symptoms, i.e., affective flattening, alogia, or avolition

B. **Social/occupational dysfunction:** For a significant portion of the time since the onset of the disturbance, one or more major areas of functioning such as work, interpersonal relations, or self-care are markedly below the level achieved prior to the onset (or when the onset is in childhood or adolescence, failure to achieve expected level of interpersonal, academic, or occupational achievement).

C. **Duration:** Continuous signs of the disturbance persist for at least 6 months. This 6-month period must include at least 1 month of symptoms (or less if successfully treated) that meet Criterion A (i.e., active-phase symptoms) and may include periods of prodromal or residual symptoms. During these prodromal or residual periods, the signs of the disturbance may be manifested by only negative symptoms or two or more symptoms listed in Criterion A present in an attenuated form (e.g., odd beliefs, unusual perceptual experiences).

D. **Schizoaffective and Mood Disorder exclusion:** Schizoaffective Disorder and Mood Disorder With Psychotic Features have been ruled out because either (1) no Major Depressive Episode, Manic, or Mixed Episodes have occurred concurrently with the active-phase symptoms; or (2) if mood episodes have occurred during active-phase symptoms, their total duration has been brief relative to the duration of the active and residual periods.

E. **Substance/general medical condition exclusion:** The disturbance is not due to the direct physiological effects of a substance (e.g., a drug of abuse, a medication) or a general medical condition.

F. **Relationship to a Pervasive Developmental Disorder:** If there is a history of Autistic Disorder or another Pervasive Developmental Disorder, the additional diagnosis of Schizophrenia is made only if prominent delusions or hallucinations are also present for at least a month (or less if successfully treated).

The DSM-IV offers the following breakdown of schizophrenic diagnostic subtypes.

Paranoid Type

A type of Schizophrenia in which the following criteria are met:

A.   Preoccupation with one or more delusions or frequent auditory hallucinations.

B.   None of the following is prominent: disorganized speech, disorganized or catatonic behavior, or flat or inappropriate affect.

Disorganized Type

A type of Schizophrenia in which the following criteria are met:

A.   All of the following are prominent:
     (1) disorganized speech
     (2) disorganized behavior
     (3) flat or inappropriate affect
B.   The criteria are not met for Catatonic Type.

Catatonic Type

A type of Schizophrenia in which the clinical picture is dominated by at least two of the following:

1. motoric immobility as evidenced by catalepsy (including waxy flexibility) or stupor
2. excessive motor activity (that is apparently purposeless and not influenced by external stimuli)
3. extreme negativism (an apparently motiveless resistance to all instructions or maintenance of a rigid posture against attempts to be moved) or mutism
4. peculiarities of voluntary movement as evidenced by posturing (voluntary assumption of inappropriate or bizarre postures)
5. stereotyped movements, prominent mannerisms, or prominent grimacing
6. echolalia or echopraxia

Undifferentiated Type

A type of Schizophrenia in which symptoms that meet Criterion A are present, but the criteria are not met for the Paranoid, Disorganized, or Catatonic Type.

Residual Type

A type of Schizophrenia in which the following criteria are met:

A. Absence of prominent delusions, hallucinations, disorganized speech, and grossly disorganized or catatonic behavior.

B. There is continuing evidence of the disturbance, as indicated by the presence of negative symptoms or two or more symptoms listed in Criterion A for Schizophrenia, present in an attenuated form (e.g., odd beliefs, unusual perceptual experiences). (Reprinted with permission from the *Diagnostic and Statistical Manual of Mental Disorders,* Fourth Edition. Copyright 1994 American Psychiatric Association)

This breakdown does not include schizoaffective disorders, which are described elsewhere in DSM-IV as disorders in which affective features and the symptoms of schizophrenia are equally prominent and occur together. Actually, the distinction between schizophrenic disorders and schizoaffective disorders is quite difficult to determine in practice. In theory, the schizoaffective disorder is distinguished from the schizophrenic illness because in the schizoaffective disorder the presence of the affective symptoms must be present for a substantial portion of the total duration of the disturbance. In contrast, the mood symptoms of schizophrenia may have a brief duration when compared to the duration of the schizophrenic symptoms which are likely to occur mostly in the prodromal or residual phases of the schizophrenic illness. The limits of "brief" are not clearly defined.

Residential care facility patients come in all shapes and sizes, although some generalizations can be made. Most of the occupants carry one of the schizophrenic diagnoses just listed. It can be safely said that most of these patients would have probably spent most of their lives in a mental hospital prior to the drug revolution. Until recently most of the patients would have been taking what we now call conventional antipsychotics—haloperidol, molindone, loxapine, pimozide, chlorpromazine, fluphenazine, perphenazine, trifluoperazine, acetophenazine, mesoridazine, thioridazine, and thiothixene.

However, since the late 1990s, many if not most of the patients have been switched to the so-called atypical antipsychotics. These are probably more accurately labeled "new generation" antipsychotics because their use is now so widespread that they can no longer be regarded as atypical. The drugs that are designated as "atypical" or "new generation" are clozapine, risperidone, olanzepine, quetiapine, ziprasidone, and aripiprazole.

Many patients, particularly those with an intractable history are taking more than one antipsychotic medication. Sometimes the combination involves two of the newer generation antipsychotics, sometimes a combination of a new generation antipsychotic medication with a conventional antipsychotic. Psychiatrists who use more than one antipsychotic medication are frequently criticized for using "polypharmacy," which has pejorative implications and which implies a reckless use of medications. Criticisms of these psychiatrists generally involve the point that the effectiveness of the use of more than two antipsychotics has never been proven experimentally and is therefore not "evidence based."

I think I can safely say that the effectiveness of two or more antipsychotics will never be evidence based for reasons cited in Chapter 8. Briefly, these reasons are that no drug company or government agency will spend millions or hundreds of millions of dollars to prove that two drugs are more effective than one drug—particularly if one of the drugs is under patent. Also, there are now at least twelve conventional antipsychotics along with six new generation antipsychotics and these provide an almost infinite number of possible combinations or permutations. Even if a specific two-drug regimen was proved to be ineffective, this would have absolutely no relevance to the effectiveness of a different combination.

Psychiatrists actively involved in the treatment of mental illness are more interested in the effective control of symptoms rather than adhering to an academic ideal based on pharmacological parsimony. In pharmacology two and two does not necessarily make four, and one may be a greater value than two. This occurs because a single drug acting on many different kinds of receptors may have a more profound effect than two drugs acting on a smaller variety of receptors. To put it another way, two drugs acting against a narrow range of targeted receptors may have a more specific effect than one drug acting as a shotgun.

For the time being, the question of whether combinations of antipsychotic medications work better than single medications must remain beyond the province of evidence-based medicine. Other unanswered questions include: Which combinations provide the best overall tolerability? Which provide the best prophylactic benefit? Is it possible to use combinations in lower cumulative doses that would otherwise be required in monotherapy?

Arguing against evidence-based medicine is a bit like arguing against motherhood and apple pie, but there is more here than meets the eye. In fact there are cogent arguments against the routine application of evidence-based medicine as routine policies governing routine implementation—with the emphasis being on routine. These arguments are rarely made in print, but they deserve careful consideration, and nobody has presented them better than Michael D. Jibson, as follows:[2]

> The first reality that confronts us is the limit of empirical knowledge in the treatment of schizophrenia. What we know with some measure of certainty is that antipsychotics are often effective at reducing active psychotic symptoms, some patients who do not respond to other medications may show improvement with clozapine, some psychosocial treatment may be helpful. We also have some data about specific medication and psychosocial treatments. Atypical antipsychotics are better tolerated than conventional agents. All first-line atypical antipsychotics are equally effective and equally well tolerated in large studies; social skills training, family intervention, case management, and vocational rehabilitation are often helpful; insight-oriented therapies rarely are.
>
> Empirical studies answer only the most rudimentary questions about treatment. The knowledge we have about medication and psychosocial treatments will get the practicing psychiatrist through the first visit of two, but what then? If the first medication is ineffective, how many more should be tried before clozapine? Are adjunctive medications appropriate? Are antipsychotic combinations ever justified? How long a course of social skills training is necessary? What level of family involvement is optimal? These are the questions that must be addressed over a lifetime of treatment. In my work on an acute impatient unit and in community mental health, I have seen few psychotic

patients who are new to treatment. Most have exhausted the standard procedures. The majority of work we do is beyond the limits of what we know with certainty. (Reprinted by permission. Copyright 2002, Lippincott Williams & Wilkins)

Be that as it may, useful guidelines are partially established by evidence-based data and partially dependent on the cumulative experiences of expert practitioners. Among these are practice guidelines established by the American Psychiatric Association,[3] the Patient Outcomes Research Team,[4] the Expert Consensus Guidelines Group,[5] and the Texas Medication Algorithm Project.[6]

That is all I want to say about the patient's role in the cast except that I should explain that in this book the word *patient* will be used to describe the role of the patient. In simpler times, men were men, women were women, doctors were doctors, patients were patients, and children—myself included—did very well on mercurochrome and cod liver oil, and that was that. That is no longer that. Times have changed, as noted by an eminent historian:[7]

> In olden days a glimpse of stocking
> Was looked on as something shocking,
> But now, God knows,
> Anything goes.
>
> Good authors too who once knew better words,
> Now only use four-letter words
> Writing prose, anything goes.
>
> The world has gone mad today
> And good's bad today,
> And black's white today,
> And day's night today,
> When most guys today
> That women prize today
> Are just silly gigolos

In the course of linguistic evolution, formerly uncomplicated words have mutated into code words that contain implications and nuances to be used in the service of people with sophisticated humanitarian agendas. As noted in the lyrics by Cole Porter, times have changed.

Take a good look at the word *patient.* Even though it is spelled with seven letters it is frequently treated like a four-letter word. Thus we now have three kinds of pseudonyms for patients, each of which tries to separate the sickness from the person.

Patients are now frequently referred to in the literature as *consumers* or *customers* or *clients.* These words are generally used in reference to patients suffering from mental disorders and are rarely applied to those experiencing nonmental illnesses. I regret this trend because it seems to me that these c-word aliases are created by the acceptance of the stigmatization that these alias creators customarily decry. Perhaps this is an unfair allegation, but the aliases create confusion where it does not have to exist. After all, we do not call surgical patients consumers or customers. We call them patients. No surgical patient minds being called a patient, and nobody takes offense. So why create this separate category of patient? I believe the answer is partly due to the misplaced democratic bias of well-meaning therapists who have a sense of guilt about being well when others are sick.

I speak with authority on this subject because at times in my life I have functioned within the role of all of the aforementioned c-words: I have been a customer to my dry-cleaning store clerk. I have been a client to my accountant. I have been a consumer as a subscriber to *Consumer's Digest.* I have even been a patient to my urologist—although I resented the fact and still do, at times—especially at night.

To put it another way and still maintain a respectable degree of vagueness, I never blamed him for the conversion (I mean converting sex from a primordial biological compulsion with its intrusive and sometimes embarrassingly intrusive manifestations to a dreary carnal obligation ritualized by marriage contracts). I never blamed him for the fact that the sinuous mystical fascinations of the night—the stuff that goes with champagne, candlelight, and saxophones with red-cushioned velveteen walls and the soft smoke of incense as it wafts upward in a slow aromatic languorous swirl—were replaced by sleep. It's not his fault that the good old days (including the nights) are gone and the hands of the biological clock hang at 6:30, either a.m. or p.m.—it doesn't matter, the whole thing doesn't matter, and that is about as specific as I wish to get without violating the boundaries of good taste. The important point is that I never felt that being a patient made me less of a valuable person, and I never felt demeaned because someone referred to me as a patient. It just doesn't matter— although perhaps it does just a little bit.

The definition of the noun *patient* as it appears in *Webster's Comprehensive Dictionary* is "A person undergoing treatment for a disease or injury." I think it is acceptable for psychiatrists and psychologists to talk about patients because they are all in the business of helping people who have a sickness. Many social workers prefer the word *client* to *patient,* but if the psychiatric social worker is helping a psychiatric patient with his or her psychiatric problem, it seems preferable (to me), to call the recipient of that service a patient rather than a client because the recipient of the service is being treated for a disease or injury. Some social workers help people who are not sick. I think under those circumstances it is preferable to refer to these individuals as clients. However, mental patients are generally referred to social workers because of the disabilities created by their illnesses, so it seems to me that they are more like patients than clients, but this is not a major sticking point and I won't argue about it except under the following two circumstances:

- If a person is so cognitively impaired by severe mental illness that he or she does not understand the implications of a relationship, that person is essentially a patient rather than a client. I say that because it seems to me that the client relationship to a professional advisor necessarily involves the patient's awareness as to the nature of the relationship.
- When the services of a professional advisor have been imposed upon a mentally impaired person rather than voluntarily selected by the person, that individual is essentially a mental patient rather than a mental client.

If my arguments about the mental patient versus client issues seem forced, consider the definition of the word *client* as it appears in *Webster's Dictionary*:

1. One in whose interests a lawyer acts.
2. Hence, one who engages the service of any professional adviser
3. Loosely, a customer or patron
4. A dependent or follower, as of an ancient Roman patrician

Is it sometimes possible for a patient to be both patient and client? In the first two definitions of client, it is clear that a patient can be a client. Many unhappy physicians are aware that under certain infelicitous circumstances a doctor's patient can be a lawyer's client, and he or she can be the same person. The answer is yes, a patient can be a client—unfortunately. However, when I was young a long time ago and had romantic fantasies about being a doctor, I did not picture myself as having relationships with clients. I can recall that as a child my first image of the physician was captured by Norman Rockwell in one of his paintings on the cover of *The Saturday Evening Post* of an aged physician seated by the bedside of a sick child—a patient, not a client—with his head cradled in his hands pondering the course of treatment. I think it was by Norman Rockwell. If it wasn't, it should have been.

I thought, *How nice of that man to be worried about the treatment of that sick child.* I identified with that child because I was sick as a child, and in my child's mind where magic and reality coalesce, I tried to reach out and touch that man and I still remember the disbelief when I felt gloss instead of garment. I thought that someday when I grew up I would like to be like that real nice man so that I could do good in the world and help sick kids grow up to be big and strong. I'm not claiming that I became a physician because of such primitively conceived monosyllabic childhood fantasies, but who knows what ignites the fires of lingering passions in a child's brain? Be that as it may, clients, as such, did not exist in the Rockwellian world. Come back, Norman Rockwell, we really need you. America needs you.

THE GENERAL MEDICAL PHYSICIAN

In addition to psychiatrists, other physicians are involved in the provision of on-site care. These are physicians who treat concurrent nonpsychiatric medical illnesses. Such physicians may come from a variety of backgrounds, but they are frequently general practitioners, family practice practitioners, or physicians who have specialized in internal medicine or some subspecialization thereof. That description is probably not sufficient to explain the rather clumsy term *general medical physician* but at the moment I cannot think of a better appellation.

In 1979 the residential care committee chaired by Richard A. Shadoan, MD, of the Northern California Psychiatric Society issued a paper titled "Medical Care Guidelines for Psychiatric Patients in Residential Care Homes" that addressed the specific needs of psychiatric patients living in residential care homes.[8] It was noted that many of these residents suffered from the chronic effects of long-term hospitalization: dependency, apathy, and social withdrawal. However, with the advent of brief hospitalization, many of the new residents were younger, more active, and disorganized. As a result, more intensive services were required. With this in mind, the following recommendations were made regarding the coordination of services among psychiatrists, other physicians, and administrators:

1. It is recommended that each RCH (residential care home) resident who suffers from a mental disorder have a personal psychiatrist. This would include all residents in RCHs, the mentally disordered ages eighteen to sixty-five and many residents in RCHs for the aged ages sixty-five and older and in RCHs for the developmentally disabled. In addition each resident of an RCH should have a general medical physician.

2. The RCH resident has a right to choose his or her personal physician. If a resident is unable to choose, assistance should be offered. When an RCH administrator has established a relationship with a physician, the house psychiatrist or house general physician who is available should become the house psychiatrist or general medical physician, respectively, for the resident.

3. When more than one physician is involved in the care of a resident, they should agree on areas of clinical responsibility and work closely together. This can usually be done by telephone.

4. When a physician assumes psychiatric or general medical responsibility for a resident, a psychiatric or general medical evaluation, respectively, should be done. Pertinent data should be recorded in the patient's RCH file. The resident's RCH file should be treated as a confidential medical record.

5. Psychiatric and medical treatment plans should be developed, periodically reviewed, and modified according to changes in the resident's clinical condition. The treatment should be discussed and coordinated with the administrator and the other professionals working

in the RCH. The treatment plan and follow-up plan should be recorded in the resident's RCH file.

6. Physicians should see the residents under their care at least once a month unless otherwise indicated. The frequency of the visits depends on the clinical needs of the resident, and acute problems may require several visits per month. Physicians should be available for emergencies or should arrange for another physician to be on call.

7. The psychiatrist should prescribe and closely monitor the dosages, the necessity, and the side effects of all psychotropic medications. The general medical physician should prescribe and monitor the dosages, necessity, and side effects of all medications in general medical care. Medication orders should be recorded in the resident's RCH file.

8. The RCH administrator may request the psychiatrist to work in active collaboration with other professionals and nonprofessionals to establish a high-expectation milieu in the RCH. This psychiatrist usually would be the personal psychiatrist of some of the residents and should have an understanding of the basic functioning of every resident. The psychiatrist's activity in the RCH may include staff meetings, group therapy, residents meetings, and ongoing consultation with the administrator and others working in the RCH.

These recommendations have held up fairly well considering they were published more than twenty years ago. There are some minor changes. Thus RCHs (the previous quoted acronym for residential care homes) has been transmogrified to RCFs (for residential care facilities).

Also I would now refer to the physician who specializes in the treatment of nonpsychiatric illnesses of chronic mental patients as a specialist in the treatment of long-term illnesses rather than a general medical physician. This is gradually evolving into a subspecialty and there is now—as is also mentioned in the Introduction—a journal called *Annals of Long-Term Care,* which reflects the issues of long-term care. Most of the physicians involved in this type of work have had additional training in geriatrics since most of the occupants of long-term beds fall within this age category.

Contributing to the problems of long-term care as a specialization is the fact that there are now legal constraints regarding the use of antipsychotic medications in nursing homes. This was legislated as part of the Omnibus Budget Reconciliation Act of 1987, otherwise known as OBRA. This is yet another acronym to worry about, and I used to wonder why medication legislation was included in a bill called the Omnibus Budget Reconciliation Act (see Appendix E). I have since looked at the cost of some of the new medications and I can now understand why some patients might have a problem reconciling their budget after paying for their medications. I shall refer more to OBRA in Chapter 15, which addresses the problem of abuses in the residential care facility industry.

The recommendations just listed encourage active coordination of treatment between psychiatrists and long-term care physicians, and represent an ideal. Nowadays with increasing Medicare and managed care problems and the increased pressure to document everything, both internists and generalists are as busy or busier than psychiatrists. In many instances the two of us are not meeting, even though we should. Many more drugs are now used by internists which have a pharmacodynamic or pharmacokinetic effect on the drugs that psychiatrists are using and vice versa. It used to be that all we had to worry about was the interactions between nonsteroidal anti-inflammatory drugs and lithium. Life was a lot easier before science discovered the interactive capabilities of the cytochrome isoenzymes.

Many nonpsychiatric medications are now known to have interactive effects on other psychiatric medications. The table of possible interactions between medications attributed to the P450 cytochrome enzyme system appears to increase weekly. I tried to memorize the table, but every month the table was extended to new medications and my efforts were soon rendered obsolete along with Bakelite pencil sharpeners and Remington typewriters.

The term *cytochrome P450* refers to a group of enzymes located on the endoplasmic reticulum in the cells of the liver and intestines. These enzymes are of particular importance when studying drug biotransformation and drug metabolism.

The primary role for the P450 system appears to be one of metabolism and detoxification of endogenous compounds after ingestion. In addition the cytochrome system acts as a protective mechanism against the possible harmful effects of xenobiotics—foreign substances that may be ingested and create a threat to the organism. More than thirty human P450 isoenzyme systems have been identified to date, although the major ones responsible for drug metabolism are the

CYP1A2, CYP2A6, CYP2B6, CYP2C8, CYP2C9, CYP2C18, CYP2C19, CYP2D6, CYP2E1, CYP3A4, and CYP3A5-7. Knowledge of the P450 system is critical in understanding drug metabolism and drug interactions.

Many drugs either inhibit or facilitate the metabolism of other medications through induction or inhibition of enzymes within the P450 isoenzyme system. Thus an individual's reaction to medications is dependent upon the administration of other medications that are affected by the P450 enzyme system. Not until the 1990s did the importance of these relationships become apparent when the combination of some nonsedating antihistamines (astemizole and terfenadine) with some psychiatric medications (such as nefazodone) resulted in arrhythmias and sudden death secondary to the inhibited metabolism of the antihistamines.

There is also an increasing appreciation of added complexities induced by other enzyme systems such as those involving glucuronidation reactions. Additional complexities are created by other enzyme systems (p-glycoproteins) that transfer endogenous substances in and out of the intestinal tract. Before the advent of molecular biology physicians did not have to worry about such matters, but as science progresses we are learning more and more about less and less until eventually we will know all there is about nothing at all. I believe it was Nicholas Murray Butler, the president of Columbia University, who first made that observation, even in the days before nanotechnology, but don't quote me on that.

However, there is a countervailing epistemological trend to learn more and more about more and more. Because of advances in all branches of medicine, much information about the treatment of hypertension, dyslipidemia, diabetes, and arthritis is not within the expertise of the psychiatrist. The era of the purely psychiatric patient—that is, the patient who is maintained on psychiatric drugs and no other medications—is now diminishing rapidly. Such patients are now a minority within a minority. Most patients are on psychiatric medications combined with other medications for concurrent medical illnesses. Thus, when I audited the medication regimens of twenty-seven patients living in a residential care facility which I periodically visit, only eight of these were limited to psychiatric drugs. When I audited another facility with fourteen patients, only four of these patients were on psychiatric medications alone. Given the qualification that this is a small sample, these ratios suggest that approximately two-thirds of the nongeriatric chronically mentally ill occupants of residential care facilities are also being treated for physical illnesses. This is of particular interest since it is not generally appreciated that in these facilities the average patient with a mental illness also has an accompanying physical illness. It remains to be seen whether this is also true of the mentally ill population at large.

At one time conscientious psychiatrists could gingerly tiptoe into the arena of nonpsychiatric medications and hardly be noticed as interlopers, but they do so now at their own risk. The days of the Renaissance physician are over. The treatment of both psychiatric and nonpsychiatric illnesses is more complex than ever before, and each requires specialists. Nor can the internist easily trespass on psychiatric terrain. Psychopharmacology is no longer tiny steps for little feet. The virus of complexity has affected psychiatry just as it has other medical specializations and the list of available psychiatric medications grows monthly and is soon rendered obsolete. (See Appendix B for the most recent obsolete list.)

Moreover, psychiatric medications can cause weight gain and/or aggravate medical pathologies associated with seizures or cardiac arrhythmias, to name only a few. Since some psychiatric medications can lead to the aforementioned medical complications, the question remains as to who should be responsible for the metabolic monitoring of parameters that might be associated with the precipitation of medical complications caused by psychiatric drugs—namely, should this responsibility fall upon the internist or the psychiatrist? The question is still being debated in medical circles—and undoubtedly it will be settled at some time in the future—but by lawyers rather than doctors. Pending the resolution of such matters, it is reasonable to presume that since the psychiatric medications may induce the pathology, it is the primary responsibility of the psychiatrist to provide the necessary oversight, especially since it is common for the internist to not know what the psychiatrist is doing and vice versa. Appendix C lists some of the recommendations made by one psychiatrist, although the listed policies are open to debate.

However, these recommendations relate to the more common illnesses affected by psychiatric medications. Some of the conditions caused by psychiatric medications may be quite rare—with a prevalence as little as 1 in 30,000 births, such as hyperammonemic encephalopathy. Even though this genetic abnormality is not common, it is still the physician's responsibility to be aware of it. Hyperammonemicencephalopathy is an example of some of the arcane but significant drug-induced medical complications that psychiatrists must be aware of in the twenty-first century. Other conditions, equally as rare, are supposed to be known to psychiatrists, and these are advertised by the FDA via boxed warnings in bold type.

Even though it is rare for a psychiatric patient to be maintained only on psychiatric medications, it is even more rare for a psychiatric patient to be stabilized on one medication. Of the aforementioned previously audited twenty-seven regimens, only one of them qualified as monotherapy. Increasing complexity has also characterized the evolution of treatment choices. An algorithm now exists for every psychiatric diagnostic category, and some of them are quite formidable. In addition to schizophrenic treatment algorithms, there are schizoaffective and bipolar treatment algorithms, which require an increased degree of diagnostic sophistication. Thus one of the recently published algorithms[9] addresses the treatment of five different types of acute manic presentations and encompasses fifteen different steps, involving lithium or divalproex either used alone or in various kinds of permutations with three other different types of anticonvulsants, calcium channel blockers, clozapine, and thyroid preparations, all of which contribute to the complexity (and efficacy) of psychopharmacology.

The treatment of patients in residential care facilities can be even more complicated because sometimes more than one physician is prescribing for the patient's nonpsychiatric problems. If an unseen third hand is pressing the mortar against the pestle, the pharmacist supplying the medication to the home will know about this. For all of these reasons the on-site services of a clinically knowledgeable pharmacist are advantageous in the treatment of psychiatric patients in residential care facilities. I discuss the role of the clinical pharmacist later in this chapter.

Because of these factors the psychiatrist and the house internist must be on speaking terms and ideally each should be aware of the ministrations of the other. Coordination of professional efforts is now more important than ever because of the increasing realization that many of the medications used to treat nonpsychiatric illnesses have an impact on psychiatric medications, and vice versa: This includes such commonly used nonpsychiatric medications as erythromycin, ciprofloxacin, diltiazem, and verapamil—to mention only a few. Entire books are now being written which focus on the interactive capabilities of psychiatric drugs with other psychiatric drugs and with nonpsychiatric medications.

Because of these developments, some of the previous recommendations may need reconsideration, especially number 8: "The psychiatrist's activity in the RCH may include staff meetings, group therapy, residents meetings, etc." The increased time demands created by documentation requirements, as well as the increasing sophistication required for the administration of new drugs, leaves precious little leftover time for participation in group therapy, residents meetings, therapeutic communities, or other variants of people's democracies.

Psychiatrists who are good psychopharmacologists should probably stick with what they do best and not venture into group therapy. I believe group therapy is best left to therapists, psychiatric or otherwise, who specialize in group therapy. However, I will concede that this is an expression of my own bias and reflects my own limitations as a therapist. I do not have the kind of radial sensitivity that good group therapists share with sea anemones and octopuses and which is an essential tool for the implementation of good group psychotherapy. I attribute this inability to the fact that I was an only child who only partially matured into an only adult. However, I can do well in one-to-one relationships in which I can empathize with an individual patient. I think of myself as having a basically linear mind with a first-in, first-out register—meaning there is room for only one patient at a time (not necessarily an only child), and when the second patient enters consciousness the first is bumped into Nevermindland.

THE SOCIAL WORKER

The residential care facility system could not function without social workers. Social workers are so important that I am not going to say much about them. Social workers negotiate with Social Security and other third-party payers to determine eligibility requirements. Social workers control the referrals to the residential care facilities from hospitals, hotels, homes, and long-term facilities; make lateral transfers from one residential care facility to another when residents are unhappy with their placement; make arrangements for patients to be released into independent living situations; and even do psychotherapy in their leftover time, which they usually don't have. A good social worker provides an extra set of eyes and ears to the psychiatrist, similar to cameras in those old Pathe newsreels.

Having acknowledged that the residential care facility system could not function without social workers, I will now make an ancillary acknowledgment. The residential care facility psychiatrist cannot function successfully without a sophisticated residential care facility placement system established by social workers. In another chapter I boasted that I was a great psychiatrist—without actually saying so—because in the course of treating over 2,000 patients I had not one who was convicted or even accused of a serious crime. There is more here than meets the eye. Actually, I'm not that great. My job was made a lot easier by the placement screening criteria for residential care facilities established by social workers. I am not privy to the formal screening criteria used by social workers for residential home placement but in general terms such criteria would include assessments for diagnosis necessitating mental health services and evaluations with respect to assaultive behavior, fire setting, substance abuse, suicide, criminality, wandering, incontinence, the presence of other chronic illnesses requiring additional care, and other factors which are unknown to me.

Obviously these admission criteria made life somewhat easier for me through the years insofar as potentially problematic violent patients were screened out. However, in recent years these criteria have not been applied stringently—mostly as a consequence of institutional facilities becoming overcrowded and also because of the high costs associated with prolonged hospitalizations.

Social workers come in all ethnicities, shapes, and sizes. The good social worker can be of great assistance to the residential care facility psychiatrist providing that the psychiatrist is nice to him or her. If the psychiatrist is arrogant or unapproachable or otherwise dismissive of the efforts of the social worker, then the social worker may not provide information that might otherwise by useful in patient care. A distinction can be made between good social workers and great social workers. Great social workers have been known on occasion to work beyond 5:00 p.m. Great social workers notice a patient's grooming and will remark upon it in ways that are meaningful to the patient. Great social workers get involved with house staff personnel and get to know them on a first-name basis so that the staff feels more at ease with him or her and can convey information more readily. Working with great social workers can be a wonderful experience. Aside from doing everything that I have already mentioned, social workers can help the psychiatrist in other ways. Social workers frequently become involved in psychotherapeutic relationships with patients and can obtain information that the busy psychopharmacologically preoccupied psychiatrist is unable to obtain. Sometimes the conveyance of such information can be tremendously useful as in the following case documented in a progress note dated November 12, 2003.

Pt. states he is ok, Staff reports no new interim mgt problems. Current meds are:

Clozapine 100 mg. Tabs 2 in AM, Tabs 4 HS.

Glyburide 5 mg. Tabs 2 B.I.D.

Depakote 500 mg. Tabs 2 B.I.D.

Norvasc 5 mg. Tabs 1 daily.

Social worker reports he is getting increasingly delusional. He tells her he works for the police and that he smells blood. He told her he thinks I am Hitler.

I then increase his HS clozapine to tabs 5 HS because I am not Hitler. The social worker has given me valuable information that helps me treat the patient and, who knows—perhaps she has saved me from an assault.

My one complaint about social workers is that they are always coming and going. I really don't mind the coming—I mind the going. No sooner have I grown accustomed to her face, as the song goes (or his face, as the song does not go), than a social worker leaves for some other place, usually described as better or higher or whatever. I have never been able to determine the location of this place, although it must be pretty crowded up there. In my fantasies I think of long lost social workers ascending to this ideal agency at the top of some big rock candy mountain where they become busily engaged applying means tests to greedy children to determine eligibility for rock candy vouchers. I think in my career I have seen about fifty of them enter and leave through this revolving occupational door, and most of them have been very helpful.

THE PSYCHOLOGIST

I do not have much to say about clinical psychologists with respect to on-site services in residential care facilities because their role has been severely limited. Most clinical psychologists are restricted to the practice of psychotherapy, which they usually practice in their offices, in university settings, or in agency settings. Clinical psychologists have also functioned very effectively as program directors. Clinical psychologists thus far—with two exceptions—have been prevented from prescribing medications. The exceptions are the states of Louisiana and New Mexico. New Mexico passed legislation in 2002 authorizing clinical psychologists to prescribe medications under certain conditions. Louisiana passed similar legislation in May 2004.

The opposition to granting prescriptive authority to psychologists comes from two sources: Organized medicine and psychiatry, in particular, have felt proprietary with respect to prescribing medication, claiming that this function is and should be dependent on a standard medical education. Academic psychology has also historically resisted this expansion as being inconsistent with the objectives of a professional education in psychology. This led to serious internal problems in psychology, and eventually professional preparatory schools specializing in clinical psychology were established in response to continuing controversies within traditional academic psychology programs, not the least of which was the reluctance of these programs to grant doctoral degrees in clinical psychology.

Generally speaking, the professional schools in psychology have granted the doctor of psychology (PsyD) degree rather than the doctor of philosophy (PhD) degree in psychology. The PhD is a more academic degree with an emphasis on research and teaching; the PsyD has a more clinical focus. The PhD generally requires a dissertation but usually not a clinical internship; the PsyD generally requires a clinical internship but not necessarily a dissertation. Obviously the role of psychologists in residential care facilities will expand dramatically if and when they achieve prescriptive parity with psychiatrists.

THE ADMINISTRATOR

Most of the residential care facilities in San Francisco were started by African-American women in the 1960s. These women, intelligent, energetic, and entrepreneurial, overcame the handicap of a poor formal education and were able to organize to obtain favorable legislation in Sacramento that would encourage the formation of a network of homes—then called board-and-care homes—that would service the needs of the chronically mentally ill. They were the pioneers of residential care, and as is the tradition of pioneers, they wished something better for their children. They got it.

The second generation of African-American would-be residential care facility administrators went to college and most of them graduated, wearing those funny-looking square graduation caps that used to be the exclusive property of the white middle and upper classes. They are no longer interested in the twenty-four-hour commitment and relatively low remuneration involved in residential care facility work. I can't blame them. Thus many African Americans have been replaced by Filipinos. Of the thirteen homes I now attend, five are administered by African Americans, seven by Filipinos, and one by a Hispanic.

Many Filipinos are ideally suited for residential care facility work with the mentally ill. They are compassionate caregivers and maintain a culturally encouraged ethic to present a cheerful face even in the presence of personal adversity. They have a respect for the elderly as well as a respect for physicians that is all too absent among native Americans—native Americans in the nonethnic sense. The exportation of caring health caregivers has been the golden export of the Philippines, not only to the United States but to other parts of the world. The biggest source of confusion in consulting with Filipino administrators is that they frequently mean "he" when they say "she." There is something about the Tagalog language that leads to an imprinted sexual misidentification in the use of the personal pronoun. That aside, they are a definite asset to the residential care system having arrived just in time, in the Japanese manufacturing sense, to facilitate productivity.

The psychiatrist helps the administrator in a number of ways in the sense that routine prescheduled visits to a residential care facility serve to upgrade the home in terms of creating a therapeutic environment. Although it is true that on-site psychiatric visits last only a comparatively short time, psychiatrists can help the administrators understand and cope with the irrational behavior of the residents. Also if the psychiatrist is able to improve or control the patient's behavior through his or her interventions, administrators will feel more secure in their management of the home. Also the administrator will grow professionally if he or she can attend the team meeting and participate in the discussions. The establishment of this kind of routine can decrease the isolation of the administrator which can be demoralizing, especially when one is confronted with situations that defy quick solutions. Administrator burnout is a problem and an accessible psychiatrist can do a lot to encourage administrators to continue their work.

Aside from the ongoing twenty-four-hour caregiving responsibility that administrators have, they are also required to take courses for annual accreditation.

One of the current requirements of the Administrator Certification Section of the California Community Licensing Division (see Appendix D) is that administrators must complete forty hours of coursework every two years. The requirements must include at least three hours in HIV/AIDS as well as one hour focusing on tuberculosis. For administrators of geriatric facilities the coursework must include eight hours of training in dementia and Alzheimer's disease.[10] For the years 2003 to 2004 the training schedule includes lectures on harm reduction, community resources, depression and creativity, fire safety and earthquake preparedness, environmental health issues, homelessness, and medication updates.

Aside from maintaining their educational requirements, administrators also have the responsibility to maintain house charts. These charts are maintained by the residential care administrator at the house and contain the psychiatrist's progress notes. The house charts also contain various documents, as is required by licensing, and also whatever historical material is made available to the administrator.

What are these documents? I will summarize one in this paragraph, an example called an "Unusual Incident/Injury Report. If an unusual incident occurs, the administrator must complete a form which specifies the date and the type of incident. Was it an unauthorized absence: Was it an aggressive act directed at self, another client, a staff person, a family member, or visitor? Was there an alleged violation of human rights? Is there an allegation of client abuse? Was this abuse alleged to be physical, sexual, psychological, financial, or neglect? Was there an incident involving rape, pregnancy, or suicide? Was there an injury? Was this injury an accident, from another client, from a behavior episode, or of unknown origin? Are there any reports of an epidemic, hospitalizations, medical emergencies, theft, fire, or property damage?

In addition to this document, many other forms are required of administrators. Following is a list of such forms available on the Web site <www.CCLD.CA.gov> and in the public domain.

I. Client Records

    A.   Preplacement Appraisal Information (LIC 603).

    B.   Appraisal Needs and Services Plan updated as frequently as necessary to ensure its accuracy. (LIC 625).

    C.   Physicians Report (LIC 602) Medical assessment including record of illnesses and medical care provided; evidence or periodic medical examination and care; and record of changes in physical, mental emotional and social functioning of residents.

    D.   Current admission agreement with authorized signatures, Admission Agreement Guide (LIC 604).

    E.   Identification and Emergency Information (LIC 601).

    F.   Record of Client's/Resident's Safeguarded Cash Resources (LIC 405), including supporting receipts of expenditures and Client/Resident Personal Property and Valuables (LIC 621), a record of each client's personal property and/or valuables entrusted to the facility.

    G.   A demand trust account for each client's cash resources if not kept in the facility.

    H.   Evidence of consultation from a dietitian, physician, social worker, psychologist, or any other consultation in determining if client needs can be met by facility or in modifying needs and services plan of client, when general facility program fails to meet an individual clients needs in Appraisal/Needs and Services Plan (LIC 625).

    I.   Centrally Stored Medications and Destruction Record (LIC 622).

    J.   Unusual Incident/Injury Report (LIC 624).

    K.   Death Report (LIC 624A)

    L.   Register of Facility Clients/Residents (LIC 9020).

    M.   Personal Rights Forms (LIC 613).

    N.   Functional Capability Assessment (LIC9172).

II. Personnel Records

    A.   Health Screening Report - Facility Personnel (with Tuberculosis (TB) clearance) (LIC 503).

    B.   TB clearance and "good health" statement from volunteer(s).

    C.   Personal Record - employment application form completed by each staff member (LIC 501).

    D.   Personnel Report - showing current roster (LIC 500).

    E.   Criminal Record Statement for persons subject to fingerprint requirements (LIC 508).

    F.   Licensee's affidavit on persons exempt from fingerprint requirements (if not on LIC 500).

    G.   Verification of education, experience, training and/or license/certificate for the administrator, staff and consultants.

    H.   Verification of training in first aid for persons responsible for providing direct care and supervision.

    I.   Valid water safety certificate for any adult giving water activity staffing responsibility.

III. Administrative Records

    A.   Employment of or evidence of regular consultation from a nutritionist, dietician, or home economist if facility is licensed for 50 or more residents.

    B.   Dated weekly employee time schedule posted in facilities for 16 or more residents.

    C.   Documentation of actual hours worked by staff.

    D.   Current and valid driver's license for each staff member transporting clients.

    E.   Surety Bond, if appropriate (LIC 402).

    F.   Menus for the most recent 30-day period.

    G.   Posted emergency phone numbers and addresses.

    H.   Emergency Disaster Plan (LIC 610) evidence that disaster and emergency drills are conducted every six months. Documentation of the drills shall be maintained for a year.

    I.   Notices of planned activities for facilities of seven or more clients posted in a central location. Copies of such notices shall be retained for at least six months.

    J.   A current written program of activities which is planned in advance and is readily available to clients and authorized representatives in facilities of 50 or more clients.

K. Documentation for Exceptions and Facility Waivers (LIC 956/LIC 971).
L. For facilities licensed for seven or more clients, posted facility license (LIC 203).
M. Provider/Licensee Rights, Appeals Procedure (LIC 9058).

Many of these forms are not easy to complete. Consider the Appraisal/Needs and Services Plan form. The form starts with the following instructions:

> Licensing regulations require that an appraisal of needs be completed for specific clients/residents to identify individual needs and develop a service plan for meeting those needs. If the client/resident is accepted for placement, the staff person responsible for admission shall jointly develop a needs and services plan with the client/resident and/or client's/resident's authorized representative referral agency/person, physician, social worker, or other appropriate consultant. In addition, the law requires that the referral agency/person inform the licensee of any dangerous tendencies of the client/resident.

The form then requires background information as follows:

> Brief description of client's/resident's medical history, emotional, behavioral, and physical problems; functional limitations; physical and mental; functional capabilities; ability to handle personal cash resources and perform simple homemaking tasks; client's/resident's likes and dislikes.

The form then goes on to list five needs, these being socialization, emotional, mental, physical/health, and functioning skills. Each of these needs must then be described in terms of four categories, objective plan, time frame, persons responsible for implementation, and method of evaluating progress.

Please bear in mind that many administrators are not college graduates and learning to spell correctly in English is hard enough even for people for whom English is a native language. The problem is that English is not spelled phonetically, Spanish is. I once had a roommate in medical school who subsequently became a pathologist. It took him two years to learn that blood was not spelled "blud." He was born in Wisconsin, an otherwise civilized state. Completing a form such as the Appraisal/Needs and Services Plan is much more difficult than spelling. Moreover, if you do not complete the form within the prescribed deadline, licensing will impose a fifty-dollar penalty. I am talking about fifty dollars *per day!* That is enough to put any otherwise smiling cheerful Filipino administrator in a bad mood.

I now understand the derivation of the word *formidable* as it pertains to forms. In the event that an administrator runs out of forms, not surprisingly, there is a special form to submit to request other forms. This list of forms is guaranteed to absorb whatever leisure time an administrator might have, which is generally not very much.

In California, the qualifications, duties, and responsibilities of the administrator are described in Title 22 of the California Code of Regulations and are included in Appendix D.

THE PHARMACIST

I have put pharmacists near the bottom of the list, but maybe they should be at the top. The truth of the matter is I talk with the pharmacist, either directly or on the telephone, more than to any other medical professional. A good pharmacist is like gold to the psychiatrist with a psychopharmacological practice. Many pharmacists are quite knowledgeable about psychiatric medications and they generally know more than psychiatrists about the nonpsychiatric medications that psychiatric patients take for the treatment of concurrent diseases. There are many concurrent diseases, as is explained in Chapter 12.

In ideal situations the pharmacist should be on the team and participate in on-site visitations with the physician. When this occurs, changes in medications can be discussed and immediately implemented without the inconvenience of telephone prompts and misunderstandings that frequently arise in telephonic communications. The problem is that pharmacists are not compensated for their on-site inputs. Perhaps they should be. It may seem that by so doing the cost of health care would be increased, but one would have to factor in the money saved by decreasing the incidence of hospitalizations that occur as a result of the rapid intervention by the Modern Psychiatric Team. I think of the Modern Psychiatric Team as consisting of the pharmacist, the social worker, and the psychiatrist. For that reason I will capitalize the concept.

The situation is somewhat analogous to the treatment of diabetes in which money is saved and the quality of lives increased by adherence to the "tight control" therapy mandates that currently exist with respect to the treatment of diabetes.

Ideally every residential care facility should be serviced by a single pharmacy. It is definitely a bad idea for a residential care facility to be dealing with multiple pharmacies because the lack of personal contact with known people will inevitably lead to misunderstandings creating otherwise unnecessary phone calls or worse. Ideally the pharmacist should arrange the medications for all the patients in the residential care facility in a Medi-set or bubble pack (I prefer Medi-set). Ideally this should not be the responsibility of the caretaking personnel at the home. The dispensing of medications should be a responsibility delegated to professionals. Also I have found that when administrators deal with more than one pharmacy, sometimes the two pharmacies wind up delivering medications for the same patient. Sometimes the same medication may be delivered by the generic label by one pharmacy and by the brand name by another pharmacy. Obviously this may cause the caretaker to administer double the intended dose. I repeat, it is definitely a bad idea for a residential care facility to be involved with more than one pharmacy.

Ideally the pharmacist should attend the scheduled psychiatric residential care facility visits as part of the Modern Psychiatric Team assuming that he or she is interested in psychiatric patients and the effects of psychiatric medications. Many times I have been helped by the suggestions of pharmacists in my on-site off-the-cuff medication management decision making although they have always couched their suggestions in such terms so as not to undermine my simulated pharmacological omniscience. The following progress note dated February 28, 2001, is an example of how the pharmacist can contribute to enhanced medical care as part of the Modern Psychiatric Team:

The patient states he wants a new medicine for depression. He is still depressed. He went to the library and found the name of a new medication for depression and it is supposed to work great—or at least that's what the book said. It is called Effexor. Patient is now on Paxil and the drug is not working very well. I am willing to prescribe Effexor. [As I said before, I don't mind patient participation in medication decisions.] I will now discontinue Paxil, start Effexor XR, as 37.5 mg HS.

Also I notice presence of a coarse tremor with 2 plus cogwheeling. Pt. on lithium with serum level of 1.1 mmol./L on 2-22-01. Will now discontinue lithium.

These instructions were transcribed by the pharmacist immediately since he was present during my interview with the patient. Thus Paxil was discontinued and Effexor started as 37.5 mg, one tab daily, and lithium discontinued. No telephone waiting, no telephone prompts. Later when the patient leaves the room the pharmacist tactfully reminds me that I tried to discontinue lithium once before and the patient did very poorly. Since I don't have a photographic memory, I review the med orders in my special handy-dandy psychopharmacological page (also described in Chapter 8), and sure enough, the pharmacist is correct. I then change the order to decrease his lithium dose by 300 mg instead of stopping it completely. No additional telephone waiting. No additional telephone prompts followed by phony messages stating that I should stand by because "Your call is very important to us." This interaction shows how pharmacists can be very helpful as members of the Modern Psychiatric Team and can help preserve the illusion of the papal infallibility of the physician. Sometimes two sophisticated psychopharmacological heads are better than one.

I keep using the term *ideally* to describe my relations with the pharmacist because in the real world the pharmacist is now a very busy professional and frequently does not have the time to attend such meetings—especially if he or she works for a chain store. A brief visit to any pharmacy is revealing: long lines of people waiting for medications (with their computerized attached instructions and warnings) and pharmacists busily engaged in typing labels, checking insurance cards, counseling patients (for which they receive no fee), answering phone calls, and preparing various Medi-sets and bubble-packs, etc.

The fact is pharmacy, as a profession, has been impacted by powerful economic trends that have had a degrading effect. Witness the decline of the mom-and-pop local pharmacies where pharmacists had intimate contacts with their patients (where patients were patients rather than mere customers) and the accompanying rise in chain store pharmacies or supermarket pharmacies. In these situations pharmacists are now employees of huge corporations and are now servicing customers rather than counseling patients. Add to this the obligation of pharmacists to check with managed care third-party payers before filling prescriptions so that pharmacists now find that they are spending more time discussing copayment issues or noncoverage complaints rather than drug therapy. Here is an example of some of the issues pharmacists are now confronting as confided to me by a pharmacist with years of experience working in the mental health sector:

Dear Dr. Fleishman:

Pharmacists are the only professionals that give away their advice for free. Many times I have phone conversations with people I don't even know, and may not even ask their name, and they call for information. Many times they are not even customers that frequent my store. Sometimes, I wonder about my profession.

I am a pharmacist with over twenty-five years of experience and I am now working in a grocery store. I am just another person in a department not looked upon as a "professional" by my fellow employees until one of them gets sick. Only then I am given some semblance of respect as long as I am accurate in my diagnostic skill, precise in my choice of pharmacological cure, and unparalleled in my ability to make the lame walk and the blind see.

I am glad you are writing about the value of the pharmacist in your next article. As I told you, I saw myself in your words. Too often, "we" hear of the negative side or the danger in the drugstore. When you wrote that a good pharmacist is like gold, you rekindled my spirit to continue my efforts to protect the health of the people that put their trust in me.

In my setting, I must perform superior service which supersedes anything else despite the workload, hours of standing, job stress, lack of space, and lack of recognition. Nevertheless, my compassion for my work still exists. As a pharmacist, I am the last connection between the doctor's order and the patient. When we consult with the patient many times we need to "sell" the patient on the need for the medicine while confidently explaining the drug's use and side effects, etc., in terms they will understand, while at the same time trying to understand some senior's position about either buying medication or doing without something, even food.

Today the most often asked questions from a patient are, "How long is it going to take to fill my prescription?" and "How much is it going to cost?" Also, managed care has brought a difficult twist for the pharmacist. No two plans are alike in the way they are placed into the patient's record or in their formulary coverage. I spend more time telling people why a drug is not covered or discussing copayment issues than I do about drug therapy and proper drug utilization.

Conversely, today's patient is much more drug savvy with Internet information abundantly available. Also, offered for our "amusement" on television we find ads for Buspar, Prozac, Paxil, Wellbutrin, etc., with "perfect people" in parklike settings acting with big bright smiles which many times mislead the public.

As you know, I have always enjoyed working with mental health aspects. I am a firm believer in seeing patients in their home environment whenever possible. One can get a whole different view or feeling about what their lives are like. Without a personal touch, a person can be reduced to just a name on a piece of paper. Without some insight into the individual, the ability of the pharmacist is compromised in offering the best assessment of drug selection and dosing in assisting the doctor in charge.

With today's telephone system, the physician can leave a verbal message on tape without even speaking to a pharmacist. I am opposed to this depersonalization, as many times information left is unclear and the patient could suffer. I enjoy the discussion with the doctor. I always retrieve the patient's record from the computer to further enhance my input in helping the doctor when necessary. We must communicate clearly to avoid mistakes. After all, the first rule of medicine is to do no harm.

Yours truly,
Steve Protzel, PharmD[11]

Regrettably, pharmacists in large corporate settings have been reduced to semi-clerkship status. At the same time, the pharmacist is underutilized in the mental health system because he or she can be a valuable asset to the system as a participant of the Modern Psychiatric Team. There should be some way of encouraging this participation, such as providing a consulting fee to his or her presence at residential care facility clinical meetings. In fact, the role of the clinical pharmacist is more important today than ever before in mental health because psychiatric patients are now living much longer, but they are living with the nonpsychiatric diseases of aging. This means that chronic psychiatric patients are frequently taking multiple medications for chronic nonpsychiatric illnesses such as diabetes, heart disease, arthritis or hypercholesterolemia. An on-site pharmacist can be invaluable in helping the psychiatrist grope his or her way through the confusing pharmacological maze that he or she may otherwise confront. Of course one can always resort to the small print in the *Physicians' Desk Reference,* but the 2004 edition has 3,533 pages, and every year the book gets heavier especially if one has to lug it to a residential care facility. Also the print gets smaller—or so it seems, and the list of accompanying medications that the patient is taking gets longer. So what is happening has not been "faster, cheaper, and better" but rather longer, heavier, and smaller.

Table 7.1 shows medications taken by a patient recently admitted to a residential care home, along with the costs of the medications.

Let me be quick to reassure those attorneys who may be reading this book that I am not the prescribing physician for these medications. Granted, this is an extreme example, but it gives one an idea as to what frequently occurs to a somewhat lesser degree. Only two medications in the above list (divalproex and risperidone) can be re-

TABLE 7.1. Medications and costs

Medications	Cost of thirty-day supply (rounded to nearest dollar)
Psychiatric medications	
1. divalproex 500 mg 2 tabs, twice daily	195
2. risperidone 3 mg 2 tabs, daily	361
Nonpsychiatric medications	
3. Isosorbide mononitrate 60 mg 1 tab daily	35
4. Glucophage 850 mg 1 tab three times a day	107
5. Catapres patch, once a week	82
6. Hydrochlorothiazide 25 mg 1 tab daily	4
7. DSS 250 mg twice daily	5
8. Lotensin 20 mg 1 tab daily	31
9. Pravachol 20 mg 1 tab daily	83
10. Betoptic eye drops, twice daily	98
11. Trusopt eye drops, twice daily	51
12. Azmacort inhalers four puffs, twice daily	69
13. Atrovent inhalers two puffs, twice daily	49
14. Aspirin 81 mg, 1 tab daily	1
15. Oyster shell calcium 2 tabs daily	3
16. Multivitamin 1 tabs daily	3
Total monthly cost for psychiatric meds	556
Total monthly cost for nonpsychiatric meds	621
Total monthly cost for all meds	$1,177

garded as purely psychiatric. On the average, a newly admitted psychiatric patient to a residential care facility is on fewer medications, only some of which are psychiatric. Table 7.2 shows an example of a more typical psychiatric patient recently discharged from San Francisco General Hospital and admitted to a residential care facility on May 9, 2002.

Of this list, four medications are for a psychiatric condition (Haldol, Prozac, divalproex, and quetiapine), one is for the side effects produced by the psychiatric medications (Cogentin), one is for the side effects of the medication used to treat the side effects of the psychiatric medications (DSS—for constipation), and six are for the treatment of concurrent medical conditions (hypertension, diabetes, and possible residual effects of tuberculosis).

TABLE 7.2. Medications and costs

Medications	Cost of thirty-day supply (rounded to nearest dollar)
Psychiatric medications	
1. Cogentin 1 mg 1 tab daily	7
2. Haldol 10 mg 1 tab daily	20
3. divalproex 500 mg 1 tab twice daily	50
4. Prozac 60 mg 1 tab daily	202
5. quetiapine 200 mg 4 tabs daily	530
Nonpsychiatric mediations	
6. Aspirin 81 mg 1 tab daily	1
7. Lotensin 5m 1 tab daily	31
8. Calcium carbonate 125 mg 1 tab daily	3
9. INH 300 mg 1 tab daily	6
10. Glucophage 5 mg 2 tabs daily	37
11. DSS 250 mg (stool softener)	3
12. Glyburide 5 mg 1 tab daily	20
Total monthly cost for psychiatric meds	809
Total monthly cost for nonpsychiatric meds	101
Total monthly cost for all meds	$910

Lest one think that the previous example is atypical, here is the regimen of the next consecutively admitted patient to a residential care facility on June 19, 2002. (The abbreviation HS stands for hour of sleep.)

The costs of these regimens raise an interesting issue, which will be discussed in a separate chapter. The purpose of listing the medications here is to illustrate the pharmacological complexity that now exists for many patients and the importance of having consultation services available with either an on-board internist or knowledgeable pharmacist.

In the previous regimen, four medications were for psychiatric illness (clozapine, Haldol, divalproex, and Klonopin), two medications

TABLE 7.3. Medications and costs

Medications	Cost of thirty-day supply (rounded to nearest dollar)
Psychiatric medications	
1. clozapine 100 mg 1 tab 1 in a.m., 5 tabs HS	599
2. clozapine 25 mg 3 tabs 3 HS	116
3. Cogentin 2 mg 1 tab, twice daily	15
4. Haldol 10 mg 1 tab in a.m.	21
5. divalproex 500 mg 2 tabs in a.m.	111
6. Klonopin 1 mg 1 tab HS	25
Nonpsychiatric medications	
7. DSS 100 mg 1 tab in a.m.	2
8. Tenormin 50 mg 1 tab daily	38
9. Levoxyl 0.075 mg 1 tab daily	10
10. Protonix 40 mg 1 tabs HS	101
11. Celebrex 200 mg 1 tab daily	83
12. Calcium carbonate 650 mg 1 tab, three times a day	8
13. Theragran M 1 tabs daily	2
Total monthly cost for psychiatric meds	887
Total monthly cost for nonpsychiatric meds	244
Total monthly cost of all meds	$1,121

were to treat the side effects of psychiatric medications (Cogentin for Parkinsonism, DSS for constipation), and six medications were for the treatment of accompanying medical problems (Levoxyl for hypothyroidism, Tenormin for hypertension, Protonix for hyperacidity or possibly gastroesophageal reflux disease, Celebrex for arthritis, Calcium carbonate possibly as a prophylactic for future osteoporosis, and Theragran M, possibly in anticipation of poor nutrition or anemia.

I previously defined the "chronic mental patient" as "those individuals who are, have been, or might have been, but for the deinstitutionalization movement, on the rolls of long-term mental institutions, especially state hospitals." By now it should become apparent that the average chronic mental patient is no longer being treated for an unadulterated mental illness. Perhaps we should dispense with the "mental" part of the "chronic mental patient" because it is too restrictive. It seems to me that we need a new term to describe the patient with a lot of mental and nonmental chronic illnesses—possibly the word "patient" is itself sufficient or "broad-spectrum patient."

THE CASE MANAGER

The utility of case management as a useful adjunct in the treatment of mental illness became apparent when the care of the mentally ill shifted from the institution to the community. Because of the increasing fragmentation of services that accompanied deinstitutionalization, many patients needed an advocate to coordinate care.

Thus far my contacts with case managers have not been extensive. I suspect that my contacts have been limited because case managers probably have a much greater involvement with patients who are not residents of residential care facilities. Such patients may need help for a variety of problems presented by the tasks of daily living, such as paying the rent and utility bills, keeping clinic and/or doctor's appointments, preparing meals, shopping, and arranging for transportation. Patients who are residents of residential care facilities are generally spared from these problems, and the problems of this nature that do arise are generally handled by the social workers who are assigned to the facility. To the extent that this is true, the role of the social worker sometimes blends into the role of the case manager, and for that reason I don't always know whether I am having social-worker contact or case-manager contact.

The one time I had extensive interactions with a case manager involved a residential care facility patient who had moved out of the residential care facility but still wanted me to follow him as an office patient. This rather simple matter proved to be very difficult, with the patient frequently forgetting his appointments or coming late and the case manager making frequent phone calls to me and even accompanying the patient to my office at times. This gave me a greater appreciation of the role of case managers, but it also gave me a greater appreciation for the role of myself by virtue of providing on-site visits and saving patients and case managers from all that bother.

It's probably best for a case manager to have a social work background, but the educational requirements for case managers have not been rigorously defined. Basically case managers function as patient coordinators and patient advocates. These are certainly important functions insofar as the fragmentation of health services is as confusing to the mental patient as it is to the nonmental patient. Advocacy has its place, but also unfortunately advocacy can be misplaced. I think one of the informal requirements of case managers should be that he or she be a wise person. Having said that, I realize that such stringencies have not been imposed upon psychiatrists, but it's too late to change the licensing requirements and even if we did, most psychiatrists would demand to be grandfathered in.

The following are standards and expectations of the case management programs which provide services to residents of residential care facilities. Under ideal circumstances the mental health providers and residential care facility staff would work together as a team to enhance communication, improve working relationships, and assist patients in achieving their maximum functional capacities in the community.

The following functions may be thought of as descriptive of their role:

1. Maintain ongoing communication with care providers.
2. Develop a care plan and a service plan jointly with care providers and clients with expectations of each party in the plan. A developed plan is to be distributed to care providers for facility record keeping.

3. Involve care providers in discussion of patient's planned or unplanned discharge placement. Inform care providers each step of the way.
4. Monitor patient progress in achieving goals during regular visits and share his or her observations with care providers in their regular meetings.
5. Link and coordinate services with community service providers to meet client's medical, mental, financial, cultural, and social needs.
6. Assist patients moving into and out of facilities.
7. Ensure patients have sufficient funds and clothing to move into a facility.
8. Assist patients to complete entitlement renewal applications in a timely manner.
9. Respond to emergency or nonemergency calls to care providers in a timely manner to prevent or to resolve crisis situations.

RELATIVES

Strictly speaking, relatives are not part of the cast, but I did not know where to place them. In fact, I would not have written about relatives at all, except that a relative called me while I was at a residential care facility and also in the midst of writing this book, and the creative thought occurred to me that I should write about this. Relatives are, after all, part of the big picture and occupy part of the time requirements involved in residential care facility work. However, if the truth be told, they do not occupy a large part of the time. The reason for this is that by the time a chronic psychotic patient gravitates to a residential care home, it is usually after multiple hospitalizations and long years of illness.

Therefore, when relatives do call, please bear in mind that you are generally dealing with long-suffering persons who are deserving of some sympathy. When they call—if they call—they are to be congratulated for maintaining their interest. Possibly this is in contrast to the calls of relatives seen in standard office psychiatry where such calls can be more frequent, more time-consuming, and sometimes fraught with possible confidentiality problems.

I think psychiatry has made great progress in recent years, not only in the treatment of patients but also in the treatment of patients' relatives. Parents of schizophrenic children used to get all the blame for the mental illnesses of their offspring. This occurred as a result of parentally induced "double binds" or imputed "marital skews and schisms" or as part of the schizophrenogenic mother philosophy that prevailed in the 1950s and 1960s. It has always seemed to me that these accusatory allegations regarding maternal etiology were more related to the impotence of the therapist than the maliciousness of the mother.

The "double bind," as described by Gregory Bateson,[12] an itinerant anthropologist with a tourist visa for psychopathology, occurs as a result of a situation in which no matter what a person does, he or she can't win. Bateson asserted that schizophrenia resulted as a consequence of contradictions in the communications between family members. Thus when children are presented with familial directives for which no obvious solutions are forthcoming, the result is an escape into schizophrenia. This theory been used as a basis for using psychotherapy as a means of treating schizophrenia. The presumption was that if schizophrenics could gain insight into their double-bind problems, the problems could then be downsized to single-bind status and the schizophrenia would be cured, or at least ameliorated. The theory was bolstered by multiple didactic homilies showing how basic misunderstandings catapulted eligible people into schizophrenia and prevented them from becoming ordinary Americans.

"Marital schisms" (when parents have contrary views which are thought to cause a child to have opposing loyalties) and "marital skews" (a pathological marriage in which one spouse dominates the other) were constructs that were devised by Theodore Lidz[13] as another way of blaming malfeasant parents for schizophrenic children. Prior to Lidz the only person blamed for schizophrenia was the schizophrenogenic mother.

Frieda Fromm-Reichmann is generally regarded as the originator of the schizophrenogenic-mother concept. In 1948 she proposed that mothers created schizophrenia in their children through cold and distant mothering.[14] As a consequence, Fromm-Reichmann produced an invidious icon which incurred the disdain and hostility of psychotherapists for a generation. She could have easily devised an opposing concept—that cold and distant mothering is an understandably protective response to a nonresponsive child, in which case the theory would have focused on the depressogenic child rather than the schizophrenogenic mother. This nonmotherly mother reputedly did not hold her babies correctly, could not maintain eye contact, did not coo at infants the way normal mothers do, and because of these deficiencies her babies became psychotic fifteen or sixteen years later. Schizophrenogenic-mother theorists with a myopic focus on the mother as a causative agent, never bothered with the depressogenic child, and rarely addressed the problem of why most schizophrenic patients were developmentally nonremarkable until midadolescence. Another relatively ignored possibility was that some schizophrenogenic mothers were schizophrenogenic because they themselves were schizophrenic—and not necessarily cold and distant, or were genetic carriers of schizophrenic vulnerabilities, or were exposed to unknown etiopathological events during their pregnancies.

In a sense Lidz was an equal opportunity employer in that he was the first to identify the schizophrenogenic father. Prior to Lidz, the mother was blamed for everything because generally speaking mothers were studied as etiopathological agents in therapists' offices. My theory is that the fathers were not fingered because they were usually unavailable for interview. Fathers could not come to the offices of therapists because the fathers were much too busy working—that is, making money so that the therapist could be paid. In those days everything was B.M. (before Medicaid). When Lidz got some of the fathers into his office, sure enough, some of them had imperfections—that is to say, had trouble communicating. Possibly the biggest mistake the fathers made was to leave work and come to the therapist's office.

I developed my reservations regarding maternal schizophrenogenicness (a word which reflects my own predilection for polysyllabic neologisms) when I was working as a clinical psychologist at Napa State Hospital and heard my colleagues berate mothers of some of the patients when it seemed to me these poor maligned mothers were trying to do a good job under difficult circumstances. Not only were the mothers feeling inadequate because of the illnesses of their sons and daughters but they also had to tolerate the accusations of therapists who saw themselves as defending the ego integrity of their patients against the onslaught of their evil schizophrenogenic mothers. The mothers, who were virtually inconsolable to begin with, became even more inconsolable. I had fantasies of these mothers going into therapy so that they could then heap blame upon their own mothers. Interestingly enough, I never heard the uncomplimentary schizophreno-genic adjective used in describing fathers, despite Lidz' attempt at sexual equality.

I recall comforting one demoralized mother, impeccably coiffed and tailored, after she was raked over the coals, read the riot act, and subjected to various other metaphorical indignities by her child's therapist who acted more like a prosecuting attorney than a therapist. Among other things, he accused her of compulsive perfectionism on the basis of her sartorial elegance using legal principle of *res ipso loquitor*—meaning the facts speak for themselves. The poor lady was almost in tears and she confided to me afterward that even though she didn't have much money, she got "all dressed up" out of respect for this person who is a doctor. She didn't know anything about compul-sions or perfectionism. I hope we have emerged from this fractious finger-pointing and fault-finding era.

I have no general policy in dealing with relatives, although I much prefer having the relatives as allies rather than adversaries. I describe in Chapter 9 the kind of relative who is virtually nonexistent until some unforeseen bad event affects the patient and then the relative springs into action like a panther going for the jugular. Little can be done about people with malicious intentions. But most people do not have such intentions, and frequently adversarial potentialities can be converted into workable relationships.

For example, consider the relative who telephoned me at the resi-dential care facility while I was visiting her sister. The relative com-plained that her sister seemed too sedated. I reviewed her medica-tions, noting that the patient was taking lithium 300 mg twice daily, carbamazepine 200 mg twice daily, and clonazepam 0.5 mg three times daily. Any one of these medications could cause drowsiness, al-though none of the doses were high and recent serum levels for lith-ium and carbamazepine were within normal limits. I told the patient's sister that the reason for her sister's sedation was unclear, but that I would stop her clonazepam. I then asked the sister to observe if there was any difference in her behavior and to be sure to check back with me about this in about one week or sooner. The point of this is that I am not only getting someone to monitor the patient closely but also converting the sister into an ally rather than a plaintiff.

Consider also the case of another patient's sister who telephoned me one day complaining that her brother was very poorly groomed and nobody was doing anything about it, and "all you do is come to the house once a month and then rush away and see somebody else." It occurred to me that the sister was really feeling guilty because she felt she should be doing more for her brother. I replied to her confrontational approach by saying that in most instances relatives lose interest in their sick mentally ill relatives, and that she was to be complimented for being a loyal and caring sister. Another potential enemy converted into an ally.

THE MODERN RESIDENTIAL CARE PSYCHIATRIC TEAM

So that's the cast—the residential care psychiatric team consisting of the psychiatrist, the pharmacist, the social worker, and in the future possibly the psychologist, depending on the laws of the land, all working in conjunction with the administrator and other caregiving personnel and all helping to increase the quality of mental health care. Possibly the proper way to describe the team is to accord it proper proper-noun status with appropriate capitalizations such as the Modern Residential Care Psychiatric Team and to designate it with an appropriate acronym (MRCPT) even though it is not pronounceable.

The MRCPT should be a task-oriented team in which each member feeds information to the psychiatrist in his or her field of expertise. The psychiatrist takes this information into consideration and then assumes full legal and ethical responsibility for making decisions regarding diagnosis and treatment. These decisions are not determined by a majority vote. Democracy is not applicable in every context. This lack of egalitarianism is good for the self-esteem of psychiatrists and also good for insurance companies because psychiatrists who bear responsibility for their decisions also bear responsibility for the adverse consequences of their decisions. That is why they buy malpractice insurance—to avoid impoverishment, which is not good for self-esteem.

The problem of who is boss has never been a problem, possibly because the team is small and each person has a defined role. One might think that a possible conflict exists between the pharmacist and psychiatrist regarding medication decisions but this is not a problem at

all. I regard myself as the ultimate authority in psychiatric pharmacotherapy, but not so ultimate in the use of medications in nonpsychiatric contexts, for which I request and appreciate the consultations provided by a knowledgeable pharmacist.

PART III:
THE PROBLEMS

Chapter 8

How It Should Be Done:
Space, Time, and Techniques

Prior to my involvement with residential care facilities, I was a conventional office psychiatrist. My own entry into the residential care system occurred in 1968. Prior to this time I was a standard office psychiatrist with a sofa, an easy chair, matching draperies, a fifty-minute hour clock, and a panoply of honorific plaques occupying every available space on my wainscotted walls. Whenever I was plagued by negative thoughts about my own personal worth, I would look at these walls. If the truth be told, I spent a lot of time looking at walls.

However, the gradual emergence of a large-volume practice, replete with unscheduled emergencies, did not adapt well to the luxuries of the contemplative one-on-one nine-to-five office life. Consequently I became dependent on techniques of rapid assessment which have served me well in the years that I have been doing residential care psychiatry. Before I describe these techniques, I would like to describe some basic differences between standard office psychiatry and residential care psychiatry.

Although the goals of the office psychiatrist and the residential care psychiatrist are the same in terms of making the patient better or well or less sick or more functional or however one wants to phrase it, the differences between office psychiatry and residential care psychiatry involve basic differences in the parameters of time, space, procedure codes, and techniques.

SPACE CONSTRAINTS

In office psychiatry, the psychiatrist arranges the room to accommodate his or her work pattern. In residential care psychiatry, the psychiatrist must adjust his or her work pattern to the limitations of the room. The kind of monastic privacy that is available to the office psychiatrist is generally not available in a residential care home. My encounters are frequently done in a living room or dining room, and occasionally the most delicate of confidences is conveyed in counterpoint to the incoming clatter of a juxtaposed kitchen and in the presence of a nosy and noisy cook. The fact is when you are a guest in someone's home—pardon me, facility—you cannot tell them where to put the kitchen. Also a nosy cook, if she is interested in people, can be much better than a non-nosy cook. Sometimes it is the nosy cook who is the first to notice a change in feeding patterns, such as when a patient stops eating, or the onset of bizarre feeding patterns, such as pouring a whole jar of sugar into a cup of coffee.

Each house is different and the modus operandi of the residential care psychiatrist should be determined by the geography of the house and the demography of the staff. In one house I was confronted with the problems created by a large population of poorly stabilized patients attended to by a kindly but disorganized staff badly in need of emergency courses in English as a second language. I sensed that communications were less than ideal and that useful information regarding the patients might be lost or inadvertently disregarded.

Because of this it became my custom to attempt to somehow observe all the patients in one visit even though it would not be possible for me to provide services to everyone. Still, observation does not have to be a formally constructed service matched to a Medicare procedure code, and I felt that it was incumbent upon me to observe without charging even though one cannot charge without observing.

With this in mind, it became my custom to arrive at the house approximately two hours before dinner and to see patients in the dining room. The fact is that in the early years of attendance, the use of a room as a private office was never proffered, so I did not have a choice in the matter. During these years, I developed the habit of dragging my office charts—with complete psychiatric and medication histories—into this rather large dining room which seated thirty-five residents around seven tables. Characteristically, I would plunk the charts down in two large stacks on one of these reliable and uncomplaining tables and attempt one-on-one interactions while surrounded by a sea of demanding and intrusive patients, each with his or her own list of priorities. To the untrained eye and unsympathetic brain, this would appear to be the essence of chaos.

Granted this was not the Sea of Tranquility, but the system worked moderately well for years. Eventually the residents learned to respect that I was working under a certain amount of time pressure but that I would try to see everyone who had an urgent problem. They learned to respect the rights of the patient who was the center of attention because they knew that their turn would come.

When I first started visiting homes in 1969 I was disturbed that frequently I did not have a separate room or office to conduct my interviews as is true in a conventional office practice. In one of those rare flashes of insight that psychiatrists frequently have in a nonrare way, I realized that I was more frustrated by intrusive irrelevant stimuli than were the patients whom I was interviewing. Presumably it is the sick ones who have the inability to exclude the intrusiveness of irrelevant stimuli—the so-called inability to gate—and at times I felt ready to join this inadequately gated community. My feelings were not without external support insofar as plenty of other psychiatrists told me I was crazy to do what I was doing.

Whether I was inconvenienced or not, the fact is I did not have a choice in the matter, and I had to make the best of what I regarded as a bad situation. I soon discovered that necessity is not only the mother of invention but it is also the father of accommodation and that there were undiscovered advantages to such accommodations. After I appreciated the fact that this lack of privacy was more disturbing to me than to most of my patients, I subsequently learned that advantages were afforded by operating in a semipublic arena. Thus I learned that I could frequently observe significant interactions of other patients on the periphery of my vision while focusing on the patient I actually interviewed. This may seem difficult to do, but the human mind has an extraordinary plasticity, and I believe the average psychiatrist would be able to do this with a little practice. After all, this is doing only what the mother of a large family of small children must do on a daily basis. This might be called the open-door system of interviewing except when the interviews are conducted in a living room or dining room there are frequently no doors, either open or closed.

That being the case, it is probably more accurate to describe such encounters as just that: no-door encounters rather than interviews. The advantages to me (and to the patients) were that I could observe other patients at a time when they felt they were not under close scrutiny and not obliged to be on their best behavior or behavior donned for the benefit of the interviewing psychiatrist. Such behavior might include manneristic gesticulations, inappropriate laughter, talking to oneself, abusive language, periodic yelling or screaming, reckless use of matches or cigarette ashes, unusual feeding patterns, as well as other inappropriate interactions with other patients and staff. A particular advantage of no-door encounters is that they allow for the expression of inappropriate social intrusiveness of people who I am not interviewing, as when a patient might repeatedly interrupt an interview with another patient with an irrational statement or demand.

It should be noted that the pattern of socially inappropriate intrusiveness is more difficult to determine when patients are seen alone in an office setting because the essence of intrusiveness is expressed by the interruption of someone else's interview. Such an interdiction might temporarily interrupt the flow of information from the interviewee, but it provides valuable information about the other patient who is also under my care. Generally speaking designated interviewees are not unduly disturbed by such interruptions—this being part of the tolerance mentally ill residents develop when living communally with other mentally ill residents.

In the following case I was not able to focus on the interview because one of the patients in the room was proclaiming in a very loud and persistent way that he was feeling so good. My initial impulse was to tell the patient to be more quiet, but upon reflection it occurred to me that this was an unusual behavior pattern for this patient and that he was, in fact, undergoing a manic episode. I had very little information about this patient because he did not have a known history of hospitalizations and the referring social worker did not have much background information. Because of this patient's apparent emerging mania and because he was a physically powerful and intimidating person, I felt the most prudent course of action would be to begin therapy with divalproex. Several weeks later I received a telephone call from the patient's sister who noted that he seemed to be taking "a lot of pills." However, she confirmed that he was feeling well. She also confirmed that in the past her brother had had periods of excitability during which he was hard to control.

Would I have been alerted to the situation if I were seeing patients in an office on the premises? I don't think so. The patient's mania may not have been that obvious to me had I interviewed this patient alone in a one-on-one office situation where intrusiveness may not have been so easily recognized. Communication between staff and psychiatrist may not have been so efficient that the staff would have suggested that I evaluate the patient. In fact, it may be too much to expect the recognition of emerging mania from a nonprofessional staff insofar as the line between emerging mania and nonpathological cheerfulness is not always easy to recognize. So this is an instance in which not having an office on the premises, served to my (and the patient's) advantage.

Several months after this episode, the administrator offered to create an office room where I could see the patients individually. I politely declined stating that this would place me too far from the patients. I had other reasons which I did not elaborate, namely that in a large, poorly organized home with many severely irrational patients and an impaired flow of communication between staff and psychiatrist, an office is not necessarily the most optimal way to deliver professional services. In this setting, the most effective way I can function is in the dining room seated at a dining room table surrounded by a covey of patients, some of them impatient, with a variety of rational and irrational demands and requests. Contributing to the impression of utter bedlam is the tabletop itself, which contains stacks of dog-eared office charts which I have dragged from my office and which contain complete medication histories. Eventually the stacked charts become unstacked—although they still remain dog-eared—as I ransack through them to obtain the proper chart for the proper patient. On this already overburdened tabletop is a large book in which I enter my current progress notes and which is the property of the house. Sometimes patients want to know what I am writing about, so I tell them. If they disagree with me, then I discuss it with them—and sometimes will even write why they disagree with me into the progress note, if it makes any sense, or even if it does not make sense.

Not only do some patients appear to adjust to this pattern, but in the course of time many of them appear to relish it, possibly because the custom of interviewing patients on a proscenium or in a theater-in-the-round situation acquires a prestigious show-business aspect, so that many of the patients will cluster close to the interviewing site insisting that they "be next." When I am in this setting, I realize that I am not distributing candy to children, yet in some way the situation evokes the memory of such pleasurable dispensations.

To the casual observer the whole picture reeks of disorganization, but it frequently works, as the previously noted case illustrates. It doesn't always work, but in psychiatry nothing always works. I might add that dining room psychiatry, if I may call it that, is not necessarily a common situation for a residential care facility, but it does exist.

When it does exist, the dining room becomes my office, but an office without walls and without doors. If this were a smaller home, I would have accepted the administrator's offer of an office. If this were a large facility with a well-organized staff and good communication, I probably would have accepted the offer. But in the setting of a large facility with poor communications between staff and psychiatrist, it was necessary for me personally to have a peripheral overview of all the patients in the facility, and the most effective way I could function was within the semipublic arena of the dining room in direct contact with the demands and complaints of the residents. Doors and walls are important in the sense of preserving privacy. They prevent others from looking in on us, but they also prevent us from looking in on them. In the situation just described, it was much more important for us to have the ability to look at them. The whole experience is analogous to having a one-way mirror but without the physical obstacle for patient-therapist interaction created by the mirror.

As a rule, patients do not seem to mind the relative lack of privacy that occurs during these interviews. Possibly such patient tolerances are enhanced because the interviewee shares the same living situation with the intruder. I would say that patients in residential care facilities generally prefer the no-door encounter to the closed-door office-type interview, and for that reason they generally do not react angrily to such interruptions. Also mentally ill patients have a greater tolerance for the idiosyncratic actions of other mentally ill patients.

Many residential care patients are not used to one-on-one interactions with therapists in private offices where the patient is alone in a room with the therapist and the pressure is on the patient to relate to a therapist. Some patients do not like to be put into this situation because it is regarded as excessively interpersonal. Other patients prefer open-door interviews because the quid pro quo for decreased patient privacy is the increased accessibility of the psychiatrist. Many patients living in residential care facilities are willing to make this trade.

In contrast, as office psychiatrists we are almost universally in favor of privacy because the question of privacy versus accessibility is not an issue in office practices. To put it into neurotransmitter language, in on-site psychiatry, privacy and accessibility are in competition for the same receptor sites. In office practice, accessibility and privacy are not in competition.

Whatever the reason, issues relating to privacy rarely occur in residential care facilities. When such problems occur, it may be desirable to see the patient in the office and this should not be ruled out as an option. At other times it may be preferable to acknowledge to the patient that certain issues are difficult to discuss, but that you, as the residential care facility psychiatrist will return to the home on a prescheduled basis, and perhaps it would be more comfortable for the patient to discuss these issues at a future time. This, of course, is one of the advantages of routine on-site visits to residential care facilities—that it is easy to punt and that by so doing one doesn't even have to give up the ball. For some patients it will take years of visits before trust accumulates and communication can flow and it frequently takes more than one or two encounters to become accustomed to the face.

The problem of the no-door encounter versus the closed door interview leads to the problem of which Medicare codes to use in describing one's visits to residential care facilities. I think one has to distinguish here between large homes and small homes. In small homes (six residents or less) where one may have the luxury of doing time-limited psychotherapy sessions lasting twenty-five or forty-five minutes with individual residents in individual one-on-one private psychotherapy sessions, the use of psychotherapy codes may be acceptable. If one were to proceed with such codes in large homes or midsized homes (ten or more), the inevitable result of such a practice would be to provide intensive services for a few patients while necessarily ignoring the needs of most of the residents because of time limitations.

TIME CONSTRAINTS

I have devoted much more time and space to space than to time. The reason for this, to put it somewhat clumsily, is that we can do something about space. In that sense, space is malleable. Time is not malleable. Time passes in an uncompromising way and we can merely segment it and allocate it.

The allocation of time is one of the principal differences between office psychiatry and on-site residential care facility psychiatry. In an office practice the psychiatrist can control time to accommodate the needs of the individual patient. Some patients bearing a wealth of information and a heavy burden of serious problems and a middle-class expectation of how much time a psychiatrist should be spending with them are fifty-minute-type patients. Others somewhat less fortunate or more fortunate, depending on how one looks at it, are twenty-five-minute-type patients, either fast talkers, people with lesser problems, or people on more restrictive budgets.

In standard office psychiatry we arrange time to fit the needs of the patient. In residential care facility psychiatry where the psychiatrist delegates a finite amount of time to the on-site visit, say two hours, the patients have to be fitted into the time rather than the time fitted to the patient. The residential care facility patients become timesharers in a zero-sum game. One patient's time surplus becomes another patient's time deficit.

The issue of time is more fully discussed in Chapter 9 as duration, which is how third-party payers measure time.

THE TECHNIQUES

At the beginning of this chapter I described how mental patients have changed my concepts of space and time, and I promised to describe rapid assessment techniques. These were not techniques produced in any one sitting, or for that matter in any other position, nor were they ever consciously planned in brainstorming sessions with myself. Rather, they gradually evolved over a thirty-year period in such a way that I was not really conscious of what I was doing. Had I been accused of any serious crime during this period, I would have pleaded diminished capacity. As fate would have it, I never received the opportunity to exercise that defense. I would like to share these techniques with you.

Actually, there's something wrong with that last sentence. Authorship requires complete honesty. I don't want to share these techniques with anybody. "Sharing" implies that I own something, and once I share it, I give away part of the product that is being shared so that I no longer can claim sole possession. It's like apple pie—if I share it with anybody, I am no longer in possession of the shared part of the apple pie. "Sharing" is not the right word. When I tell others about these techniques, I can still utilize them fully. I am not giving anything away. What is the right word? The right word was said two sentences ago. The right word is "tell." Since there are ten of these techniques I have decided to call them the Ten Commandments of Residential Care Psychiatry.

The Ten Commandments of Residential Care Psychiatry

  I. Thou shalt make routine home visits to evaluate patients on the premises and not wait for crises to occur.
 II. Thou shalt accumulate as much historical information as you can from external sources utilizing hospital summaries and/or other sources of information and place this information in the office charts.
III. When making a visit to the residential care home, thou shalt *schlep* the office charts with you.
 IV. Thou shalt focus on prodromal signs of relapse.
  V. Thou shalt enhance communication with administrators and other caregivers regarding ongoing problems.
 VI. Thou shalt enhance communication with social workers and other mental health workers.
VII. Thou shalt segregate psychopharmacological orders into separate progress notes for each patient.
VIII. Thou shalt segregate laboratory test reports into separate folders for each residential care home.
 IX. Thou shalt practice psychoperambulation when indicated.
  X. Thou shalt involve patients in medication management decisions when indicated.

Although these principles are popularly known as the Ten Commandments of Residential Care Psychiatry, they are only popularly known only to me, since I coined the phrase and didn't tell anyone. I hope that might change once this book is published. The principles are so important that I have designated them with Roman numerals. They are there for the guidance of those psychiatrists who hope to become engaged in residential care facility work. If they choose to ignore them, so much the worse. I am like the signpost that points the way to weary psychiatrists but does not accompany them to their destinations.

I will now elaborate on each of these points:

I. Thou shalt make routine home visits to evaluate patients on the premises and not wait for crises to occur.

It is important to establish a routine schedule when administering to residential care facilities. This should be done in cooperation with the administrator. Administrators have time commitments just as physicians do and it is important for the psychiatrists to respect this in their scheduled appointments. Administrators will appreciate that you consider their time valuable and such consideration will carry long-run dividends in facilitating communication. Also if the psychiatrist is committed to a certain appointment time, and he or she is late, then he or she should call the administrator and explain that he or she will be late. The first time that I did that, the administrator was absolutely astonished. She had never had the experience of a doctor calling her and explaining that he might be late. I think she may have had the impression that possibly I was not a real doctor. I insisted on showing her my license to allay whatever misgivings she might have had.

The establishment of a routine will also be respected by most patients, who generally will make an attempt to be at the home when you visit. If the opposite happens and patients are deliberately avoidant, that is also useful information.

The timing of the visit should not be dependent on crisis situations, although sometimes extra visits may have to be made in response to such situations. One of the advantages of routine visits is that the observations and medication changes made during these visits can generally prevent crisis situations from emerging. I provide specific examples of such incidents in Chapter 9.

II. Thou shalt accumulate as much historical information as thou can from external sources utilizing hospital summaries and/or other sources of information and place this information in the office charts.

Residential care facility work can be made much easier if the psychiatrist uses a little creativity. Using a combination of guile and charm, I have been able to convince experienced professionals to interview my patients for me. Also I have successfully persuaded skilled typists to type the interviews so I can review the information very quickly—and all this virtually free of charge. I get this information by writing to hospitals and requesting discharge summaries. Thus, in addition to guile and charm, I needed to lay out money for postage stamps and envelopes to enclose my release of information forms. Starting January 1, 2001, I have had to spend thirty-four cents and later thirty-seven cents to obtain a hospital summary, but in past years my overhead was much cheaper. You win a few, you lose a few. I do not understand why some psychiatrists still do not do this, but, as is well known, not all psychiatrists are understandable.

Generally, I have had no problems getting patients to sign release-of-information forms. I would like to say that this is because I establish rapport with my patients, but this is an untrue statement. The truth is that when I encounter a new patient, my first statement is not a statement at all; it is a question. Before I say "Hello," I ask, "Is it okay if I write to hospitals to obtain background hospital information about you?" Ninety percent of the time patients will sign unhesitatingly on the dotted line. Actually, I am not sure if the line is really dotted on my forms, but I think you catch my drift. In the past, when I was younger (as most of us were in the past), I used to first introduce myself to the patient as a somewhat civil person. I would say something like, "Hello. My name is Dr. Fleishman, but you can call me Marty." However, I eventually learned that once I said that and established rapport, frequently patients would refuse to sign the form. They would say something like, "Sorry, Dr. Fleishman, or Marty, or whatever you call yourself, I am not going to sign the form." After a while, I no longer worried about rapport, and I no longer tried to establish a first-name relationship with any of my patient-buddies. And my mother still calls me Martin.

When it comes to signing forms, there are two prodromal patterns to worry about. The first occurs when the patient actually attempts to read the form. I realize this is within his or her civil rights or duties or obligations, or his or her Miranda rights, or it occurs because he or she is reading consumer-activist newsletters such as Dr. Sidney Wolf's *Public Citizen* (just kidding, Sidney) and trying to be an educated consumer. I know all that and I don't dispute the fact that we all have rights, but from the standpoint of predicting a good response to the residential care facility environment, that patient is a troublemaker.

The second prodromal pattern occurs when the patient actually refuses to sign the form. Aside from validating the diagnosis of paranoia, either in its pure form or the adulterated schizophrenic variety, that behavior is an absolute predictor of a failed placement. I know because I used to attempt to cope with it, but I invariably failed in helping the patient make a good adjustment to community living. When it happens now—now that I am not living in the past and have acquired the wisdom that sometimes accumulates with age and replaces other things that were a lot more fun—I indicate that if the patient does not sign the form, I cannot be involved in his or her treatment. If patients do not take any responsibility for their treatment, then they cannot be well served. I call these prodromal signs the Fleishman signs, in the hope that someday I will get eponymic credit in one of those large books on psychiatry periodically published by Harvard University.

Sometimes it is not easy to access important information. Consider the following case:

A patient was admitted to a residential care facility with a background case history from the hospital, but someone had forgotten to provide her with medication, and there was no medication information in her records. At this point it became necessary for the residential care facility psychiatrist to telephone the hospital psychiatrist. The latter was unavailable, so the former was told to call the ward clerk. The ward clerk stated that the patient's chart had been transferred to Medical Records. Medical Records could not find the chart immediately but offered to call back, which they subsequently did. Included among the patient's medications were lithium and lorazepam. It then became necessary to contact the clinical laboratory to make routine follow-up visits for serum lithium determinations. Also, it was then necessary to include CBC, BUN, creatinine, T3, T4, and TSH since these should also be drawn at least initially for patients on lithium. The pharmacy was contacted regarding refilling these medications, but there was one obstacle: since lorazepam was not then in the Medicaid formulary, a treatment authorization request had to be made to the Medicaid consultant. The consultant's office was then contacted. The authorization clerk had to know the patient's birthday, Medicaid ID number, pharmacy phone number, pharmacy address, and so forth. The consultant then came to the phone; he had to know which formulary drugs had been used in the past and why they could not be used now. What did I forget? Oh, yes—the telephone prompts, the ones that say, "Your call is very important to us. Please hold."

Such events are not typical insofar as most patients do come to residential care facilities with a greater degree of preparation. But they still happen occasionally, and they illustrate the extent to which residential care facility psychiatrists must be reasonably tenacious in order to obtain information and ensure proper care.

To work most productively, the psychiatrist should have an intimate knowledge not only of the patient's case history as provided by the patient and the external sources of information as described above but also of the patient's historical response to medication. The vast majority of schizophrenic patients cannot provide such a history. In many instances such information is unavailable. However, in other situations such information is available but obtaining it requires extra efforts, such as writing to the hospitals for case history information and then reviewing and digesting this material within the silence of one's office so that it becomes part and parcel of one's professional expertise. Third-party payers do not reward one for such solitary lucubrations, since compensation is dependent on face-to-face contacts. There is much more to residential care psychiatry than meets the face.

III. When making a visit to the residential care home, thou shalt schlep the office charts with you.

Schlep is not an acronym, acrimonious or otherwise, but a Yiddish word that includes the concepts of pulling, dragging, dredging, commandeering, and conscripting, all of which requires considerable muscular exertion—all of this in a one-syllable word with numerous consonants. Actually the word derives its onomatopoetic impact from the energy required to schlep all those consonants and all those nuanced interpretations of awkward dragging into one single monosyllable vehicle. I think it is appropriate to use a Yiddish word since we are talking about the Ten Commandments of Residential Care Facility Psychiatry, although a Hebrew word would have been even more appropriate. Unfortunately there is not a Hebrew or English word quite equivalent to *schlep*—possibly for the aforementioned reasons. *Schlep* will have to do. In some texts *schlep* is no longer italicized, which is analogous to acquiring naturalized citizenship. We will encounter *schlep* in future chapters, either in its italicized or unitalicized homolog, to describe the phenomenon of unwilling exertion combined with awkward dragging.

When entering the all-important progress note, the progress note shall duly be entered in the house chart. The house chart, as the name implies, is the chart kept at the house for each individual patient. What is in the house chart besides your progress notes? The house chart is full of forms as required by licensing. There is a form explaining the patient's personal rights, a form for emergency procedures, a physician's report form for community care facilities, a community mental health form for the annual plan of care, a form explaining the admission agreement, a form explaining eviction procedures, a form describing the house rules and regulations, a form containing a record of cash deposits as well as additional case history information.

If the house chart is so all encompassing why do you schlep the office charts with you? You do this for all the reasons mentioned under Commandment II. Also it is very difficult to make intelligent psychopharmacological decisions without the histories that are in the office chart, as will be explained in Commandment VII.

Commandment III also has implications regarding one's filing system. It is the usual and customary practice (a phrase I shall come back to later in this book) for physicians to file all their charts alphabetically by the patients' last names. The best filing system for a residential care facility psychiatrist is to alphabetically file by homes—that is to say, Facilities with the capital F, and then file the patients alphabetically behind the Facility folders. In this filing system the Facilities come first followed by the patients. It is best to use different colored folders for the Facilities, preferably orange. In case you are ever lost in a snowstorm with the folders, orange will show up the best. This is not a problem in San Francisco, but for psychiatrists visiting adult psychiatric facilities in places like Fargo, North Dakota, there might be some problems. I know this because I like to tape the programs on the Weather Channel. Then when I awaken at 2:00 a.m. and need something to relax, I watch the tape. I know a lot about snowstorms. I even know a lot about Fargo.

Actually, I have two orange folders for each house. One of them contains the Health Care Financing Administration (HCFA) 1500 claim forms in red dropout ink (in case I suddenly decide to drop out) for each of the patients in the facility. The other contains the lab tests for the patients. I discuss this issue under another commandment.

This filing system has several advantages. By using this method it will enable the physician to more readily appreciate which patient is in which house. This should be not a problem for the psychiatrist while he or she is on the premises (at least I hope it's not a problem), but a lot of adult psychiatric facility related work does not occur on the premises. What am I talking about? I am talking about the telephone. If the psychiatrist uses the above filing system, he or she will have an immediate knowledge about who is where—possibly because memory engrams are facilitated by behavioral operations, as when pigeons push levers—this being another subject I discuss later in this book. In this case the behavioral operation is the operation used to push the patient charts into their proper sequences behind the Facility charts.

Another advantage of this filing system is that it saves time. Let's say you have twenty patients in a facility. Because you have read this book you now have an office chart for each of these patients packed with relevant information that will help you make significant clinical decisions when you are at the house. Also you have read the Ten Commandments so you know about the importance of schlepping the charts with you to the facility. With a regular filing system, every time the psychiatrist went to the house, he or she would have to riff through the charts trying to remember which patient was in which house. This is a deplorably pedestrian way of doing things, even if it is the fingers that are doing the walking. Filing by facility allows one to unthinkingly grab a bunch of charts and be on one's way. As I said, it saves lots of time. And time is important for physicians to conserve, because they don't have a lot of it.

This raises another issue that I do not discuss at length in this book. Did you ever notice how conservationists never talk about the importance of conserving time? Why is that? I don't know either. So let's ignore the digression and return to the Commandments.

IV. Thou shalt focus on prodromal signs of relapse.

The psychiatrist working in the residential care facility setting is in a good position to decrease rehospitalizations. This is especially true of the psychiatrist who is schooled in the early detection of relapse. Sophistication in this area is dependent on knowing the idiosyncrasies of the sickness cycle, particularly if individual patients demonstrate a prodromal sequence. For instance, a psychiatrist who waits until a patient becomes belligerent before increasing a maintenance dose may be waiting too long. Frequently, harbingers of relapse precede aggressiveness and hallucinations which can be used as signals for changing maintenance regimens, such as complaints of poor appetite, nervous tension, deteriorating sleeping patterns, complaints of being talked about or ridiculed, diminished feelings of self-esteem, and increased religious thoughts. To be sensitive to the sickness cycle the psychiatrist has to be familiar with the individual case histories of each patient. For those with a predictable prodromal sequence, and this would comprise about 70 percent of schizophrenic patients, the psychiatrist is able to intercede earlier in the prodrome and prevent a rehospitalization.[1]

The optimal use of medications involves much more than pill pushing and shot giving. When the patient is violent, hallucinating, and obviously bizarre, the psychiatrist should have intervened before this regrettable point. By understanding the prodromal antecedents to an acute exacerbation, the skilled psychiatrist is in a position to intercede so as to abort the episode and avoid a hospitalization.

The schizophrenic patient is generally not a good source of prodromal information, possibly because the change or deterioration in habit patterns preceding an exacerbation is not regarded by the patient as unusual or worthy of note, or possibly because there is defective registration of experience secondary to impaired concentration.

Sometimes the pattern is not obviously related to deterioration but merely appears to be an idiosyncrasy that characteristically appears before an overt break, much as an aura might precede a convulsion. The importance of such idiosyncratic harbingers of exacerbation has only recently been acknowledged in the treatment of manic-depressive illnesses in the promotion of life-charting systems in which such preexacerbation patterns are aggressively pinpointed. However, I wrote about the importance of such information a long time ago as an important technique to minimize relapses in schizophrenia.[2]

Thus, I know that when a certain patient talks of the importance of losing weight, she is not on the verge of getting better; instead, she is about to undergo a depressive exacerbation that has been associated with suicide attempts in the past. All of her attempts thus far have been trivial, but I have been forewarned.

When another patient talks of becoming the recipient of a large charitable endowment, I know he is not taking his medication and will go on to develop overt paranoid delusions if there is no intervention.

I know that if a third patient starts having nightmares, she will soon start burning herself with cigarettes unless her medication is increased. The cycle has happened many times, and in this instance her medication has been titrated using IM fluphenazine decanoate in weekly doses that have been gradually escalated to 3 cc per week. Attempts to retreat from this high plateau have always resulted in a dysphoric decompensation associated with self-mutilation, usually with cigarettes but sometimes with razors.

In the home situation such cosmetic and eleemosynary prodromal preoccupations might first become apparent to a patient's relatives. In residential care facility settings it is the administrator who has this role. It is the psychiatrist's responsibility to communicate with the administrator and to act appropriately. Nor can one overlook information supplied by cooks and housekeepers. The cook may be the first to notice an increase in inappropriate dietary habits which may signal a coming exacerbation of illness. The housekeeper may be the first to notice the patient throwing clothes on the floor or developing nocturnal incontinence.

Frequently it is the administrator who may be first aware of a deterioration in the activities of daily living such as refusal to bathe, or change clothes, or poor appetite or increased irritability. Patients do not always fess up to the psychiatrist that they are undergoing an increase in irritability because that may not be subjectively acknowledged. Patients may not complain about a poor appetite because it may not bother them. However, when both psychiatrist and administrator are sensitized to the early detection of prodromal sequences, rehospitalizations can frequently be avoided. Naturally this requires a free flow of information between psychiatrists and administrators and other caregivers, which logically leads us to the next commandment.

V. Thou shalt enhance communication with administrators and other caregivers regarding ongoing problems.

This commandment is intimately related to Commandment IV focusing on prodromal signs of relapse. This is true because in order for a patient to improve after showing signs of incipient relapse to caregivers, it is necessary for the caregivers to communicate this to the psychiatrist. My experience in residential care facilities has made me appreciate that relapses frequently occur in stages. An early stage may occur as a deterioration in one of the activities of daily living and may be as simple as a patient starting to neglect brushing his or her teeth. Psychiatrists may not notice this but caretakers very well might. The caretakers are the radar-screen watchers when it comes to the early warning signals of ADL deterioration.

The ADL approach represents a good way to systematically approach administrators and other caretakers to obtain information. All caretakers are attuned to the problems of the activities of daily living. These activities involve ambulation, bathing, continence, dressing, eating, hygiene, and toileting. These activities are listed in almost alphabetical order, making it easier to address these issues in a progress note. These again are issues evident to caretaking personnel. Generally ADL issues are not addressed by patients when seen by the psychiatrist in office settings and this once again illustrates the shortcomings of standard office psychiatry in the treatment of patients in the residential care facility system.

Consultation with the administrator is especially valuable in that the administrator may be aware of changes in behavior that occur over the course of a twenty-four-hour day which are not evident during the psychiatrist's visits. This may occur in the context of the administrator's knowledge of the patient's ADLs, such as observing deteriorations in the patient's capacity to bathe, change clothes, eat, or attend to personal hygiene.

These may precede more obvious changes such as complaints of tension, nervousness, complaints of being laughed at or talked about, or diminished feelings of worth, and increased religiosity. At this point it may be wise to consider changing medication regimens. This can be done before the occurrence of more dramatic exacerbations involving hallucinations, delusions, mood changes, and bizarre behavior. The psychiatrist's knowledge of symptomatic progression and the administrator's knowledge of the patient's twenty-four-hour pattern represent a complement of understandings which, if communicated, can be extremely useful in the area of medication management.

The phrase *if communicated* probably should be italicized. There can be numerous impediments to a free flow of ideas. If the psychiatrist is aloof or otherwise unapproachable, the administrator may not feel free to convey his or her impressions about a patient. Patient care will suffer accordingly. Also, if the administrator is too busy to be involved or is otherwise unavailable or feels the psychiatrist should make people better but does not feel he or she has the obligation to provide input, the relationship has serious problems which require more than the services of a marital counselor. Not all unions are felicitous, and sometimes both parties are better off if they seek other mates.

Here is a good example of coordination by administrator and psychiatrist involving the treatment of someone who demonstrated an unusual reaction to psychotropic medication:

MS, a sixty-five-year-old Chinese female with a history of lobotomy, violence, and delusions of poisoning, was able to leave the hospital in 1968, twenty years after having been started on fluphenazine decanoate as 1 cc q 2 weeks. Eventually this was discontinued because of pacing problems. Attempts to treat with chlorpromazine and trifluoperazine were similarly unsuccessful. Eventually, thioridazine was substituted. She was able to make a successful adjustment, with good control of violence and delusions and with minimal adverse side effects for four years, but eventually started having hypotensive episodes. Afterward mesoridazine was substituted in minimal doses, as 10 mg daily, but even this was poorly tolerated. Patient described by the administrator as falling and refusing to stand up. Thereafter, all antipsychotics were discontinued with the subsequent emergence of agitation, tongue protrusions, pacing, and dysphagia. It was presumed that patients had symptoms referable to both tardive dyskinesia and exacerbating psychosis. Because of an intolerance to all known antipsychotics, a decision was made to attempt to treat the patient with chlordiazepoxide. MS was started as 25 mg BID but shortly thereafter the patient manifested muscle stiffness, although agitation and tongue protrusion decreased. It was then decided to discontinue the chlordiazepoxide and resume this medication with a smaller dose. This was done with chlordiazepoxide as 10 mg BID, which she could tolerate without side effects for about four days after which the administrator noted the recurrence of muscle stiffness. The chlordiazepoxide was again discontinued but with a return of agitation, tongue protrusions, and dysphagia. After one week I then restarted the chlordiazepoxide as 10 mg BID with the amelioration of the above symptoms and continued this for four days. I then withheld the chlordiazepoxide for one week before starting on another cycle. The patient has been well stabilized on this schedule and her agitation, tongue protrusion, pacing, and deglutition difficulties have not been a management problem in recent years.

This is an old case[3]—cited before the advent of the newer minor tranquilizers and the boxed FDA warnings regarding the QTc prolongations of thioridazine and mesoridazine, but it is a good illustration of how coordinative efforts by psychiatrist and administrator were instrumental in the treatment of an unusual and difficult case. Here it spelled the difference between survival in a community facility and placement in a long-term facility. In psychiatry, as in most fields of medicine, it is the unusual case that creates difficulties. The usual is usually not a problem.

VI. Thou shalt enhance communication with social workers and other mental health workers.

Social workers are not only important to the residential care facility psychiatrist, but they are also important to the residential care facility system. The entire residential care facility system could not function without social workers, as I discuss in Chapter 7 on the cast. They are important to the psychiatrist in a personal sense in that they provide the psychiatrist with valuable information regarding the clinical status of patients. These workers, some of whom may be involved in therapeutic interactions with patients, may be among the first to note signs of relapse. By maintaining open lines of communication with social workers and other professionals, the psychiatrist can acquire an extra set of eyes and ears without incurring a profound physiognomic deformity.

In addition to the aftercare social worker, the psychiatrist may find it necessary to communicate with and/or receive information from pharmacists, hospital social workers, hospital physicians, day treatment center workers, conservators, disability evaluators, rehabilitation workers, recreation therapists, licensing workers, mobile EKG technicians, psychiatric nurses working in hospitals, public health nurses working outside of hospitals, Medicaid consultants (as when requesting nonformulary drugs or extension of hospital days), phlebotamists (as when requesting serum lithiums and TSHs and T-3s for patients on lithium or serum valproic acids for patients on divalproex or WBCs for patients on clozapine, serum potassiums and magnesiums for the thioridazine and mesoridazine patients), etc. Who did I forget? Oh yes, I forgot relatives, and, oh yes, other nonpsychiatric physicians involved in other aspects of patient care. Also, psychiatrists sometimes have to remind themselves that the legal constraints of confidentiality pertain to the dissemination of information rather than to its reception.

VII. Thou shalt segregate psychopharmacological orders into separate notes for each patient.

The residential care psychiatrist with a large caseload should have at least a nodding acquaintance with all major antipsychotic medications in current use. The reasons for this are at least twofold. To begin with, in a large practice there will be an active inflow, as well as outflow of patients. Patients will be referred to residential care facilities from many different sources—halfway houses, long-term locked facilities, and local hospitals that render acute care, as well as state hospitals. Patients being referred will have been treated by a variety of physicians using a variety of medications. Usually it is preferable to continue the medications the patient has been taking on release from the referring institution for the obvious reason that in most instances patients are discharged with the medication or combination of medications that appear to be most effective in facilitating remission, hopefully.

Another reason why the psychiatrist should be familiar with all the major antipsychotic medications lies in the fact that some patients may be relatively nonresponsive to most antipsychotics but selectively responsive to one or two. Sometimes this selectivity does not extend to the more widely used antipsychotics but is restricted to those that are used infrequently, such as acetophenazine (Tindal) or chlorprothixene (Taractan) although they are no longer manufactured in the United States. The psychiatrist who is aware of all of the pharmacological options is in a better position to treat difficult cases. In some instances, patients who have been refractory to treatment for many years may respond to exotic combinations, as is illustrated in the following case.

R.W. is a fifty-five-year-old single woman whose chief complaint is that she is feeling very nervous and very agitated, and that she wants to be admitted to the hospital.

Present illness: This patient has been gradually becoming more agitated in the past two weeks. Over the weekend, she started to complain about hallucinating and was at the Mount Zion Crisis Clinic on two separate occasions requesting to be hospitalized. Today she called me from her home and repeated the request. I saw her briefly at the board-and-care home, and I agreed that her symptoms might best be controlled within a hospital setting. Upon being interviewed at the board-and-care home, she appeared oriented to time, place, and person. She did not appear to be depressed, and she denied suicidal intent; however, she did appear to be extremely agitated. She spoke with a great deal of pressure, and she appeared to be preoccupied with hallucinated experiences.

Past illness: This patient has a long-standing history of mental illness, starting at the age of sixteen and a half. About this time, she quit school and remained at home. She says that she spent most of six months in a corner of her kitchen, sitting in a straight chair. During this time she closed all the windows, put towels in the cracks of the doors, turned on all the gas jets, and put her head in the oven. Following this, she was sent to Napa State Hospital, where she remained for seventeen years. During this time she received many shock treatments, probably in excess of 100. I have been following her since 1969. She has required multiple hospitalizations during this interval, but only for fairly brief periods of time. Generally her hallucinations are controlled with medications, although usually it is necessary to use combinations to control them. However, episodically she appears to go out of control, and in these circumstances it is necessary to change her medications and sometimes to hospitalize her during this period of change. Consequently, I am recommending that she be hospitalized so that we can obtain a greater degree of control over her psychosis. She is consenting to come to the hospital as a voluntary patient.

A review of this patient's medication history revealed that since 1969 she had been on multiple medications including chlorpromazine, thioridazine, mesoridazine, trifluoperazine, fluphenazine, thiothixene, haloperidol, molindone, loxapine, and acetophenazine, singly or in combination, with only borderline and transient periods of remission. Not until acetophenazine was combined with loxapine did the patient manifest a sustained recovery, although she had some difficulties after Tindal was withdrawn from the market. This occurred in 1981, before the advent of the newer generation of atypical antipsychotics, and the patient has remained stable ever since.

At the time when I first quoted this case in the literature many years ago, life was somewhat more difficult for psychopharmacologists than it is today.[4] This is because although there were many drug options, there were no outstanding options. Thus at that time we were limited to the antipsychotics within five major antipsychotic drug categories (phenothiazines, thioxanthines, butyrophenones, dibenzoxepines, and dihydroindolones) but today, with the advent of the atypical (or novel) antipsychotics, we have more therapeutic options with less side effects and greater therapeutic efficacy.

This case also illustrates the principle that it is important to classify a patient's response to ongoing medication and to have this information available at one's fingertips. In real life, medication decisions are usually made hastily and standing on one foot. For this reason it is important to maintain drug doses and responses in a separate log, not to have them interspersed with general progress notes. By so doing one can more quickly arrive at optimal medications, optimal doses, and even optimal combinations.

Some authorities assert that the concurrent use of two or more antipsychotic medications necessarily constitutes "irrational polypharmacy."[5] The routine application of this parsimonious one-man, one-drug philosophy can only lead to grief in the long run. By grief I mean suboptimal outcomes. Indeed it may be irrational, but what if it works? There are many instances in the history of medicine when an apparently irrational treatment has worked better than any other previously constructed approach based on rationality. This can occur for unknown reasons, but when it does occur the reasons underlying the effectiveness of an apparently irrational approach is generally worked out later, after the fact. Such fortuitous events are not unheard of in medicine. The process is called serendipity.

It is generally acknowledged that some patients are refractory to all known antipsychotic agents. Under such circumstances, it is not unusual for psychiatrists to use more than one antipsychotic agent, although the authors of the just-referenced article cite the use of "several antipsychotics at the same time" as an example of "irrational polypharmacy." Moreover, this allegation of irrational polypharmacy as dependent on the number of drugs being used is simplistic bean-counting. A single broad-spectrum drug interacting with a large number of different types of receptor sites may actually be more "polypharmaceutical" than the simultaneous use of two or more drugs that have a narrower receptor focus.

Psychopharmacology is not an exact science. Psychiatrists and other physicians vote with their feet. They will walk toward whatever combination works. They will walk away from whatever regimen does not work. Therefore, it is not surprising that polypharmacy is widely employed domestically and also on a worldwide basis. Thus, in a recent study in Austria it was reported that 47 percent of patients received two antipsychotic medications and 8 percent received three antipsychotic medications.[6] A study from Japan documented even

higher rates of polypharmacy with more than 90 percent of schizo-
phrenic inpatients receiving two or more antipsychotic medications.[7]
The prevalence of polypharmacy has also been documented in the
United States.[8]

To make matters even more complicated, polypharmacy is not only
used to treat psychiatric illnesses but is also used in the therapies of
cancer, hypertension, tuberculosis, congestive heart failure, seizure
disorders, and a host of other illnesses. Polypharmacy has been round-
ly condemned by some academicians in the past because the utility of
using two or more antipsychotic agents in the same patient has never
been proven experimentally. It has never been disproved either. It will
never be proved or disproved in an experimental design in which the
responses of a control group are compared to the responses of an experimental group.

The reason for this is that there are currently twelve conventional
antipsychotic agents in use in the United States. These are haloperidol (brand name Haldol), molindone (brand name Moban),
loxapine (brand name Loxitane), pimozide (brand name Orap), chlorpromazine (brand name Thorazine), fluphenazine (brand name Prolixin), perphenazine (brand name Trilafon), trifluophenazine (brand name
Stelazine), acetophenazine (brand name Tindal), mesoridazine (brand
name Serentil), thioridazine (brand name Mellaril), and thiothixene
(brand name Navane). These drugs are the conventional or typical
antipsychotics. In addition to these drugs, an additional six newly
minted antipsychotic medications are available sometimes designated as "atypical" or "new generation" or "second generation." The
emerging consensus seems to be in favor of using the term "second
generation antipsychotics" using the acronym SGA, and designating
the conventional antipsychotics as "first generation antipsychotics"
using yet another acronym (FGA). However in this book I will use
any three of these terms to describe the new generation antipsychotics depending on my mood, since all three terms are in current usage. Also, I will scrupulously avoid the use of additional acronyms. In addition, I shall adhere to convention and call conventional
antipsychotics conventional. The six new drugs new drugs are clozapine (brand name Clozaril), olanzepine (brand name Zyprexa),
risperidone (brand name Risperdal), quetiapine (brand name Seroquel), ziprasidone (brand name Geodon), and aripiprazole (brand
name Abilify).

In this book I shall generally use generic names to identify the new generation antipsychotics, but will usually refer to conventional antipsychotics by their brand names, because the conventional antipsychotics have been in use for a long time and as such are generally referred to by their brand names. Thus Thorazine has become the lingua franca for chlorpromazine. Also generic names can be somewhat clumsy and misleading. Thus, fluphenazine (Prolixin) can easily be confused with trifluopherazine (Stelazine). Use of the brand names avoids this sense of confusion. Also brand names are frequently used in the progress notes, and when I quote from my progress notes as they are written I prefer the verbatim translation.

The other abbreviations in progress notes that might not be obvious to the nonmedical reader are BID standing for twice a day, TID standing for three times a day, and HS standing for meds to be administered at bedtime. In medicalese shorthand, DC stands for discontinue.

Following is an example of how entries on a psychopharmacological log (accompanied by brief descriptive notes) helped to obtain an optimal therapeutic combination on a patient who might otherwise have not responded:

8-3-89 Admitted to house

    Current meds: Navane 20 mg. 2 tabs TID
    Cogentin 2mg BID

6-25-92 Increasing confusion

    Increasing hallucinations
    Switch to Haldol Dec. 50 mg
    DC Navane

7-23-92 Pt. better for 1 wk. after Haldol Dec.

    Increase Haldol Dec. to 100 mg q. 2 wks.

12-16-97 Pt. yelling, up at night

    Augment with Mellaril 100 mg HS

11-24-99 DC Mellaril (recent boxed FDA warning re: QTc problems)

12-08-99 Pt states he feels "crazy" without Mellaril therefore restart Mellaril. Obtain EKG

1-8-00 QTc interval on EKG = 390 msec. OK to continue

The patient has since made an optimal adjustment on a combination of Haldol Dec. and Mellaril. The previous example is a bare-bones summary of all the entries made on the psychopharmacological log. Also during this interval unsuccessful attempts were made to use atypical antipsychotic meds to control his symptoms, which I have omitted from this recitation in the interests of brevity. Also let me emphasize that these psychopharmacological entries are meant to supplement progress notes, not to replace them. Progress note problems will be discussed in Chapter 14.

The problems grow in geometric progression when one is treating multiple patients rather than an individual patient. In the previous case it would not have been possible to arrive at a therapeutically effective (albeit exotic) combination of medications without a systematic way to eliminate past drug failures.

With this in mind there is a special place in my office chart where I note each medication in shorthand notation and in a small script. When a medication is discontinued because of side effects, this is similarly noted. The net effect of this is that the response to medication over a period of many years is compacted into a single psychopharmacological diary that can be quickly reviewed, thus facilitating future decisions about medication changes. When such a history is available, the physician will avoid the inadvertently repetitious administration of medication found to be ineffective in the past.

The advent of the new generation antipsychotic drugs has only added to the importance of keeping an updated, easily accessible, segregated psychopharmacological file in which responses to medications can quickly be accessed and evaluated. The reason for this is that the new drugs are not "me too" drugs. Each of the new drugs has a different receptor-blocking profile, and response or lack of response to one drug cannot be inferred as predicting the response to another drug.

The new generation antipsychotics entered the market in seriatim fashion after the FDA approval of clozapine in 1989. Clozapine is now produced by several manufacturers, although the remaining five new generation antpsychotics are still under drug patents in 2003— these being risperidone (manufactured as Risperdal by Janssen and FDA approved in 1993), olanzepine (manufactured as Zyprexa by Lilly and FDA approved in 1996), quetiapine (manufactured as Seroquel by AstraZeneca and FDA approved in 1997), ziprasidone (manufactured as Geodon by Pfizer and FDA approved in 2001), and most recently aripiprazole (manufactured as Abilify by Bristol-Myers Squibb and FDA approved in 2002).

The new drugs represent an advance in the treatment of schizophrenic psychoses and probably other psychotic disorders in that they generally cause fewer side effects than conventional antipsychotics and are generally more efficacious in controlling symptoms—although there may be individual exceptions as I shall describe later in this book. This is a huge market involving billions of dollars, and there is a literal marketing frenzy among the major players—meaning the rich and powerful drug companies just listed—to prove which drug is the best. All of the aforementioned pharmaceutical companies have sponsored expensive scientific studies to prove that their products are the best. This does not necessarily make life easier for the prescribing psychiatrist.

Drug marketing strategies involve presentations to physicians' offices by drug company representatives, sponsoring of lectures at dinner meetings, placements of elaborate ads in medical journals, television ads pitched to consumers, and gifts to physicians—sometimes inconsequential items such as calendars and pens, sometimes not-so-inconsequential, such as covering travel expenses to distant locations for the purpose of attending educational meetings. I condemn this in the abstract, although as an individual I love it. This is a little like being courted, and since I am seventy-five nobody else seems interested in me. In terms of the results of such marketing, I doubt that it affects my objectivity. No amount of seduction will induce me to prescribe a drug that is ineffective, and I think I speak for most physicians when I say this. In truth, there does not appear to be one drug that is best for everybody—but there is a best drug for individuals which may be any of the atypical antipsychotics—which again emphasizes the importance of meticulous record keeping. Also, some individuals respond better to conventional antipsychotics.

Did I say there was a special place for pharmacological notations in my chart? Not exactly true. There is a special place on my charts: on the outside of the manila folder, to be precise. This enables me to scrutinize years of medication orders without opening the chart in much the same way that terrain can be viewed from a helicopter. One doesn't have to traverse the trails in order to understand the topography. In complicated cases with many changes, the front cover can be completely occupied with these notes. I then insert the old folder into a new folder, staple the two together from the back covers, after which I am able to open the folder like the leaves of a book, but with the spine on the bottom rather than to the left.

Although these are office charts in the sense that they are kept in the office, I do take them with me to the residential care facilities when I make visits, because the information they contain facilitates on-site medication decisions immeasurably. However, they are office charts and when not accompanying me on my visits, they reside in the office. It is important to have this information available in the office, because patients do not necessarily restrict their exacerbations to the times that psychiatrists are actually on the premises of the residential care home. Residential care psychiatry is not a portal-portal enterprise in which the obligations of the psychiatrist begin and end coincident with his or her presence on the premises. Many crises and incipient exacerbations can be aborted through telephone contacts when the psychiatrist is in the office provided he or she has pertinent historical information at fingertip availability. Refusal to accept this as a fact of life in board-and-care psychiatry will simply result in an increased incidence of untoward events and hospitalizations.

VIII. Thou shalt segregate laboratory test reports into separate folders for each residential care home.

There was a time when I could not distinguish a granulocyte from a granola bar. There was a time when I thought a "shift to the left" represented nothing more than a political preference. I now have mended my ways. I now know that this "shift to the left" in the hematological sense describes a significant number of early neutrophilic precursors as compared with segmented neutrophils. I no longer have a problem with granola bars.

All of this is by way of introducing the concept of those carefree days of yesteryear when psychiatrists could frolic in the sunshine of their practices with nary a thought of serum chemistries. Those days are over. Psychiatrists are now big-time laboratory players. Adequate psychiatric pharmacotherapy now mandates many different kinds of laboratory tests. Thus psychiatrists now find themselves frequently ordering liver panels, thyroid tests, electrolytes, EKGs, weekly or bi-weekly hemograms (for patients on clozapine), and serum determinations for lithium, carbamazepine, or valproic acid, as well as various other tests once thought to be irrelevant to the practice of psychiatry. I am now on a first-name basis with many of my phlebotamists and while it would be an exaggeration to say that we are pen pals, it is not an exaggeration to say that we are fax pals.

When laboratory tests are ordered, laboratory results are received. These cannot be thrown into a wastebasket. They must be read and assimilated into one's fund of knowledge. It is also advisable to memorialize many laboratory tests in progress notes. In standard office practice it is customary to place these laboratory test results directly into the patient's charts.

In residential care facility practice this is a rather pedestrian method. When this is done psychiatrists find that they spend an inordinate amount of time leafing through progress notes to get at relevant laboratory tests. Also an impressive amount of intervening notes might well obscure trends in serum values that can only be detected through serial determinations. These can be very important, such as a gradual diminution in the white blood count with clozapine therapy, or a gradual increase in serum lithium values with lithium therapy.

My experience in residential care facilities suggests there is a better way to do this bookkeeping. A more efficient method is to create a separate laboratory folder for each residential care home. Thus all laboratory results for the residents of the Hilton Residential Care Facility would then be placed in the folder titled Hilton Residential Care Facility Laboratory Results. It is important that one keep them in chronological order, which is easy enough to do. This might be considered a cross-sectional approach rather than a longitudinal method in which each laboratory finding is posted in the patient's individual charts. Then prior to the visit to the residential care home, it is an easy matter to review the laboratory findings for all the patients in the facility for any significant values or trends. This is not to say that one should wait until just before a visit to make this review. Laboratory findings should be reviewed upon receipt, but trends are more evident when values can be compared with previous values if the lab tests are unobscured by intervening progress notes.

I then schlep this folder along with my other office charts to the residential care home, where I can then combine lab results, clinical impressions, and caretaker information for the purpose of creating a meaningful progress note. After I devised my special laboratory folder, I found it essential that it accompany me on all my residential care home peregrinations. By performing the operation of inserting a lab value report into its very own house lab folder (instead of a patient's folder), I was better able to remember its values.

The utility of this system can be inferred from the following progress note entered by me on March 6, 2001.

A sixty-one-year-old chronic schizoaffective woman who I have been following at the Waldorf Residential Care Facility since 1995. Her current meds are

> Lithium 300mg daily
> Olanzepine 10 mg daily
> Carbamazepine 200 mg daily
> Clonazepam 1 m. daily

Pt. has a long history of hospitalizations described in the note of 10-10-00 dating back over a period of thirty years. However, she is much improved on this combo even though the dosages are low. Her serum lithium on 2-22-01 was only 0.3 meq./L but I know from past experiences that if she does not get lithium she gets maniclike episodes. However, if she gets a conventional lithium dose yielding a conventional therapeutic serum level, she tends to get a severe and disabling tremor.

It is unusual that a patient would react this way, but usually it is the unusual that causes grief in psychopharmacology. It is true that most psychiatrists would have been able to make this connection, but the previously described charting system enabled me to do it quickly and with a minimum of paper shuffling. The fact is that more can be accomplished in two minutes of focused attention to an organized psychopharmacological log than in twenty minutes of frantic paper shuffling through unorganized progress notes.

So there you have it. For generations physicians have been placing laboratory results in the charts of individual patients. By not insisting that a patient's laboratory test results be placed in the patient's very own chart, I have challenged one of the hallowed traditions in medicine, maybe even the hallowedest, if that's a word. Was it not Dr. Semelweiss who contested one of the equally hallowed traditions of the physicians of his time—that you are not supposed to wash your hands in the assistance of childbirth? It is gratifying to know that in the twenty-first century there is still room for iconoclasts.

IX. Thou shalt practice psychoperambulation when indicated.

In addition to the previous commandments the ideal residential care facility psychiatrist should practice something more than psychopharmacology. Do I mean psychotherapy? I do indeed, but there is something more than psychotherapy or psychopharmacology. What I mean is psychonetworking and psychoperambulation. No one word with a psycho prefix indicates this. Psychonetworking involves the facilitation of communication with anyone who is involved in patient care—administrators, social workers, pharmacists, and other caregivers such as cooks and housekeepers. I have already described psychonetworking as part of Commandments IV and V.

Perambulation is defined in *Webster's* dictionary as the act of perambulating. *Perambulate* is defined as "to walk through or around as to inspect." Psychoperambulation is not defined in the dictionary because it is a neologistic formulation, but essentially it means to walk through or around as to inspect in a psychological way. Perhaps I should say in a psychiatric way.

Psychoperambulation is a form of psychowalkingaround. But psychoperambulation is not just any walking around, but walking around in a residential care facility in a casual way, noticing what goes on. While noticing what goes on, you are also making yourself available in an informal way to patients who might want to approach you while you are not busily preoccupied as a scribe in order to accommodate Medicare progress note requirements. The ever-present obligation to produce the written word compels me to use the term *psychoperambulation* rather than *psychowalkingaround*. Psychoperambulation sounds more professionally impressive and therefore may be a potentially compensable procedure.

Psychowalkingaround or psychoperambulation is the best time to engage the invisible patient—the patient who will not come to the psychiatric workplace to be evaluated. Some individuals get lost in the shuffle and are rarely noticed until they are found hanging from the ceiling. At that point the psychiatrist is also noticed as are his or her progress notes or the absence thereof. Absence sometimes makes the heart grow fonder, but this is not true in the case of the absent progress note. An absent progress note may be interpreted as an indication of an absent psychiatrist. Some of us, given to disputation, might aver that an absent psychiatrist is a negligent psychiatrist. In that event, absence may need to be explained and may even be the subject of litigation. Thus absence may not make the heart grow fonder, but it could make the heart beat faster.

When dealing with the withdrawn isolated room-bound patient, it is well to remember the wise parables of other cultures. Thus, if the mountain won't come to Mohammed, Mohammed must go to the mountain. In this case the mountain is the patient's room and the psychiatrist is Mohammed—even if he or she is an atheist. While the psychiatrist is in the room he or she should notice how the room is kept. Is it messy? Is clothing piled on the floor? Are there irrational notes posted on the wall? Are there cigarette ashes strewn about?

Psychoperambulation is, in a sense, looking for work and, in another sense, puts the psychiatrist in touch with his or her patients as constituents rather than patients. Sometimes much can be learned as a consequence of this change of roles, such as consumer-type complaints: Is the food quality poor? Is the room too cold? Psychoperambulation sometimes invites gossipy observations by patients about other patients and such gossipy observations sometimes have psychiatric utility, such as when a patient notices that another patient has stopped eating and this has escaped the notice of the administrator, or when a number of patients state that they are afraid of a newly admitted patient and relay information that was not previously available from the papers that accompanied the patient. This can happen because harassed discharge workers are sometimes under pressure to facilitate community placements of long-term hospital patients because certifications for continued hospitalizations are denied. Under such circumstances important information can sometimes be omitted or attenuated so as to facilitate placement. This psychowalkingaround type of information might not ordinarily be transmitted by the patient in formal sessions where the focus is on the patient expressing his or her problems, rather than on problems encountered by or created by other residents.

Psychoperambulation and psychonetworking are two reasons why it is difficult to assess time limits on residential care facility services. Medicare does acknowledge the concept of billing for "floor time" when the psychiatrist is working in the hospital setting. Floor time is time spent on patient care but not in face-to-face encounters with the patient, such as time spent on charting, on working with the nursing staff, or ordering or interpreting lab tests. The concept of floor time as previously explained does not exist in residential care facilities. The concept of floor time is also not applicable to psychiatrists' offices. This is understandable since average office psychiatrists will be spending practically all of their billable time in face-to-face encounters with their patients. Residential care psychiatrists, however, will find that much of their office time will be consumed taking care of patients who are not in their presence. I will cite specific examples of this in Chapter 9.

X. Thou shalt involve patients in medication management decisions when indicated.

Here is an example of such a negotiation, but first a little autobiographical information to tell you where I am coming from—but not in the colloquial sense, because I hate colloquialisms, but in the literal sense. My father owned a secondhand clothing store in a run-down neighborhood in Los Angeles near skid row—near Third Street and Main, to be precise about it, where he would sell his goods to poor people who could not afford to pay retail prices. We were not exactly wealthy ourselves. The store was called Ben's Clothing Store, which pretty well says it all in terms of ownership and function. So, despite my undeniable eloquence in the use of the English language, I was not to-the-manor-born. Many of the patients—whoops—customers, were Spanish speaking and monolingual. My father was bilingual, but Spanish was not part of the bi. He was bilingual in English and Yiddish, a language that was rarely spoken by people in uniforms, a language that has never tasted the intoxicating elixir of power. Under such circumstances, a dialogue might have proceeded as follows:

CUSTOMER [in Spanish]: I would like to buy a shirt. [He then points to the shirts].

FATHER [in Yiddish]: Try this one on.

CUSTOMER [in Spanish]: I like it. How much is it?

[Father then writes a number down on a slip of paper using Arabic numerals.]

CUSTOMER [in Spanish]: Too much. [Writes another number down consenting to use Arabic numerals.]

FATHER [in Yiddish]: I would have to go out of business with that price. [Writes another number down.]

CUSTOMER [in Spanish]: It's too much. There is no button on the sleeve. [Comes up a little bit from his initial offering.]

FATHER [in Yiddish]: I don't charge for the missing buttons. [Comes down a little from the initial offering price.]

CUSTOMER [in Spanish]: It is still too much. The collar is bad. It's frayed. [Comes up a little more.]

FATHER [in Yiddish]: Okay, I'll lower the price a little more.

CUSTOMER [in Spanish]: Okay, it's a deal.

The Yiddish version of "okay" is very similar to the English and Spanish renditions so they would understand each other. Then they would shake on it. Everyone would smile and be happy. So there you are—negotiations carried on in Yiddish and Spanish using Arabic numerals which were originally invented by the Indians—not the American Indians, the Indian Indians. Globalization as it was practiced sixty years ago.

End of nostalgic story which, unaccountably, brought tears to my eyes when I wrote it. Perhaps it's not so unaccountable. Maybe I reacted that way because my father endured a hard life so that I could have an easy life and I never had a chance to thank the man, except that I will do it now: "Thanks, Dad. I know it's a little late to say it, but thanks anyway. I could never tell you that while you were alive because I was always too busy. Thanks for giving me a good life." I have to go now, typographically speaking, because I hate to see a grown man cry, even if it's me looking at my image in the mirror of life—especially if it's me. I will tell you something else. A lot of us had fathers like that. A lot of us were "too busy."

The interactive merchant-customer episode just described is an example of why this book, which is essentially a how-to-do-it manual, is necessarily autobiographical. Since I am describing how to interact with patients as well as caregivers—in a sense, how to win friends and influence patients—I cannot do so effectively without describing my own life experiences: how I became the kind of person that I became. Here is how this father-customer scenario plays out in the doctor-patient setting.

Actually, what my father called bargaining I call psychopharmacological negotiations. My interactions with patients are pretty similar to my father's mercantile transactions with customers, but with the following minor changes in dialogue, only he didn't need twelve years of an intensive education to prepare him for his role. In the following script the patient plays the role of the customer and I play the role of me:

PATIENT: It's too much [Addressing dosages rather than dollars].

ME: You would have to go into the hospital with that dose [Instead of father's "I would have to go out of business with that price"].

PATIENT: It's too much. My hands are shaking so much I cannot button my sleeve [Instead of customer's, "It's too much. There is no button on the sleeve"].

ME: Okay, I'll lower the dose a little more [Instead of father's "Okay, I'll lower the price a little more"].

PATIENT: My color is bad. I'm afraid. [Instead of customer's, "The collar is bad. It looks frayed].

ME: Okay, I'll lower the dose a little more [Instead of father's "Okay, I'll lower the price a little more"].

PATIENT: Okay, it's a deal [Instead of customer's, "Okay, it's a deal"].

The main difference in the two transactions is that I generally do not shake hands with the patient when the deal is consummated—although that's probably not a bad idea. The next time it appears appropriate, I will attempt to do so. Much can be learned from a handshake, as I have briefly described in Chapter 5 and will explain more fully in Chapter 15. Also another difference is that in my negotiations with monolingual Spanish-speaking patients, I generally have a Hispanic social worker present to provide me with some assistance. Sometimes monolingualism has its advantages. This whole business is somewhat similar to the transactions on priceline.com but without the intervening cyberspace.

I realize that the principle of allowing some patient involvement in psychiatric pharmacotherapy may raise some psychiatric hackles, but it is not as unreasonable as it first appears. Let me first explain that I am not someone who strives for political correctness and I do not believe that democracy is applicable in every context. However, in looking at this principle do not forget the two little words "when indicated." Obviously there will be many instances involving many patients where involvement is not indicated. However, in some cases it is the preferred option because it can enhance patient cooperation. I use the word *cooperation* rather than *compliance,* because compliance suggests that the patient is taking medications as directed and little else. I want more than that. I want cooperation in the sense that the patients will level with me regarding their true feelings, even if they want to conceal them from other people.

In fact *compliance* and *noncompliance* as words and as concepts are in danger of being nuanced out of business in medicine. I think this is true because the concept of noncompliance suggests violating the provisions of powerful penalty-levying federal organizations with acrimonious acronyms such as OSHA or IRS. It has been estimated that at least half of all schizophrenic patients do not comply with treatment.[9] This ratio appears to hold true for the treatment of other chronic diseases such as seizure disorders, diabetes, hypertension, and asthma.[10] Some have suggested that *adherence* and *nonadherence* should replace *compliance* and *noncompliance.* I don't like *adherence* because it has a kind of sticky quality associated with Band-Aids or Elmer's Glue, but this is undoubtedly an idiosyncratic reaction. Others have suggested that *compliance* be replaced by *concordance,* the reason being that *compliance* suggests that the patient passively obey the advice of the doctor. I don't like the word *concordance* either. It sounds too supersonic. Still others don't like the word *patient* and prefer the word *client.* Someday we might be talking about *client concordance* rather than *patient compliance.* If this will come to pass, you heard it here first. This chapter addresses the problem of patients as customers, clients, and/or consumers.

The advantage of making repeated visits to the patient's place of residence allows the psychiatrist certain freedoms—even the freedom to make mistakes, because these mistakes can be corrected in subsequent visits. This is not necessarily true in office practices or clinic practices in which inadequate or misguided dosages may simply lead to the patient not keeping future appointments. (I shall describe more fully the advantages of residential care facility visits in Chapter 10). Follow-up visits can be made even if the patient-therapist relationship deteriorates and the patient would not wish a follow-up visit. This creates the freedom to engage in psychopharmacological negotiations with patients regarding medications and dosages that might not exist in other places of service.

In brief, the residential care facility psychiatrist should think of himself or herself as working as a ship's doctor on a nonluxury cruise ship interacting with both passengers and staff to make the voyage as pleasant as possible. The voyage is the voyage of life because most of the passengers will be there for life. On-site visits are preferable because on a cruise ship one doesn't have other viable options.

So there you are, the Ten Commandments of Residential Care Facility Psychiatry that have served me well in my career as a residential care facility psychiatrist. At one time I thought of publishing them and marketing them as the basis of a rating scale called the Fleishman Rating Scale for the Purpose of Evaluating Psychiatric Services to Residents of Residential Care Facilities. I intended to publish it under the acronym of FRSPEPSRRCF. Psychiatrists could then rate compliance with each of the commandments on a one-to-five scale. The publisher refused to publish it unless I could find an acronym that rhymed with PANSS (acronym for Positive and Negative Symptoms Scale, this being the standard clinical rating scale used in most clinical trials). However, I was unable to do this because of a shortage of creativity, so it never developed into something worth bragging about.

When all is said and done, the bottom line is, do these techniques enhance the physician-patient relationship, or are these techniques simply gimmicks that have no real use in residential care facility psychiatry? Who can say? Perhaps I can say. My answer is that in my prolonged history of visiting patients in residential care facilities, I can think of only two instances in which I was fired because a patient demanded individual psychotherapy sessions. Perhaps I suffer from selective amnesia and there are more patients who opted out, but there really weren't very many. In the rare instances when patients have requested other psychiatrists, I encourage them to make the contact. I assure them that my feelings are not hurt. That being the case, many patients prefer to see me in my office after they leave the residential care facility, and I generally accommodate them. When I see them in my office I may code for medication management or psychotherapy, depending on how much time we spend together. One code blends into the other quite imperceptibly, and patients do not generally know whether I am doing psychotherapy or medication management, and it's none of their business. Frankly, there are lots of times when I don't know either.

The Ten Commandments of Residential Care Facility Psychiatry are not exactly Koch's postulates, but I will call them Fleishman's postulates. I do this not for any egocentric reasons, but because ever since I was a child I have always craved an eponymic set of principles immortalizing my father's name. After all, he was the one who pioneered in the use of one of those principles, and this is my only chance to have him achieve the recognition he richly deserves.

Chapter 9

The Problems of Frequency and Duration

How often should visits be made? The literature is quite sparse about this point and obviously much depends on the status of the patient. It is easy to misinterpret the status of the patient if a long time has elapsed between visits. Sometimes patients who need attention are the very same patients who avoid attention. In an earlier chapter I stated that sometimes the most important part of a residential care facility visit is represented by the patient who is not there—that is, the patient who does not show up in the office or dining room but stays in his or her room and continues to withdraw and exacerbate. Under such circumstances the psychiatrist would do well to furnish room service by knocking at the patient's door, somewhat aggressively if necessary, and intrude himself or herself into the patient's private world. I suppose the question can be raised whether such patients should be followed at all, or with what frequency. Patients have to be followed even when not much is happening. If they are not followed and something happens (as it usually does when someone is not followed), then lawyers or relatives might ask embarrassing questions, such as when was the last time the psychiatrist visited the patient.

VISITATION FREQUENCY IN RELATION TO THE UNPREDICTABILITY OF ADVERSE EVENTS

In this respect two incidents come to mind. Many years ago I saw a patient at a Mission neighborhood residential care home. He seemed fine and I could not detect any recent significant psychiatric changes. Shortly after I saw him he jumped out of a third-story window into a garden. As it so happened a severe rainstorm had occurred the night before which transformed the garden into a muddy swamp. The patient left foot-deep indentations in the mud for both elbows and both knees but otherwise was none the worse for wear. Later that day I received an angry phone call from his brother—whom I had never spoken to before despite the fact that I had been treating the patient for years. He demanded to know when I had last seen the patient. I told him about fifteen minutes before he jumped. I never heard from him again, although I believe that if I did not make routine visits to the residential care facility or if the visits were very infrequent, I would have heard a lot more from him or his lawyer. I suspect there is a certain category of relative who sits around waiting for an adverse event and when it happens this relative springs into action. I have this image of a panther patiently watching its prey from the treetops and going for the jugular at the opportune moment. No jugular for this relative.

The other incident did not end so happily and involved a successful suicide attempt by a fairly young patient. At some time in the past the mother visited me and asked me how frequently I intended to visit her son. I said about every two weeks. She said, "If you visit him every two weeks, what will you do for him?" I said that seemed like a fair question and the purpose of my visits was to get to know him and follow him as necessary. She seemed satisfied with that, and never raised any question that I was neglecting her son despite the unhappy ending. I think if my visits were infrequent or only focused on crises, she might have questioned my actions or the lack of my actions. The fact is that the patient's suicide was entirely unexpected. No outward signs of crisis were evident from my progress notes which had been recently entered and which indicated no unusual changes in this patient's behavior.

So the lesson in this is that periodic visits at a certain frequency may seem unnecessary when there is no trouble. However when trouble occurs, people—meaning relatives and lawyers, among others—will ask why routine visits were not made prior to the trouble. The problem with trouble is that it cannot always be anticipated. So there should be no question that periodic visits should be made even when nothing much is happening. But how often should these visits be made? This is important because there is a Medicare penalty for rendering unnecessary services. That may be as high as $10,000 per occurrence. If there are many occurrences, as might well be the case in a residential care facility where multiple patients are seen, then the penalty may be as high as $10,000 times that many occurrences. This may be hard to believe but that penalty was specified in a law passed by Congress, as I have described in Chapter 8.

Just as there is a penalty for rendering services that are medically unnecessary, there is also a penalty for not rendering services that may be regarded as having been medically necessary after a retrospective investigation of medical necessity. This penalty—which can amount to millions of dollars—is not determined by Congress but by lawyers—malpractice lawyers. The fact is that there is not a universally accepted rule regarding an optimal frequency of visits to residential care facilities. Much depends on the size of the home, the kinds of patients in the home, and the kinds of medications being used.

Obviously, the larger the home, the greater the necessity for an increased frequency of routine visits—either weekly or every two weeks. An increased frequency of visits is also obviously necessitated where there is a disproportionate number of severely mentally ill or poorly controlled patients. What may not be obvious is that the issue of visitation frequency is also dictated by the kinds of medication the patient is receiving. Increased visitation frequency is advisable when the medications being used have the capacity to induce a toxic reaction even when therapeutic levels are only slightly exceeded.

The following case is an example of this:

I had been following a sixty-two-year-old Caucasian woman for years in a residential care facility where most of the residents were geriatric patients. The patient had a history of multiple hospitalizations with multiple bizarre delusions and agitation. A previous admission history described her as "frightened, delusional, and tangential with fears of being punished by Satan who wanted to control her and that her hair and skin was about to fall off."

I had been taking care of her for about twenty years and her current medications were olanzepine 7.5 mg two tabs HS, lithium 300 mg three tabs HS, haloperidol 10 mg one tab twice daily, and diphenhydramine 50 mg one tab twice daily.

She did marginally well on this regimen, although she still continued to be delusional. However her agitation and hyperactivity were somewhat controlled to the extent that it allowed her to continue to reside in a community facility. During one of my biweekly visits to the home, I noted the presence of dysarthria and a moderately coarse tremor accompanied by upper extremity rigidity. I suspected emergence of lithium toxicity even though the patient had been on the same lithium dose for years and previous serum lithium levels were always within the normal range. None of her other medications had been recently changed. The patient was then referred to an emergency room where her serum lithium was determined to be 3.5 mmol/L. This is described in the texts as "severe toxicity" and can result in seizures, coma, and even death. However, in two days the patient's lithium level had normalized and she did not manifest any severe symptoms or residual effects. What had happened?

A review of her Medi-set box revealed that there had been a mistake in the dispensing of her medications which was recently taken over by a new pharmacy. Human error will always be with us as long as there are humans. Instead of receiving her lithium as three tablets at bedtime, she was receiving it as three tablets per bedtime plus three times a day. Since Medi-set boxes contain only a one-week supply of medications and since she was only halfway through the box, the overdoses were limited to a four-day period. This explains why there was such a rapid reduction in serum lithium levels after the very high serum level on admission. Had the overdoses continued for a longer period of time, there would have been a prolongation of high serum levels with possible irreversible neurological sequelae.

This case illustrates the importance of an appropriate frequency of visits. It is true that lithium is monitored through the application of periodic serum lithium determinations, preferably every two to three months, but this routine would not have uncovered the rapid rise in serum lithium that occurred following the brief period of overdosage. The lesson is that although it is necessary to monitor serum lithium levels it is also necessary to monitor patients. Every two or three months is sufficient for monitoring serum lithium levels, but insufficient for monitoring patients. I had been visiting this primarily geriatric home every two weeks for many years, and not much was happening, so I was thinking of decreasing my visitation frequency to once every three weeks—possibly only monthly, and spend some extra time in Hawaii. This incident, which occurred during the writing of this book, has made me think twice about such fantasies. My vacations will have to wait.

My own experience is that once every two weeks is generally adequate in nongeriatric non-DD (developmentally disabled) homes with active schizophrenics who are either young or middle aged. However for very large homes weekly visits might be necessary because many unanticipated events can happen in a large home. This doesn't mean that one sees the same patients every week. It means that new problems can arise on a weekly basis. For other types of homes, I would think that monthly visits would be sufficient. I know that at times in the past I have visited homes for the developmentally disabled every two weeks and abandoned doing this because I felt I was not doing any work. However, it is quite possible that when the focus is on psychotherapy or behavior therapy rather than psychiatric pharmacotherapy, a two-week interval might be justifiable.

THE STANDARD OF CARE IN THE COMMUNITY

So what can be said about optimum frequencies? One would think that the best estimates of appropriate frequency should be existent community standards. The problem is that not much is written about community standards addressing the question of visitation frequency to residential care facilities. In fact, not that much has been written about residential care facilities, much less about visitation frequencies.

Be that as it may, I think we should establish the expectation that routine visits at certain frequencies are to be expected. The reason for this is that it may be impossible to defend against the allegation of rendering a "medically unnecessary" service for any given visit if there is no obvious crisis situation. The medical necessity of visits is relatively easy to prove in the treatment of acute states or crisis situations, but difficult or impossible to prove in the treatment of chronic conditions. With respect to community standards, the previously quoted reference by VanPutten and Spar stated that the average schizophrenic board-and-care patient was visited by a psychiatrist 1.72 times per month.[1]

This reference goes back to 1979. Other references state that visits should be made at least on a monthly basis,[2] but all of these references predate the arrival of the new antipsychotic medications, the tendency of the newer generation of antipsychotics to complicate or contribute to the development of other chronic diseases, the tendency to release increasingly irrational and violent offenders into the community after only short hospitalizations, the new understandings with respect to the cytochrome P450 enzyme interactions, the increased reliance on lab studies, the use of medications with a narrow therapeutic window, and the increased prevalence of rational polypharmacy and complex algorithms[3] in the treatment of chronic mental illness.

Given all of these factors, what can be said regarding general rules addressing the appropriate frequency of visits? Since there is not much in the literature addressing the problem, I can only describe what has evolved from my own practice. I have found that in the early course of a relationship it is more important to follow a patient more frequently than might be true in the later phases of a relationship. This is understandable because in the course of time, the psychiatrist gains a greater degree of understanding of the patient and can be less vigilant without sacrificing quality of care.

As a general rule—and with the stipulation that general rules are not uniformly applicable in every instance—it is desirable to see the patients about once every two weeks early on and later shifting to about once a month in the well-stabilized patient. Thus, most of my patients are seen on a monthly basis, even in those large houses where weekly visits are advisable as a way of keeping abreast of the general problems of the house. I frequently see the patient without seeing him or her in the formal sense that generates third-party insurance compensation. One might say that under such circumstances I oversee patients without seeing them. I believe that by so doing I have decreased the incidence of rehospitalizations (something I cannot prove) and I have also decreased the incidence of nonhospital criminal incarcerations (something I can prove and will describe at length in Chapter 10). In that sense, besides providing good care I have saved the state lots of money. I shall return to the problem of economics in a separate chapter but I now wish to describe some of the Medicare service codes that are useful in the provision of services to the occupants of residential care facilities and which can be considered in the context of the prevailing standards of care.[4]

> 99331*: Domiciliary or rest home visit for the evaluation and management of an established patient, which requires at least two of these three key components:
> * A problem-focused interval history
> * A problem-focused examination
> * Medical decision making that is straightforward or of low complexity
>
> Counseling and/or coordination of care with other providers or agencies are provided consistent with the nature of the problem(s) and the patient's and/or family's needs. Usually the patient is stable, recovering, or improving.

Generally speaking two other Medicare service codes are commonly used for the pharmacological treatment of mentally ill patients. These codes are distinct from the aforementioned E&M codes because their usage is not dependent on the documentation of interval history, problem-focused examination, and medical decision making. These elements may be part of the service rendered, but they do not have to be documented. They are as follows:

M0064*: When the medical record indicates that a patient is stable from a psychopharmacologic point of view but still requires pharmacologic regimen oversight.

90862*: Pharmacological management including prescription, use, and review of medication with no more than minimal medical psychotherapy.

The difference between the two codes is that 90862 should involve an in-depth assessment because the drugs that are used are considered potent medications with serious side effects but should not be used to bill for a simple dosage adjustment of long-term medication. On the other hand, M0064 is to be used when the patient is stable but requires routine pharmacological oversight even though the drugs being evaluated are the same. Psychiatrists can also use psychotherapy codes when attending to occupants of residential care facilities. Briefly these are 90805, standing for a psychotherapy session of twenty to twenty-five minutes, and 90807, representing a psychotherapy session of forty-five to fifty minutes. I shall address the economic implications of these codes in the chapter focusing on economic problems (Chapter 24).

That is all I want to say now about the essentially boring subject of Medicare service codes except that it is possible for a subject to be boring and interesting at the same time. How is such an oxymoron possible? It is possible because Medicare service codes became interesting after passage of the Health Insurance Portability and Accountability Law of 1996 (HIPAA) which specified fines for "upcoding." If a physician uses a service code that pays more than the service code that should have been used, this violation is called "upcoding" by Medicare. Upcoding violations may result in a denial of payment, or in the imposition of penalties. Where the upcoding violations are systemic, the physician may face fraud charges. Such charges may be entertained if it is determined that the physician is acting in reckless disregard of the truth or falsity of the information conveyed or out of deliberate ignorance, even though there may be no specific intent to defraud. These legal problems will be more fully addressed in Chapter 12.

THE PROBLEM OF DURATION

How much time should be allocated for an on-site visit? The answer to that question is that it varies between minus ten seconds and infinity. Before I explain that answer, let me say that it is the answer to the wrong question. The question really should be "Should time values be assigned to on-site medication management visits?" I briefly discussed this issue in the chapter on how to do it, but will now use some examples from my own practice to illustrate a point. Time is intrinsic to psychotherapy—but not necessarily to psychopharmacology. In my opinion the psychopharmacologist who is well organized and keeps all the medication regimens and changes on a separate psychopharmacology med sheet, can work with much greater accuracy and speed than the physician who does not do this. The physician who does not have the assistance of a segregated medication sheet must then study all of his or her progress notes for a half hour or more to try to make sense out of all the medications changes which may be interspersed with other progress notes that may not be relevant.

Leafing through such notes is a bit like trying to determine the topography of a jungle by bushwhacking. It can be done but it is pathetically pedestrian and it generally involves turning many pages just as bushwhacking involves whacking many bushes. By the time one is finished turning pages or whacking bushes, the arms get tired and the mind becomes exhausted. The trees may be sighted but the sight of the forest is lost. Working from segregated medication notes is much easier on body and mind. When I do this I get the impression that I am looking down on psychopharmacological topography from a hovering helicopter. I know how to proceed because within minutes I can discern the crevasses of past dangerous reactions, and the barren terrain of previous ineffective drug strategies. Many times the five-minute medication management decision based on an organized chart, is much more effective than thirty minutes of frantic paper shuffling through a poorly organized chart. That is one reason why I am against Medicare imposing time parameters for medication management service codes.

THE EFFECTS OF OFF-SITE WORK ON ON-SITE VISITS

I find the quality of the work which I do on-site is dependent on the quality of the work that I do off-site. In my office I accumulate and review all the background information regarding the patient, as when I write to hospitals requesting old records. I review these in my office. I note which medications have been used in the past, which are effective, and which are ineffective. I also update the patient's current meds in my office chart and so get a more complete picture of the patient's reaction to medication. This time is not spent at the house yet this contributes to quality of care. Thus it may appear that I have spent only a short time with a patient in an on-site situation, but this does not represent the true time spent in patient care. That is another reason why I am against time parameters for medication management.

Thus in clocking a doctor, a time-and-study man (or woman) could say that the doctor spent only ten minutes per patient—instead of the recommended twenty minutes—while on the premises, and not have the slightest idea that additional work is involved, nor is there any reason why they should have a prior knowledge of this. I will cite an actual example of this by talking about one day in the life of Ivan Denisovich—I mean Martin Fleishman. In doing this I describe the actual events but have changed the names of the residential care facilities and the mental health workers. The patients will be referred to by initials, but the initials have been changed to prevent recognition. What follows is a verbatim reproduction of events recorded that day in real time, February 8, 1999, without any follow-up:

A TYPICAL DAY IN THE LIFE OF A RESIDENTIAL CARE FACILITY PSYCHIATRIST

On Monday morning, February 8, I spent two hours at the Argus Residential Care Facility seeing approximately twelve patients. Several medication changes had to be made. I called the pharmacist from the home, but the pharmacist who services residential care facilities was not scheduled to come to work until the afternoon. I know from personal experience that it was unwise to speak to the other pharmacists. Some lessons are learned only from experience and one of those lessons is that pharmacists generally do not make mistakes but in the rare instances when miscommunications occur it is usually with a substitute pharmacist. Consequently, all the calls were made from my office after I had left the premises and were as follows:

Pt. K. I.: This is really a fascinating situation. K. I. is a chronic schiz. African-American male whom I have taken care of in the past in other residential care facilities. On Friday, I had received a call from a day treatment staff person stating that pt. K. I. was actively hallucinating and had attempted to start two fires in the bathroom. They then instituted a 5150 commitment and had the patient transported to the county hospital. Apparently pt. was seen for approximately one-half hour (or so he reported to me later) and then sent on his merry way—back into the community, as they say, where he is the community's responsibility—meaning the responsibility of the residential care facility psychiatrist, meaning me. The administrator then called me on Friday asking me what to do. I decided the safest bet was to flood the patient with higher doses of Navane, increasing his dose from 30 mg to 60 mg. I knew it was safe to do this since in my office charts I have all of the old hospital records obtained by me by writing to the hospitals which I then review in the office—this is off-premises time not recorded by clockwatchers and not covered by proposed 90862 time guidelines. By reviewing the chart I could determine that the patient had received this dose in the past with good results.

When I saw the pt. on Mon. he had improved somewhat but his facial expression indicated that he was still excessively preoccupied. I could make this judgment in three seconds even without talking to him. How can I do this? Because I know him very well and have been following him for years. Also I generally kid around with this patient, and he is generally able to roll with the punch and smile and reciprocate. On this day he was neither smiling or reciprocating. If you know patients very well and have been following them for years and have documented case history information in your files, you generally don't need to spend twenty minutes evaluating the patient as is required by Medicare when one bills for a psychopharmacological evaluation—coded by Medicare as a 90862 service code. So what I did at that point was to start patient on risperidone and continued the Navane and the patient rapidly improved.

What can we say in general terms about this situation? I believe this sink-or-swim policy of hospitals wherein patients are dropped back willy-nilly into the community ocean is probably occurring nationwide and possibly accounts partially for the increased incidence of use and the perception of widespread abuse of 90862. In my opinion this is really the most useful code in the treatment of severely disturbed schizophrenics who may be too disorganized to profit from psychotherapy. I can understand private hospitals doing this—although I do not approve—since it is possible for a private hospital to go bankrupt because of certification problems, but I don't understand why the county hospital should do this. Perhaps they are under pressures which I am not aware of.

Pt. X. N.: This pt. is a schizoaffective schiz. with a history of severe alcoholism. He actually has been doing well in the past year and has controlled his drinking problem with only one setback in recent months. However, he is complaining now about being depressed. I would like to start him on citalopram because of its allegedly minimal interactive capabilities with other medications, but this is still nonformulary and Medi-Cal will not approve unless we have had some failures with formulary preparations so I will start him on Paxil and hope for the best.

Pt. C. M.: This pt is a chronic schiz. Asian woman who is only semi-coherent. Lately she has been shouting at dinnertime for unexplained reasons. She is on risperidone as 4 mg BID, and not currently on an anti-Parkinsonian agent. There are two routes to go here. Possibly switch to quetiapine starting low and gradually titrating up or supplementing with an anti-Parkinsonian agent because she may have some EPS secondary to this moderately high dose of risperidone and the shouting may occur as a result of inner restlessness or inner akathisia, which the patient is unable to verbalize because of her semi-coherent state, which may be partially attributable to language barrier and partially to mental illness.

Pt. S. M.: Pt. now having constipation problems. States he has BMs once every two weeks—possibly less. Pt has been on Prolixin decanoate injections, 75 mg every week. Okay, so why such a high dose? Because this patient has a history of irrational criminality and has been very well controlled with this pro. dec. dose without apparent adverse side effects except for this pesky constipation. When I say well controlled I am talking about acting out, no recent episodes of assault or rape, which have been problems in the past. However, when I do see him he is generally talking to his voices but responds appropriately when addressed as if he is at a cocktail party and now pays attention to what I am saying because I am close enough to bend his ear. And he is even capable of kidding around as when he calls himself a real *mishigginer*—which is Yiddish for crazy. So I have to think about stopping his Pro Dec. which I am reluctant to do because possibly thanks to Pro Dec. he is only a *mishigginer* instead of a rapist. Also when on Pro. Dec. he is forced to see me every week, and in his case there is a real psychotherapeutic aspect to this injectable interlude insofar as he seems to enjoy our encounters and respects what I have to say. But we can't continue this forever, especially when faced with the continued possibility of severe constipation or worse, such as obstipation secondary to paralytic ileus or megacolon, so I will bite the bullet and switch to olanzepine. However, I will provide the appropriate warnings to him and the administrator—that if he feels aggressiveness coming on he should let us know. Actually, I have come to trust him and vice versa, which is why I have been talking psychotherapy.

So these are the off-premises in-office calls made for patients at one residential care facility while I am not on the premises. One has to allow time for the calls, time to review the office charts, and time to think about the issues, and none of this time is observable to our hypothetical clockwatching whistleblowers at the residential care home. So much for off-premises work at Argus.

Well, not exactly. Actually there was still another call for an Argus patient after I left the facility. This one was from intern Mary Rogers at a private hospital. Regarding patient K. B., I didn't see K. B. at the Argus facility today because he is in the hospital so I cannot bill 90862 for him or use any other code, but that's not Dr. Rogers's problem, is it?

Pt. K. B. is at a community hospital for medical reasons, part of which involves an inability to walk. He is a chronic schizoaffective marginally stabilized with lithium, Navane, Artane, and Symmetrel. He is on two anti-Parkinsonian agents because of severe EPS which is not unusual in patients on both lithium and typical antipsychotics. Also possible problems with diabetes insipidus. Dr. Rogers is a nice lady, and very smart of her to call me, because now that pt. is in the hospital there are several things we could do that I was reluctant to do with this patient as an out-patient because of his marginal and at times semi-coherent status. In the first place this is a good time to get off lithium because of his possible diabetes insipidus problem and attempt stabilization with valproic acid. In the second place this is a good time to dump the typical antipsychotic and try for stabilization via an atypical—preferable quetiapine, because pt. has done poorly in the past with risperidone and olanzepine—as sometimes happens with manic patients, and also because I have had some good luck in the past treating this type of patient with quetiapine. In the third place after a few days we can try stopping the Artane. In the fourth place we can then try titrating down and stopping the Symmetrel. In the fifth place I invite her to call me back in a few days to tell me how it's going. In the sixth place there is no charge for this—not 90862 or any other number. This is what is known as a freebie—in the oldest profession, which is not medicine.

So what else is new? As it so happens other patients in other homes have problems:

W. M.'s mother called. W. M. is a Chinese pt. at the Acme Board-Care Home. He is completely mute and has a history of unprovoked aggressiveness—including choking family members and assaulting strangers, but as long as he is on a combo of Pro. Dec. 50 mg IM q. week plus oral Haldol plus Artane, he is a pussycat—albeit a mute pussycat. W. M. now spends much time at his mother's house where he hasn't tried to choke anyone lately, but she tends to stock up on Haldol and Artane in case there's an earthquake. So anyway Mrs. M. calls. Can I please call the pharmacy so she can pick up the "blue" pills and the "white" pills?

Because I am such a genius, I know what she is talking about. So I do it.

Anything else? Miss Carter called. Miss Carter is a coordinator. Coordinators are people who go to college and major in coordination. Either that or they watch a lot of videotapes featuring Jane Fonda jumping up and down. Anyway Miss Carter is coordinating patient N. H. as he leaves the Farley Board and Care facility to an independent living site. I have been aware of this plan for some time and have allowed patient N. H. to monitor his own meds, which he does by keeping them in his room in a locked box and taking them on his own. I have indicated this plan in the progress notes so that Mr. Farley, the administrator, will not have to go to jail for violating the oath he has taken to licensing. Patient N. H. has been doing fine, I tell her. She wants to know what meds he is on and we talk about this for a while. Miss Carter was under the impression that N. H. takes Prolixin as 5 mg, once daily—well, not exactly. He does take a 5 mg Prolixin tablet but takes three daily instead of one daily. She is very grateful for the info. Another freebie.

Anything else? Oh, yes. Mario called. Mario is a staff person at La Quinta Halfway House. Pt. E. P. is a new admission to La Quinta. The person who is coordinating him—not Miss Carter—felt it might be a good move because he was exacerbating. Anyway, Mario called because he wanted to know when E. P. was scheduled to receive his next Prolixin injection. I tell him that E. P. was scheduled to receive his "next" Prolixin inj. three days ago, which of course is news to Mario. He asks when I can schedule him and heaves a sigh of great relief when I tell him I can see him later today. At least this one will not be a freebie, assuming E. P. will keep his appointment, which doesn't always happen.

Anything else? Mrs. Jones called regarding patient E. K.

E. K. is a lovable Down's syndrome patient who always embraces me when I come to the house. It would seem that I am very important to him. He tells everyone he has a twin brother and that he is Elvis Presley. Anyway, today E. K. told the social worker at his program that he couldn't walk and that he had no doctor. How could he be so ungrateful? How quickly they forget. Anyway, the worker called Mrs. Jones in a huff demanding why E.K. does not have a doctor. Mrs. Jones then took E. K. to the county hospital where he remained overnight and was observed to indulge in unencumbered ambulation despite his continuing protestations to the contrary. Nevertheless I decided to change his meds switching him from olanzepine to risperidone. Some developmentally disabled patients do great on risperidone. Others do better on olanzepine, and there is no way to determine who will respond to what. One can argue all night about who has the right to do what and how and to whom, but what it boils down to is that it's all empirical.

So the point of all this is that a lot of 90862 is off premises-type work and not amenable to clockwatching or timecard punching. Actually, I think the record time for a 90862 is minus ten seconds. This occurred on January 6, 1999, and this should appear in the *Guiness Book of World Records*. I remember the date exactly because it was on the same day that representatives from the county psychiatric society met with Dr. Evans, the clinical director of the insurance company, to discuss the possibility of utilizing time guidelines for 90862. I kid you not.

On that historical date there is a progress note entry for patient S. H. at Jones's Residential Care Facility in which I discontinued the patient's olanzepine and put him on 800 mg of chlorpromazine (brand name Thorazine). Does that seem like an unenlightened move? Well, not exactly. The patient had been well stabilized for many years on Thorazine at 1,000 mg daily after years of hospitalizations and failures on lower dosages and other meds. Several months ago I decided it was time for a change. The newer antipsychotics are working miracles—I mean, they really are, and everyone and his or her cousin knows about tardive dyskinesia. Tardive dyskinesia describes the tendency of some of the older antipsychotic medications—such as Thorazine—to cause irregular movements of the lips, fingers, toes, and trunk after prolonged use. Even pt. E. K., the previously described devopmentally disabled wanna-be Elvis Presley, knows about tardive dyskinesia, so it was time for a change. So several weeks before the record-breaking day of January 6, 1999, the patient's Thorazine dose was decreased to 400 mg and 10 mg of olanzepine was added.

Now we return to January 6, 1999, and here is patient S. H., seated on the doorstep of the residential care facility in plain view of all the NIMBY neighbors, talking to himself, giggling to himself, spitting, dirty, and disheveled. The administrator, Mr. Jones (no relation to the aforementioned Mrs. Jones), didn't like it and the neighbors didn't like it and what is more, the neighbors didn't even like Mr. Jones. And at that point Mr. Jones didn't even like me, so aside from the fact that the patient had a problem, the entire community—including me—had a problem. To make a long story very short, in the ten seconds that had elapsed between the time I saw the patient and the time I entered the portals of the residential care home, I had all the information I needed for an in-depth reevaluation of this patient's medication. So if time guidelines were in effect I would rate this 90862 service as minus ten seconds. Now I realize that the *Guiness Book of World Records* affords no accolades to the shortest length of time spent in an in-depth psychopharmacological examination, but if there were such a category, I would submit my name in nomination. Incidentally (and in violation of my initial promise earlier in this chapter that there would be no follow-up regarding the events of February 8, 1999) almost immediately after this regressive reversion to Thorazine, the patient made a rapid improvement.

Chapter 10

Why Do It?

The value of home visits by mobile crisis teams in response to emergency situations was briefly discussed in the Introduction. The focus of this book is more specialized in that it concentrates on the role of the psychiatrist in providing routine maintenance visits (in contrast to visits necessitated by emergencies) to a particular kind of home. In the absence of routine visits, patient contacts with psychiatrists might be limited to clinic appointments, office appointments, emergency room contacts, the aforementioned visits by mobile crisis teams, or those contacts that occur during the course of a hospitalization.

Sullivan and Cohen have described evaluation and home treatment when rendered by such teams based on the experiences of a mobile crisis team operating from a public general hospital in an inner-city community.[1] They note that the team, working closely with families, agencies, and hospitals, has found the home visit to be a valuable addition to the treatment resources of the community. They note that there is a general lack of training among psychiatrists for this type of service and that mental health practitioners have multiple excuses for not being involved, such as "if the patient were really motivated for treatment he or she would get to the clinic," or "it's too intrusive," or "the patient will become too dependent." They describe the home visiting teams as having the general goals of (1) brief intervention to restabilize the patient in the community, (2) long-term treatment to provide ongoing treatment in the home for the patient who is chronically resistant to more traditional treatments, (3) brief crisis intervention to restore the patient to equilibrium without immediate need for further treatment, and (4) hospitalization of the patient when hospitalization appears advisable.

Many residential care facility residents are unreliable appointment keepers. They either confuse the hour of the appointment, or forget the date of the appointment or lose the appointment card or miss the bus or take the wrong bus or lose the transfer coupon, or they may not feel like going to the psychiatric office on a particular day because they didn't feel like going that day. There are, of course, many reasons for missed appointments. Some psychiatrists might attribute this to resistance, and there are traditional psychodynamic strategies of dealing with resistance—such as charging for missed appointments. Since most chronic psychotics are covered by third-party payers, including Medicare, these techniques of overcoming patient resistance might in itself create resistance—resistance from these payers, resistance which can lead to hostility which can lead to allegations of fraud.

It is not an exaggeration to say that those patients who can keep their psychiatric office appointments tend to be the better functioning residential care facility patients. If office appointments were the only psychiatric source of treatment for residential care facility patients, many of them would never be treated, and these would be the more severely impaired patients who are more likely to be hospitalized. Just what the incidence of rehospitalization might be is very difficult to estimate because nobody follows patients who are not followed. This is one of the reasons why residential care facility on-site visits are very important: they provide psychiatric services to those patients most in need who might otherwise not receive any services.

I cannot really prove that the residential care facility system is an effective system by referring to the literature because no literature exists that provides this proof. I am unable to find any article that proves hospitalizations were decreased by having psychiatrists making on-site visits to residential care facilities. But I did find one recent article indicating that the incidence of hospitalization was decreased if on-site visits were made by case managers.[2] The sample consisted of 321 patients identified by hospital records as living in one of twenty-four board-and-care homes in the Los Angeles area that were approved by the community residential care program. A total of 214 subjects who received monthly home visits from case managers (program group) were compared with 107 subjects who did not receive monthly home visits (comparison group).

Among subjects in the program group, the median number of psychiatric bed-days used decreased significantly, from fifty-nine days to fifty days. No significant change in the median number was observed for comparison subjects. Comparison subjects were rehospitalized 1.7 times more often than program subjects.

THE VALUE OF ON-SITE VISITS BY PSYCHIATRISTS AND THE "CONTINUITY OF CARE" ISSUE

If on-site visits by case managers can really decrease the incidence of rehospitalization, then I say more power to case managers and their on-site visits. Thus far I have not been able to find any comparable studies addressing the efficacy of on-site visits by psychiatrists to residential care facilities. Sometimes the effectiveness of on-site care can be inferred from studies which address the problem of "continuity of care" as a desirable treatment modality.

Continuity of care has been defined as "a process involving the orderly, uninterrupted movement of patients among the diverse elements of the service delivery system."[3] The continuity of care model implies the continuity of caregivers. The continuity of caregivers "implies that the same mental health team will be responsible indefinitely for a given chronic mentally ill patient no matter where the patient is—hospital, foster home, shelter, family, own apartment—and no matter what the patient's needs."[4]

Some studies have indicated that chronic schizophrenic patients when followed by the same treatment team, score better on self-ratings and show less psychotic symptoms when compared to a control group followed by a succession of different mental health professionals.[5]

Continuity of care has geographical implications in that the same mental health professionals are involved in the provision of care no matter where the care is rendered. Thus according to this concept the same professional team would be involved whether the patient is in the hospital or out of the hospital. According to this model the people on the home visiting team would be the same people on the hospital treatment team.

Ideally the continuity of care team is envisaged as

> taking responsibility for seeing to it that a chronically mentally ill person's needs are met. . . .The team members do not necessarily meet all the client's needs themselves (they may involve other persons or agencies). However they never transfer this obligation to someone else . . . the buck stops with the team . . . the team remains responsible for the client no matter what his or her behavior is. This fixed point of responsibility means that the client always has a consistent resource.[6]

E. Fuller Torrey offers a graphic example of the differences between the continuity of care model and the conventional method of service delivery which is called the "availability of care" model in an article titled "Continuous Treatment Teams in the Care of the Chronically Mentally Ill."[7]

> An analogy to bus systems will clarify the differences in the availability of care, the continuity of care, and the continuity of caregiver models. In the availability of care model, a bus system is available that the person can use with a timetable and a willingness to transfer from bus to bus. In the continuity of care model, the person is given one or more case managers who ensure that the person has a timetable and is given instructions on how to negotiate transfers; case managers also keep track of the person within the bus system. In the continuity of caregiver model, the person is assigned a specific bus whose drivers accept ongoing responsibility for ensuring that the person reaches all destinations; the person may be left off at various locales for specific services, but at the end of the day the same bus and drivers will pick the person up. (Reprinted with permission from American Psychiatric Publishing, Inc.)

Despite its advantages, continuity of care with continuity of caregivers may be difficult to implement for a variety of reasons. Hospital salaried staff are not likely to be granted the time to make home visits because this would necessarily subtract from the time they had to make hospital visits. In this sense time is a zero-sum game. What goes into one pot comes out of another pot and hospital administrators do not like their pots depleted.

Moreover, hospital personnel undergo frequent job changes in the course of time. The members of such treatment teams are usually social workers and psychiatrists in the early course of their careers or residencies. Social workers frequently change positions either via promotions or lateral transfers to other agencies. Psychiatrists as psychiatric residents necessarily change their job focus as part of their training. Psychiatrists in hospital service in the early part of their careers frequently drift into private practice or positions of greater administrative responsibility. Whatever the reason, the personnel responsible for caregiving rarely remains stable. In fact, the most permanent caregiver in residential care tends to be the residential care administrator who is sometimes overlooked as a caregiver.

There are other problems in implementing a continuity of care program as described by Dr. Torrey.[8]

The most formidable obstacles were job descriptions, union rules, and matters of professional turf. Outpatient staff members who had worked hard to achieve their Monday-to-Friday, 8:30 a.m. to 5 p.m. workday were distinctly uninterested in discussing other shifts or being on night call. For continuous teams to work, members must be flexible and be willing to go into the community regularly; such a prospect did not seem inviting to staff whose horizons had not extended beyond the walls of the hospital.

Nursing supervisors became anxious about how they would know what nursing staff were doing when not on the ward, and all disciplines were reluctant to consider being supervised by a professional from another discipline. To encourage effective continuous team members to remain in service positions and not migrate to administrative roles for promotion, career ladders clearly had to be restructured.

Another issue raised by some of the hospital professionals was whether continuous treatment teams foster dependency in patients. The ideal for American mental health for many years has been cure and independence: chronic mental patients are ultimately supposed to get well and be able to live without extensive support systems. The realization that many patients with chronic mental illness will not be able to achieve this idea has only reluctantly been accepted by many mental health professionals.

Administrative problems also arose concerning what to do with chronic mental patients who wander from city to city. They could theoretically be followed by a special continuous care team that coordinates efforts with similar groups in other regions. Such an arrangement would raise civil liberties issues, including how much information could be disclosed across jurisdictions without the patient's permission, as well as the problem of outpatient commitments becoming void by the patient's movement from state to state. (Reprinted with permission from American Psychiatric Publishing, Inc.)

I favor continuity of care but in the historical rather than the geographical sense. Thus I have been the psychiatrist for many of the occupants of the residential care facilities for decades; as a consequence I know them very well. In the past when my patients had to be hospitalized, I would then assume care for them in the hospital, so in that sense the continuity of care that was rendered was geographical as well as historical. The continuity of care was not rendered by a team—it was rendered by me. I did this by being on the psychiatric staff of three local hospitals.

However, for a variety of reasons, I no longer do hospital work. Part of this disinclination is a function of the decreasing energies associated with increasing years. I no longer have the energy required to do all the heavy-lifting legal paperwork that is now part of hospital treatment procedures. As a result, I leave that to my younger colleagues (the hewers of wood and the carriers of water), but when my patients are now hospitalized, hospital doctors frequently contact me to solicit my opinion about what should be done. Basically I do not believe much is lost when the responsibilities for care are partitioned in this way, and sometimes something is gained in the sense that two heads may be better than one—even two psychiatric heads. Sometimes a new psychiatrist can suggest an alternative mode of treatment that I had overlooked and that has good therapeutic possibilities. In this context, it may be that the continuity of care model has some unrealized disadvantages in that an unchanging treatment team may not be accessible to new ideas.

I have quoted Dr. Torrey at length to support my view that it is probably best that the psychiatrist rendering services to residential care facilities be in private practice—no union rules, no 8:30 a.m. to 5:00 p.m. allegiances, no clenched-teeth exchanges with naive and unsophisticated team members with their exasperating misdirected democratic agendas about fostering patient dependencies, no professional turf battles about who is doing what and why and to whom, no federal case problems with litigious civil rights attorneys defending the rights of paranoid patients or paranoid civil rights attorneys defending the rights of litigious patients because communications have crossed state lines. The psychiatrist in private practice can avoid such problems unless he or she seeks them out. The only problem for the private practitioner is how he or she will be paid. (This problem is addressed in Chapter 24 on coding.)

Aside from these reasons, I am in favor of the residential care facility psychiatrist being in private practice because it facilitates a permanent commitment to this type of work. However, if a salaried psychiatrist is dedicated to his or her job, likes his or her work, and wants to stay put, more power to him or her. The problems arise when residential care is a job assignment rather than a professional preference. The psychiatrist in private practice is free to come and go in the sense that he or she can choose the kind of work and the kind of patients that he or she can best treat—to put it monosyllabically. Under those circumstances the kind of psychiatrists who will succeed in residential care facility work are the kinds of psychiatrists who enjoy the work. It goes without saying that private practice psychiatrists who do not enjoy the work will leave for sunnier climes. In psychiatry the sunnier climes are usually located in private practice offices. In private practice a process of natural selection occurs in which professionals do what they want to do (and hopefully what they are good at doing) and not what they are told to do. We may all be thankful for natural selection and differences in personal preferences. Without these variables, proctologists might never have evolved.

The stable, nonchanging, permanent type of residential care facility psychiatrist (one who does not look for another job and is not upwardly mobile) is of great advantage to patients and facility caretakers because sometimes it can take years to establish a good relationship. The longer the psychiatrist knows the patients, the better he or she can treat them. Under such circumstances, familiarity does not breed contempt. It breeds a greater degree of understanding of the patients' impairments. After a period of years the psychiatrist may achieve the distinction of being the world's greatest expert in treating a certain restricted segment of humanity. The negative aspect of this distinction is that eventually it will become difficult to retire. Many people will request that the psychiatrist not retire, and the psychiatrist may correctly anticipate that the adulation he or she receives at the residential care facility will not be forthcoming on the golf course. It is not easy to make the transition from being the world's greatest expert to being an ordinary person. As a rule, psychiatrists do not aspire to be ordinary.

Obviously this book is a pitch for the effectiveness of on-site visits by psychiatrists. I cannot prove that I decrease the incidence of hospitalizations by virtue of my on-site visits because there is no comparable control group. All I have are anecdotes, and my anecdotes are not related to hospitalizations but to criminal convictions. I am able to write about criminal convictions because I have kept close track of them in the course of my career as a residential care facility psychiatrist during which I treated over 2,000 patients. No incidents of serious violent crimes were committed by any of my residential care facility patients when I was actively involved in their treatment. Some of them had serious problems before they were in treatment, and a few of them undoubtedly had problems after we terminated treatment.

I feel confident in saying this because I keep very accurate records of events that never happened. This is not to say that encounters with the police did not occur. Such encounters did occur, but when they happened they were limited to offenses such as drinking or urinating in a public place. Some patients, despite all our efforts in psychopharmacology, psychotherapy, and social skills programs, are still too disorganized or irrational to succeed in a residential care facility setting. Serial urinators generally fall within that category.

It can be argued that the more than 2,000 patients I have seen in my career are little more than 2,000 anecdotes, and can only suggest the effectiveness of a system rather than prove it. Nor do I have statistics on a control group of 2,000 patients who were not followed by on-site visits. Such a group would be difficult to follow because the members would move around a lot—from doctor to doctor or clinic to clinic or hospital to hospital or city to city or even state to state. Under such circumstances, follow-up would be impossible.

Nor do I have statistics on the extent to which the residential care facility system has decreased hospitalizations, or for that matter prevented suicides. Still a zero incidence of incarceration is pretty good considering that in 1999 the Department of Justice reported that as much as 16 percent of the population of state jails and prisons suffer from mental illness.[9] In California more than 10,400 persons who are diagnosed as seriously mentally ill are booked annually into county jails across the state, usually for a short length of stay.[10] They are then released due to their relatively minor crimes, and repeatedly brought back to the criminal justice system after being arrested for new offenses. However, not all crimes committed are for nonviolent felonies and misdemeanors. A California Department of Corrections report indicates that 43 percent of its Enhanced Outpatient Program are incarcerated for a violent crime. The most frequent offenses in order were robbery, assault with a deadly weapon, assault and battery, second-degree murder, and first-degree murder. In addition to the costs inflicted upon the victims of violence, the cost of housing 21,000 prisoners with mental health problems in state prisons and 2,500 offenders in county jails probably exceeds $500 million annually.[11] This sum does not include the additional costs or treatment while incarcerated or the costs to local law enforcement agencies and courts to deal with mentally ill offenders caught in the revolving door of the criminal justice system.

I repeat, a zero incidence of violent crimes is a pretty good record. The fact that I have what might be called a good criminal record is not necessarily attributable to my personal brilliance as a psychiatrist, although if someone were to argue the point I would not engage in bitter disputation. The fact is that I have been helped immeasurably in my efforts by the Modern Psychiatric Team.

Aside from my good criminal record, I would like to assert that my efforts in residential care facilities have led to spectacular rehabilitative results in that many of my patients resumed their schooling or obtained a job. I would like to say this, but this is not true with respect to a majority of patients. For many patients residency in the protected setting of a residential care facility does not presage a return to true independence in which one's status as a tax recipient is converted to that of taxpayer. Such conversions face an almost insurmountable barrier, especially if the newly converted taxpayer is obligated to pay a high price for the medications that facilitated the conversion.

Possibly this failure to fully proceed on the road to independence is partially attributable to the dependency style of life fostered by the residential care facility, and partially to the social stigmatization process that is part of mental illness. More likely the most important factor that prevents the achievement of full economic independence is the severity of the illness itself. Even when the illness abates and/or responds to medications, frequently the residual impairments such as poor judgment and poor grooming militate against a successful work career. Also, what is equally important is the loss of job skills that inevitably occur as a result of an illness that crests in early life, when learning capabilities are at their greatest. In addition, one must not underestimate the limiting effect created by the lack of a job history, even in someone who has made a very good recovery.

For all of these reasons, placement in a residential care facility may be regarded as rehabilitative in the sense that it prevents exacerbations of illness and resultant hospitalizations, but in most instances it is somewhat less than rehabilitative in the sense of facilitating success in the world of work. Perhaps it might best be thought of as maintainative (even though this is not a word) in the sense that residential care facility placement maintains a style of nonproductive stability in which hospitalizations and exacerbations of illness are avoided but improvement is not of sufficient quality to allow for true independence. Improvements in "social and occupational functioning" are frequently descriptively joined as if they were inextricably intertwined, but in truth adequate social functioning may be achieved in the absence of occupational success. Residential care facility occupants frequently enjoy an improvement in social functioning but only more rarely an improvement in occupational functioning.

CLINICAL EXAMPLES OF THE ADVANTAGE OF ON-SITE ENCOUNTERS

Some events are more likely to occur in residential care facilities than in other types of treatment settings. Here is a progress note on a patient seen in a residential care facility on February 19, 2001. This was President's Day, but I was working anyway. Here is my progress note that day which I entered into the house chart:

> Refuses to take Haldol inj. today. I discussed inadvisability of doing this with pt., but he is adamant. So will not administer, but he promises to contact staff if he feels worse and staff has been alerted as to above. I will administer inj. in my office before next two-week interval if indicated.

How could the nonadministration of a long-lasting haloperidol decanoate injection be therapeutic, and why should this type of situation be limited to a residential care home? I knew this patient fairly well since I had been treating him for over ten years and had established a therapeutic relationship. It may be difficult to imagine how such a relationship could be established as the result of injections, but if the injections have been helpful, the patient's trust in the administering doctor increases accordingly. Eventually the trust that accompanies the injection lingers after the injection and becomes as long-lasting as the effect of the medication.

In the course of several years the patient had been making steady progress and was now able to function as a supervisor in a janitorial setting. I believe the patient thought that in order to continue making progress he could now function autonomously—without the aid of IM administered medication. Had I strongly insisted that he consent to the injection, he would have consented, but he would have felt defeated and demoralized. Mental patients have lots of experiences in defeat, and I did not wish him any more experiences of this kind. I would allow him this victory. But I knew him well enough to know that when he felt worse, he would tell the staff person who would then contact me.

My verbal contract with the patient went something like this:

> I don't want you to take shots if you don't need them, but you must promise me that if you feel worse in any way you will tell the staff and they will let me know. You can then come to my office instead of waiting for the next time I come to the house, and I will give you the shot in my office. Is that okay with you?

When oral understandings with patients are phrased this way, in which the involvement of the patient is invited, and in which the thrust is not solely on compliance, agreement frequently follows. Contracts like this are best honored if the language is clear and the commitments are stated in one-syllable words—unlike my literary style.

The patient readily agreed to this and was not once again defeated in his quest for autonomous health. Will it work? I don't know. I am allowing him to take some responsibility for his own health, which is not really such a bad idea. Also I am promising my availability even if he does not follow my instructions to the letter. Admittedly one cannot do this with every patient. One must know one's patient, which is one of the advantages achieved by the residential care facility psychiatrist who follows his or her patients longitudinally.

But why is such an encounter more likely to occur in a residential care home rather than in a clinic setting or private office? Because the patient under these circumstances would simply not miss the appointment and might then be lost to follow-up. What would happen in a hospital setting if the patient refused the treatment? He or she would either be discharged against medical advice (AMA) or be discharged on a non-AMA basis (with or without some kind of lots-of-luck discharge instructions) or forced by some legal means to receive treatment even without his or her consent. However, in the residential care facility setting, the refusal to cooperate with treatment does not result in a follow-up treatment loss. By allowing him to win this encounter or win in his own eyes, I incurred a short-term treatment loss for a long-term treatment gain.

The long-term treatment gain would have been this patient's increased sense of self-esteem that he was no longer dependent on injectable medication for a continuing good adjustment. Unfortunately, that is not the way it happened. Here is my progress note for this patient dated April 2, 2001, after the administrator called asking me to make a special visit.

Now is increasingly irritable, complains of hearing voices, is easily upset. Told staff that if they wanted him to leave he could leave in three days. Staff has noticed that he is increasingly active and cannot stay still. Pt. states that he feels bad because his "bronichal tubes" are bothering him and he is afraid he might get cancer. He is very concerned. Also he is concerned that OSHA will fine him for doing a bad job. Pt. is overtalkative and disconnected in his speech pattern. He states he plans to live another forty-nine years. Will restart IM Haldol as 150 mg R. deltoid.

Basically very little was lost by acceding to this patient's wishes. He had a week of diminished productivity but did not lose his job and quickly improved back to his baseline. But the reason why not much was lost is because he was monitored by the staff of the residential care home, and I made it clear to them that in the event the patient started relapsing I was willing to make a special visit. The experience may have contributed in the long run to the patient's acceptance of the current treatment plan.

Undoubtedly there are many reasons why on-site visits contribute to more efficient patient care. What I have not described thus far is how on-site visits contribute to increased caretaker care. Admittedly it is not the primary function of the psychiatrist to take care of caretakers. Yet this function is extremely important. There is such a phenomena of caretaker burnout, and when that happens caretakers can either leave the field entirely or become less conscientious in terms of administering optimal care. This is particularly true for caretakers who deal with difficult patients—patients who are bizarre or belligerent or demanding. When faced with constant unrelenting day-and-night pressure to render conscientious care, it is easy to understand why some caretakers become demoralized. If caretakers resign from the field, sometimes institutionalization is the only option for their patients.

One of the ancillary benefits of helping psychiatric patients improve is that caretaker attitudes can also improve, so that there is an indirect salutary effect on the atmosphere of the residential care home. But in addition to that, a direct beneficial effect is realized when the psychiatrist has a consultative relationship with the caretaker.

THE EFFECT OF ON-SITE VISITS ON THE ADMINISTRATOR

While it is true that on-site psychiatric visits last only a comparatively short period of time, the psychiatrist through consultation can help the administrator understand and cope with the irrational behavior of the residents that can occur on a twenty-four-hour basis. Also if the psychiatrist is able to improve or control the patient's behavior through interventions, the administrator will feel more secure in the management of the home. Also the administrator will grow professionally if he or she can attend the team meetings and participate in the discussions. The establishment of this kind of routine can decrease the isolation of the administrator. Isolation can be demoralizing, especially when one is confronted with situations that defy quick solutions. Also this pattern of periodic prescheduled consultations or meetings should help to upgrade the home in terms of creating a therapeutic environment.

By helping the caretaker understand the meaning of a patient's symptoms, the psychiatrist is better able to help the caretaker cope with the obligations of caretaking. Sometimes helping the caretaker can be an apparently simple matter—such as providing the patient with a hypnotic so that he or she can get a good night's sleep— thereby enabling the caretaker to get a good night's sleep, thereby enabling the physician to get a good night's sleep. One should never underestimate the importance of a good night's sleep either for patients or caretakers or even for physicians. Taking care of caretakers is very important even though it is not the primary function of the psychiatrist.

On-site residential care facility psychiatric visits help the administrator in many ways besides consultation if only that it saves them from the agony of accompanying patients for clinic visits. Have you had the misfortune to be a clinic patient lately? I have not had this experience for personal reasons, however I recently accompanied my mother for her clinic appointment although she was under the impression that she made an appointment to see the doctor in his private office. What a revelation! Long lines of people waiting to be registered, long lines of people waiting for an elevator, long lines of people waiting for their turn in those little examination rooms with no pictures on the walls and those outdated and boring magazines which I will describe in boring detail later in this chapter.

Finally after about an hour's wait she saw the doctor and the doctor saw her. This exchange of visual images took about five minutes. If there is an adjective in the English language that indicates both harassment and boredom, I would use it to describe the doctor, but I haven't found it so I am unable to utilize it. The fact is I know the feeling and probably conveyed that impression to some of my own patients.

After the doctor had completed his stethoscopic adventures accompanied by facial expressions indicating deep thought, he ordered a flu injection. The injection was given at another floor requiring another registration with more lines and more waiting. The clerk completes an additional registration form. She instructs us to follow the blue line to receive the injection. We follow the blue line. At the end of the blue line is a desk. Nobody is behind the desk but at the top of this desk is a box. The instructions on the box tell us to to put our form in the box, which we do. Something then is supposed to happen but after a while nothing happens. The form just lies there—in the box. Other forms, equally unprocessed, are also lying in the box. More people are waiting. Everybody and everything is waiting—people, forms, boxes, and still nothing is happening.

It is lunchtime. I suspect the nurse is out to lunch but I don't really know. I notice a busy clerk apparently busy with busy paperwork. Because I am a physician and somewhat fearless when it comes to confronting medical bureaucracy, I ask her where the nurse is. The other people are too intimidated to ask. "She is out to lunch," the busy clerk tells me without looking up. I say "Thank you." (That will teach her who is boss). Incidentally, my mother is ninety-five years old. She admits to eighty and would kill me if she knew I revealed this publicly.

Actually the problems started long before the day of the appointment—the problems started in the making of the appointment. In the interests of brevity I will not describe in detail the exhilarating antipasto experience of negotiating an appointment date via the formidable telephone prompts that inevitably end with a "please hold" command accompanied by the boilerplated phrase "your call is very important to us" blah blah blah, you are very important even though they don't know who you are and don't really care even if they say they do. Actually this is really little more than the telephonic equivalent of the box at the end of the blue line. I think there should be a federal law against telephone prompts although it might violate the freedom of speech provisions of the Constitution—but then again it might not. (I don't think the Constitution has any provisions protecting freedom of recorded speech.) This whole telephonic version of a Byzantine maze seemed cleverly designed to discourage appointments. I did not understand the reason for this until I realized that doctors in capitated practices are paid by the head and not on the basis of a fee-for-service system.

I think this requires some explaining. Physicians in capitated systems are paid a set amount based on the number of patients in their case load that they are responsible for but do not necessarily see, and the expenses the patients incur are deducted from the kitty based on the size of the caseload. One could have a long discussion as to whether this is a conflict of interest. I choose not to engage in such discussions because the answer is pretty obvious. Only then did I understand the rationale of the final prompt—the "Please hold" instruction delivered in English and three other languages. The real meaning of "Please hold" is really "Please don't hold" or possibly, "Don't call us; we'll call you," in the show business sense of the word. In my mind's eye I see these doctors comparing their practices as Texas ranchers with big hats and lots of cattle might compare theirs: "I run a spread with three hundred head. What are your holdings?"

The whole experience reminded me of my own hitherto repressed memories of unpleasant experiences in a doctor's office as an impatient outpatient scantly clad in a sterile paper hospital gown open at the backside while seated on an uncomfortable chair in the solitary confinement of a cold tiny waiting-room cubicle while awaiting the arrival of his eminence with my only surcease provided by outdated editions of *Ferret Digest* or *American Angler* with such stimulating articles as "How to Choose the Right Fly Every Time"—articles which neither titillate my curiosity nor express my preferences. I have absolutely no interest in choosing the right fly every time.

Anyway, getting back to the administrators—that's why administrators love residential care home visiting psychiatrists, because we save them from such experiences. In truth, they love us not for our minds but for our on-the-premises bodies.

Shortly after I wrote this paragraph an administrator telephoned me on a Friday night. She was very concerned because one of her residents had ingested another patient's medications and she didn't know if she should call an ambulance or take the patient directly to an emergency room. I was certain that the extra medication would not have harmful effects and I was able to reassure her about this. A follow-up call by me on the next day was greeted with a strong degree of appreciation, and I can understand why. A visit to a busy emergency room on a Friday night in a big city by a psychiatric patient who is not in acute distress can easily require an all-night stay on the part of the administrator.

Chapter 11

The Residential Care Facility First-Aid Paperwork Reduction Kit

I first thought of including this chapter in the how-to-do it chapter, but I changed my mind. The first-aid paperwork reduction kit does not really belong with the Ten Commandments of Residential Care Facility Psychiatry. Rather it is a device which enables the Ten Commandments to be implemented more effectively. It is to residential care facility psychiatry what a utility is to an operating system for a computer.

The average psychiatrist is flooded with paperwork. The average residential care facility psychiatrist, if such an entity exists, is flooded with even more paperwork than the average office psychiatrist. This is because he or she has more patients, and residential care facility inhabitation requires residential care facility documentation. For this reason the residential care facility psychiatrist schleps with him or her a special paperwork emergency first-aid kit, so that paperwork obligations can be done on the premises and immediately. This is infinitely preferable to waiting until you get to your office insofar as when that happens, other obligations will inevitably intrude themselves into consciousness. What then happens is that paperwork obligations to distant patients in faraway residential care facilities will soon be forgotten.

The best way to control paperwork obligations is to prepare boilerplated forms under one's letterhead that will minimally satisfy the requirements of the situations one is going to confront. It is best to prepare the forms in such a way that the only items that need to be completed are the patient's name and the date. What am I forgetting? Oh, yes—the signature of the physician, we do need that. Here is an example of such a form, excusing a patient from jury duty.

Date

To whom it may concern:

This will certify that _____ is currently in psychiatric treatment, and is unable to serve on a jury. The disability is permanent.

If you need any additional information, please contact me.

_____, MD

Jury letters can be quite important. A patient once told me that she liked to be on juries because she liked to find people guilty because it made her happy to make other people unhappy. The Germans have a name for this. It is called *schadenfreude,* which means experiencing pleasure from other people's pain, and I believe this lady had a rather severe case. I offered to write the letter exempting her from jury duty and I even offered to send it special delivery, but she politely declined. So far I have not been approached by the producers of *American Justice* about this matter which I like to watch on the A & E channel.

The fact is I receive many letters attempting to conscript mental patients for jury duty, but most patients will request exemption letters. This is indeed fortunate because if exemptions were not requested, the juries would be overrun with mental patients. To put it bluntly, I don't know if this would be good or bad for the justice system but I do know this: When a psychiatrist is asked to complete such a letter, he or she should be a sport and shell out the money to buy the stamps. This is not as painless as it used to be, since the average letter now costs thirty-seven cents, but for some patients this is a big production and they may even lose the envelope after investing in the postage. Also don't be surprised if when you do this, someone will accuse you of "infantilizing" your patients. Common decency has always had its critics and, besides, "infantilizing" is a dumb word to describe this situation.

The most important boilerplated letter which you should have in the paperwork reduction kit is the authorization release-of-information letter:

AUTHORIZATION FOR RELEASE OF INFORMATION

I hereby authorize _____to disclose to
_____, MD, my records obtained in the course of
the diagnosis and treatment for medical and psychiatric illnesses, and/or alcohol and/or drug abuse.

This disclosure of information is required for evaluation and treatment planning.

This consent shall become effective on _____
and shall terminate on _____.

_____   _____

Signature of patient   Date of signature

_____

Birth date

_____, MD

I have already commented in Chapter 8 on the inestimable prognostic
value of the authorization release form.

Another release-type letter is the progress note release letter to
Medicare. It probably is not necessary since Medicare apparently has
the right to monitor progress notes but I carry it in my bag just for
emergencies.

I authorize Dr. _____ to release copies of
my progress notes to Medicare for the purpose of evaluating the adequacy of medication management services. This authorization is good
until canceled. I have been informed that I may cancel this authorization at any time.

_____   _____

Signature of patient   Date of signature

Another important letter is the geriatric letter. Following is an example of a geriatric letter.

Date

To whom it may concern:

In my opinion _____,
a geriatric patient, is compatible with the other residents of the
_____Residential Care Home and can safely
continue to reside there.

_____, MD

The purpose of a geriatric letter is that the licensing laws mandate that when patients reach age sixty, they should be transferred to a geriatric home. In many instances this is not a good idea, and licensing will consent to continued placement in the same facility if the physician writes something similar to this letter. Many geriatric patients are not really geriatric at all in the sense that they have the energy and desire to socialize with nongeriatric patients. Prematurely transferring such a patient to a geriatric facility can have extreme consequences and in some instances it can spell the difference between life and death for a geriatric patient.

I like to write a special progress note when I first see a patient. Following is the form I use for the initial interview:

Date: _____
Name: _____
Insurance: _____
Previous Residence: _____
Prior Hospitalizations: _____
Closest Relatives: _____
Relative's Phone Numbers: _____
Current Medications: _____
Helpful Past Medications: _____
Medical Problems: _____
Allergies: _____
DOB: _____
M S W D (married, single, widowed, divorced): _____
Children: _____

What you see is what you get in the initial interview letter. Obviously one can add to it or subtract from it, but this boilerplate has stood the test of time for me.

What else is in the first-aid paperwork reduction kit? I always carry an extra supply of HCFA 1500 forms in red dropout ink, in the event I decide to drop out because of recurrent Medicare audits, or even worse in case I lose or misplace some forms, and a dire emergency might occur because I might forget to submit a claim. What is worse, I might remember to submit the claim but forget the actual date the service was rendered and then be docked for submitting a claim for a service that was not rendered. This doesn't happen if I have a just-in-time inventory of extra claim forms which I complete on the premises.

What else is in this bag? We need an extra folder for letterhead stationery and envelopes, just in case we run into a form that we have not anticipated. Sometimes it is necessary to write a letter for a patient should some unanticipated event occur, as sometimes happens. This is illustrated in the following progress notes:

> 12-18-00. Says "I feel depressed." Social Security is asking her to refund overpayment of $1,350 for the year. The social worker told her she had a form and will appeal to them. I offered to write a letter for her if that will help.

> 01-08-01. Says she is still depressed because she has to pay the government money every month and she doesn't have it. She has to pay them $83 every month. She still has her job at Civic Center where she helps the security team monitor the metal detector. She says the social worker looked into the problem and Social Security does not want to waive payments.

The patient tells me she cannot sleep and is very depressed because she is afraid that she might have to go to jail. Of course this is unrealistic, but as a consequence of spending her nights without sleep and her days looking for bombs, she is headed for the hospital rather than jail. This is not unrealistic. Were that to happen, the poor government would have lost the anticipated $1,350 refund within two days. Clearly something had to be done and be done fast.

Enter Dr. Fleishman with his emergency residential care facility first-aid kit and his letterhead stationery.

I addressed a letter to Social Security which read as follows:

To whom it may concern:

> Miss S has suffered from a severe mental illness for many years. She does not have a work history and is very inexperienced regarding money matters. A rehabilitation counselor convinced her that if she were able to work she would feel better. For the past year she has arisen at 4:00 a.m. so she could arrive on time for her job at the Civic Center. The problem now is that as a wage earner, her income has risen, but she did not declare it so she is now obligated to return $83 per month to the government. However, she is unable to do this and she is afraid she might have to go to jail and cries herself to sleep every night. Is it possible to decrease her monthly obligation or even cancel it entirely?

Shortly after I sent the letter with my brazen request, her obligation was rescinded. Miss S thinks I am a great psychiatrist. I hope she will testify in my defense if Medicare ever asks me what I do in residential care facilities. Never underestimate the power of letterhead.

What else is in the bag? Special progress paper with my name printed on it. The reason it is special is a long story, but I will tell it anyway because this is a long book.

There was a time when one could submit a claim to Medicare and they would pay, no questions asked—unless, of course, one was audited years later, in which case lots of questions were asked about services rendered years earlier. However, I will get to that story later in the book.

Later in my career Medicare started asking me for copies of progress notes—no note, no payment. Now progress notes on residential care facility patients are kept at the residential care facility and are the property of the residential care facility, which is as it should be, so in order to send Medicare my progress notes, I started making carbon copies of my notes.

That turned out to be very unwieldy because soon my fingers would reek of carbon paper. After a while I would leave smudgy fingerprints on the deltoids of the patients I had to touch in order to administer decanoate injections, and sometimes the fingerprints would be on the gluteus, which might be difficult to explain to some people. The whole experience was very messy and I could see why some of my professors in clinical psychology were so dedicated to not touching patients; obviously they had all been working with carbon paper.

So I had to think of something else. I then started disassembling the residential care facility charts, removing my progress notes and taking them to a commercial source for photocopying, and then reinserting them the next time I visited the home. Now residential care facility charts are generally bound at the top with metal binders, much like hospital charts, so disassembling them is no mean trick. It gets very messy, especially when dealing with multiple charts, and administrators don't like this because stuff can get lost or misplaced or put out of sequence. Then when licensing workers visit for their annual evaluation, they inspect the charts and say things like "Why is page seven followed by page nine?" and there is some sort of horrendous fine levied against the administrator for this type of transgression and the doctor gets off scotfree. Obviously this could have an adverse effect on the psychiatrist-administrator relationship. So I had to find some other solution.

Fortunately about this time when I was trying to think creatively about this highly technical problem, I was changing addresses and I asked one of the furniture movers for an estimate. He scribbled a number down on his pad, tore the sheet off, and handed it to me, and still he had *two additional copies remaining on his pad with copies of his estimate.* Well, everyone knows the story of James Watt and how he saw steam lifting the lid of a cooking pot and how he immediately invented the steam engine. (Smart fellow that Watt.) It was that kind of epiphany. So I bravely asked, "Where do you get those things?" He responded, somewhat annoyed, "Actually, I don't know. Everybody has one." Actually he didn't say actually. Actually it's called invoice paper or something like that. It even has two holes at the top to accommodate top-loading metal binders. I get my invoice paper from a company called New England Business Services, 3,000 miles away, but nobody seems to mind. They even pre-imprint my name on each copy for a small fee and that solved the problem.

I now write my progress notes on invoice paper. I tear off the copies of my progress notes just like a real furniture mover, although thus far I have resisted the impulse to dress in OshKosh B'Gosh coveralls. I then send my invoices to Medicare with the attached claim form. The only problem with the invoice paper is that it says "Specifications" at the top of the page. I asked New England Business Services if they could remove this, but they said it would cost several thousand dollars to do this, or something like that. What's the name of that comedienne who use to say "Never mind"? Anyway, never mind, that's what I said. If push comes to shove and Medicare insists on specifications, I will list the height and weight of each patient on each progress note. Never underestimate the creative power of us Americans when it comes to solving problems.

The OshKosh B'Gosh method of accounting had some unanticipated advantages. Many psychiatrists receive long forms from various disability evaluation divisions of various departments of social service, the purpose of which is to make sure that the patients are not cheating the welfare department and not receiving checks to which they are not really entitled. In my experience, most of these inquiries refer to patients who have been continuously and severely ill for decades, and who could not possibly work. In fact, employers would pay them not to work; it's that bad. But never mind. Somebody thinks of them as welfare cheats, so the form addresses problems pertaining to general observations: Please describe posture, gait, mannerisms, and general appearance. Once one passes that barrier one is asked about the details of the present illness, the past illness, the family, social, and environmental history, the current mental status, the current affective status, the current level of functioning including present daily activities, social functioning, concentration and task completion, adaptation to work or worklike situations, current medications, diagnosis, prognosis, and competency. I used to pay serious attention to these forms and dutifully completed most of them and at times received as much as twenty-five dollars for my efforts. Well, you know how it is—a dollar here and a dollar there; it all adds up.

Now when I receive such forms I generally tear off one of my handy OshKosh B'Gosh duplicate progress notes, underline certain key elements of the progress note to call it to the disability evaluator's attention, and everyone is happy.

While I am on the subject of unsolicited mail, I should mention this, although for reasons that will become obvious I hesitate to do so. Many state-funded centers throughout the country focus on the specialized needs of the developmentally disabled. I will frequently get letters from them with the following message:

As you may know, the above-named person, who we understand has been seen by you, is a client of this agency and we are writing at this time for a report of your evaluation. This evaluation will be coordinated with other information from schools, psychologists, etc., to provide us with a comprehensive evaluation which will be useful in total planning for the client. Unless specified to the contrary, this information will be shared with the client, the family, and other involved professionals.

Have you got that so far? Now the next paragraph is in bold print, because that is generally how it appears in the letter:

Enclosed is a signed consent form authorizing the release of information to the _____ Regional Center. Being a nonprofit organization funded by the state of _____, we do not have the financial resources to reimburse you for this information.

The letter is then signed by a physician who works for this boldface nonprofit tax-supported organization who in addition to receiving a salary and paying no overhead, presumably receives sick leave, and vacation benefits—perks that are not ordinarily available to private-practice physicians. Interestingly enough, the letter contains not a trace of the conventional socialized rituals that lubricate the wheels of communication in both Western and Eastern societies, such as "please" or "thanking you in advance for your time." Naturally I cooperate with this agency as much as possible, although I am not ecstatic about cooperating with an agency that demands I volunteer my services and doesn't even say "please."

What else is in the bag? I also stock additional consent forms allowing me to release progress notes to Medicare. This is probably unnecessary since Medicare has a right to inspect the forms even if no release is signed, or so my lawyer tells me.

What else is in the bag? A generalized informed consent form for antipsychotic medications. This is what it looks like:

IMPORTANT INFORMATION ABOUT YOUR MEDICATION:

This medication will help you to relax, think more clearly, keep your thoughts together, and reduce the frequency and intensity of hallucinations. The medication does not produce a high feeling (euphoria) and is not addictive. The medication is usually tolerated well. However, please be aware of possible side effects and precautions (most side effects go away within one or two weeks).

Side Effects/Precautions:

1. You may experience drowsiness, blurred vision, dry mouth, or constipation while taking this medication. Dry mouth may be relieved by chewing sugarless gum. Regular brushing of the teeth is important. The medication may cause blurred vision and/or constipation. Drinking plenty of water, eating fresh fruits and vegetables, and engaging in regular exercise can be helpful in relieving constipation. In addition, use of a stool softener can help prevent constipation.
2. Do not use alcohol or other depressant drugs while taking this medication.
3. Do not drive a car or operate dangerous machinery until you are sure the medication does not make you drowsy.
4. You may experience dizziness or lightheadedness. Get up from a lying position slowly, as standing quickly can cause dizziness. In the morning when you awaken, sit up in the bed for one full minute before standing.
5. If you develop a sore throat without other cold or flu symptoms, this should be reported to your nurse or doctor.
6. You may experience periods of muscle stiffening or restlessness (feeling like you can't sit still and have to move around).
7. Your skin may become more sensitive to the sun. If you are going to be outside, be sure your skin is covered or use a sunscreen lotion containing PABA (para amino benzoic acid) and wear sunglasses.
8. This medication may rarely cause women to lactate or miss menstrual periods.
9. It is important to take this medication exactly as directed. Do not stop taking the medication or change the dosage without contacting me. If you forget a dose during the day, you may take that dose later in the day.
10. Notify me if you have difficulty urinating.
11. Do not take antacids (Maalox, Mylanta, etc.) within an hour of taking this medication.
12. High doses of antipsychotic medication over a long period of time might produce an irreversible movement disorder, characterized by involuntary jerking and twitching, called tardive dyskinesia. Therefore, it is very important that we establish the minimal effective dosage of medication required to maintain symptom relief and prevent relapse of your illness.

This form has both advantages and disadvantages. The advantage of a generalized medication consent form is that it saves one from the nuisance of having to complete separate forms for each medication. I left hospital work after an overly-conscientious hospital administrator insisted that I complete a separate medication consent form for every psychiatric medication, even though some of them are very safe. I knew it was time to leave when, after explaining the side effects of a medication that was only used to treat the side effect of another medication, an impatient inpatient told me that I had just explained that to him and I was repeating myself. I explained that my purpose in doing that was to test his alertness, which of course was an outright lie. After that happened I looked around for a towel to throw in. Once I found it, I threw it.

The disadvantage of this kind of generalized form is that patients might read it. Once having read it, they might say something like this:

> Doctor, you are telling me that this medicine causes drowsiness, blurred vision, a dry mouth, dizziness, lightheadedness, muscle stiffening, restlessness, sensitivity, difficulty in urinating, and an irreversible movement disorder characterized by involuntary jerking and twitching. Doctor, a person has to be crazy to take this medication.

This would be the reaction of a rational person. Fortunately people who take antipsychotic medications are not necessarily rational. Speaking more seriously, the disadvantage of preparing a laundry list of possible adverse reactions can frighten many patients away who might ordinarily benefit from the administration of these medications. This laundry list was plagiarized with some modifications from the consent form of a mental health agency. It is only now, as I write this book, that I realize one interesting omission. Nowhere is there an explicit reference to tremor. The lesson here is that if one tries to list all the possible adverse side effects of a medication, one might omit the most common adverse side effect.

Fortunately, many of the newer so-called atypical antipsychotics do not have many of the side effects listed, so the job of informed consent should be much easier, although I am not sure about how the wording should be constructed and I prefer not to make any suggestions at this time.

What else do I have in the residential care facility paperwork reduction kit? I have a copy of the Global Assessment of Functioning Scale. This is a rating sheet used to assess psychological, social, and occupational functioning in which numerical ratings are used to denote degrees of impairment. These ratings are widely used and are popularly referred to as GAS ratings. There was a time when I didn't know about this and when a social worker told me that one of my patients had a high GAS rating, I promptly ordered antiflatulent medication in accordance with my self-concept of being a renaissance physician practicing enlightened holistic medicine whose therapeutic efforts were not restricted to the provincial demands of psychopathology. Now I know what GAS ratings are, but I can never remember whether 100 is a good score or a bad score, and it is for that reason that I carry an emergency copy of the GAS ratings with me at all times.

Also sometimes I will get calls from other mental health workers who apparently are as inundated with forms as I am, asking me about the meaning of a GAS rating of a particular number—say 50. I am then able to respond quickly, referring to my emergency copy of the rating scale with something like

> A GAS rating of fifty means serious symptoms such as suicidal ideation, severe obsessional rituals, and frequent shoplifting or any serious impairment in social occupational or school functioning such as no friends and unable to keep a job. This of course, is in contrast to a GAS rating of forty, which indicates some impairment in reality testing or communication, such as illogical, obscure, or irrelevant speech, or major impairments in several areas such as work or school, family relations, judgment, thinking, or mood—such as a depressed man who avoids friends, neglects family, and is unable to work—or in the case of a child who frequently beats up younger children, is defiant at home, and is failing at school.

In the recitation of this it is very important to avoid the impression of reading and to simulate complete spontaneity so as to create the perception of encyclopedic knowledge. This will enhance the image of the physician as being a competent and even omniscient professional and will undoubtedly stimulate referrals. If you forget this advice and mnemonic assistance, try to remember the phrase "simulation leads to stimulation." In my case the presence of an emergency GAS rating form is particularly important because I can never remember whether 100 is good or bad—or did I already say that?

Now I take all of these forms and put them in separate folders identifying which form is which, and put all the folders in a professional-looking black bag which I schlep with me (along with the office charts) to the residential care facility, and I am on my way.

Actually there's something else in the bag I almost forgot about because it doesn't fit into a folder. I carry extra vials of fluphenazine decanoate and haloperidol decanoate. I keep extra vials in the bag even though they do not fit the paperwork imagery. These medications are generally kept at the residential care home, but that does not mean they are always found there. In addition, the pharmacy may have forgotten to refill the order. A remote possibility is that the doctor may have forgotten to notify the pharmacy to refill the order, which in actuality is the more likely possibility. (Sometimes when I type remote, I don't mean remote.)

I believe that's enough stuff for one bag. Actually, it's getting rather heavy.

Chapter 12

The Legal Problems

Some of the material in this chapter appeared in an article I wrote for the March 2001 edition of *Psychiatric Times.*[1] I wrote it because of the emerging problems surrounding the issues of medication management and medical necessity which I encountered in a Medicare audit. I believe these issues impact the residential care facility psychiatrist even more than office psychiatrists, because, for previously described reasons, residential care facility psychiatrists are more likely to be targeted for audits. Also, for reasons described below, it is advisable, if not necessary, that the American Psychiatric Association amend its definition of "medical necessity."

As stated in the Introduction, it is estimated that one-third of chronic psychotic patients in California are taken care of in residential care facilities.[2] Also extrapolating from the HCFA statistics on nursing homes, it was estimated that almost 166,000 patients are living in licensed residential care facilities nationwide. One may argue with the methods in the Introduction used to arrive at these statistics, but the exact numbers are not important. Undeniably, this is a large population. However, despite this fact, very little recent literature exists regarding this population. Are these patients best treated in psychiatrist's offices or in clinics or at their places of residence by visiting psychiatrists? If treated on-site, professional organizations and third-party payers will want to know what the appropriated parameters are regarding the problem of visitation frequency. In a previously cited classical study done before the advent of atypical antipsychotics, VanPutten and Spar reported that the average board-and-care resident was visited by a psychiatrist 1.72 times per month and received an average dose of 760 mg of chlorpromazine or chlorpromazine equivalents.[3]

RECENT CHANGES
IN RESIDENTIAL CARE PSYCHIATRY

The nature of residential care psychiatry has undergone a rapid evolution in the past ten years. In a series of articles I described the characteristics of board-and-care psychiatry as well as recent changes which have added to the complexity of the medication management of patients in these homes as well as in other settings.[4] Among these changes are the development of new medications, many of which have the capacity to accelerate or inhibit the metabolism of other drugs; the rise of atypical antipsychotics now regarded by many as the first line treatment for schizophrenia; the increasing necessity to follow drug treatment with laboratory tests (some of which are legally mandated); the emergence of more sophisticated treatment algorithms in which polypharmacy is presented as a viable alternative when patients do not respond to single drugs[5]; the increased frequency of FDA boxed warnings for rare side effects; and the tendency of some of the newer antipsychotic medications to precipitate illnesses. These illnesses include obesity, prediabetic hyperglycemia, osteoporosis, and adverse cardiovascular side effects associated with drug-induced conduction defects (i.e., prolonged QTc interval) such as syncope, ventricular arrhythmias, and ventricular fibrillation (Torsades de Pointes syndrome).

In addition to these medications, many patients require additional treatment for nonpsychiatric concurrent diseases which may or may not have been aggravated by psychiatric medications. In many cases it is difficult to distinguish the psychiatric cart from the nonpsychiatric horse. These nonpsychiatric illnesses, such as arthritis, diabetes, heart disease, hypertension, and hypercholesterolemia—to name only a few—also require treatment with medication. Despite this, the cost of treating mental illness is frequently based on estimates restricted to psychiatric medications while ignoring the added costs incurred by accompanying nonpsychiatric illnesses.

Unfortunately, these increased costs are coming at a bad time, considering the growing requirement to reduce costs because of other priorities, such as additional defense spending. Regrettably, world events have had a negative impact on mental health spending. In addition, more provincial financial demands remain necessitated by the need to balance the federal budget and the perceived threat of Medicare insolvency in the next decade. The combination of these factors has increased the urgency to control costs on the part of managed care providers, third-party payers, and government agencies. As a consequence, all health care providers will come under increasing pressure by federal agencies to justify their role.

THE IMPACT OF HIPAA

The legislative mechanism for such oversight was created in 1996 in the form of the Health Insurance Portability and Accountability Act, otherwise known as the Kennedy-Kassebaum Act, otherwise known as HIPAA acronymically. This act requires that the secretary of Health and Human Services set up a health care fraud program to coordinate the efforts of federal, state, and local law enforcement agencies with the authority to investigate the delivery of health care to all health plans—both public and private. Moreover, the act establishes an account that is funded by civil monetary penalties, criminal fines, and other penalties collected as a result of successful prosecutions and authorizes the use of these funds to finance additional health care fraud prosecutions. The act also provides for whistleblower rewards based on a percentage of recovered moneys. In addition, the act enables the agency to impose civil monetary penalties for certain actions including upcoding, providing unnecessary services and false certification of home health services. These penalties are described as modifications of the Social Security Act in language that is not notable for its clarity.

Here is a good example of what I am talking about. Under section 231 of the act is a section titled "Social Security Act Civil Monetary Penalties" and after that paragraph (c), from which I now quote word for word.

(c) MODIFICATIONS OF AMOUNTS AND ASSESSMENTS.—Section 1128A(a) (42 U.S.C. 1320a-7a(a) as amended by subsection (b), is amended in the matter following paragraph 4—
(1) by striking "$2000" and inserting "$10,000"; (2) by inserting "; in cases under paragraph (4), "$10,000 for each day the prohibited relationship occurs" after "false or misleading information was given"; and
(3) by striking twice the amount and inserting "3 times the amount."

(d) CLARIFICATION OF LEVEL OF KNOWLEDGE REQUIRED FOR IMPOSITION OF CIVIL MONETARY PENALTIES—

(1) IN GENERAL—Section 1128A (a) (42 U.S.C. 1320a-7a(a) is amended—

(A) in paragraphs (1) and (2) by inserting "knowingly" before "presents" each place it appears; and

(B) in paragraph (3) by striking "gives" and inserting "knowingly gives or causes to be given."

(2) DEFINITION OF STANDARD—Section 1128A(i) 42 U.S.C. 1320a—7a(i), as amended by subsection (h) (2) is amended by adding at the end the following new paragraph:

"(7) The term 'should know' means that a person with respect to information—

"(A) acts in deliberate ignorance of the truth or falsity of the information; or

"(B) acts in reckless disregard of the truth or falsity of the information, and no proof of specific intent to defraud is required."

This is very hard to understand and even more difficult to type. It is not easy to get all the capital letters, the upper case A's and B's (each with their own parentheses), the lower case c's and d's (each with their own parentheses), the quotation marks, and the apostrophes all in the right places and in the proper sequence—especially if one has finger agnosia, which I have. The reason why I went to all this trouble is to give the reader a feeling for the aforementioned governmentese, and also to bring to one's attention for future reference the phrase, *"and no proof of specific intent to defraud is required."*

This quote represents a novel concept of fraud. In the past it was necessary to invoke three tests to prosecute a physician for fraud. First, the physician had to make a material misrepresentation of fact. Second, this misrepresentation had to be made with a knowledge of its falsity. Third, that knowing misrepresentation had to be made with the intention that the payer would rely upon that falsity as the reason for payment.

Under the new HIPAA law, a physician engages in health care fraud whenever he or she recklessly or knowingly submits a false, fictitious, or misleading statement of material fact. Fraud also is alleged if the physician omits a material fact from any record, bill, claim form, or other document submitted for payment. In fact, every time such a claim is submitted, a separate crime is inferred. It is not necessary for the government to prove a specific intent to commit fraud. A physician's knowledge of the falsity of a claim can be inferred from the physician's signature on the claim form. The signature itself is sufficient to infer that the physician has read and reviewed the claim. A physician cannot escape culpability by attempting to shift responsibility to administrative staff or billing agencies. Prosecution for fraud can result in draconian financial penalties, criminal conviction with imprisonment, and permanent loss of the physician's license to practice medicine.

To fully understand the evolution of fraud law one must add a pinch of FCA to the HIPAA broth. FCA (standing for False Claims Act) is yet another acrimonious acronym in common use in the twenty-first century, yet the law was passed at the time of the Civil War. The facts underlying its schlepped provenance were as follows: In 1863 Congress passed the FCA in response to widespread fraud by contractors providing goods to the Union Army. One of the first applications of the law was to prosecute horse traders who cheated the government by mixing mules into the herds of horses that they delivered to the army. However, FCA stipulated that in order to be convicted, violators had to commit the acts "knowingly," and this was somewhat problematic because "knowingly" was difficult to prove. Apparently some of the horse traders pleaded innocence because they claimed that they did not know a mule from a horse. Because of this, FCA was amended in 1986 in which "knowingly" was interpreted as the state in which someone had actual knowledge of the information or acted in reckless disregard of the information or acted in deliberate ignorance of the information. In other words, physicians could no longer claim immunity from fraud because they do not know their ass from their horse—not only metaphorically speaking but also in the literal sense. So that is how the concepts of "reckless disregard" and "deliberate ignorance" came to be incorporated into the HIPAA modifications of Medicare fraud.

It seems to me that these concepts carry intrinsic difficulties in enforcement because ignorance implies lack of awareness and deliberate means to consider carefully. That being the case, one might well ask how it is possible to carefully consider something that one is unaware of, even if it means ending the sentence with a preposition. Possibly it is for this reason that the phrase "no proof of specific intent to defraud is required," was inserted into the HIPAA law. Since HIPAA stipulated that "no specific intent to defraud was required" to invoke the $10,000 penalties mentioned in the act, violations that were not actionable under FCA became actionable under HIPAA. What we have here are complementary acronyms. Incidentally, ladled on to these $10,000 penalties like a gratuitous dollop was an additional penalty of three times the charge for the unnecessary service. This is somewhat like adding insult to injury except that in this case it is adding injury to injury, or if you prefer metaphors, being walloped with a dollop.

The problem of upcoding (this being a violation incurred when a physician uses a code that pays more than the code that should be used) and the problem of rendering unnecessary medical services were not addressed by FCA because of its Civil War origins. Following the Civil War there were no codes to up, and it is quite possible that the majority of medical services administered at that time were unnecessary considering medicine's state of development. Thus one couldn't pass a law against rendering medically unnecessary services. If they did this, every physician in the country faced the possibility of incarceration—not a good idea for a developing country.

I now call your attention specifically to how HIPAA handles the problem of medical necessity. These violations are covered under section 231 of the act in the section titled "Social Security Act Civil Monetary Penalties." Within this section is a paragraph titled, "Modification Of Amounts Of Penalties And Assessments—Section 1128A(a) (42 U.S.C. 1320a-7a(a) as amended by subsection (b), is amended in the matter following paragraph 4—(1) by striking '$2000' and inserting '$10,000.'"

Please note that the term *upcoding* is not specifically used in the above paragraph, so it may be safe to assume that the $10,000 penalties for using the wrong code do not necessarily apply to upcoding errors, even though intent is not a necessary precondition for the implementation of this penalty. However, such penalties could be levied on a per service basis for providing services that may be regarded as "medically unnecessary." Obviously the problem of defining medical necessity is quite important. Defining "medically" is not much of a challenge, but defining "unnecessary" is quite another matter and will be directly addressed shortly. But before I do that, other aspects of HIPAA merit serious consideration in relation to prosecutions for fraud.

Under the new law, the secretary of the Department of Health and Human Services (DHHS) and the attorney general are mandated to establish a health care fraud control program to coordinate antifraud activities of local, state, and federal agencies with respect to both public and private plans. Most physicians believe that such antifraud programs are specifically restricted to the government programs of Medicare and Medicaid. This is not so. As part of the health care fraud control program, HIPAA requires that state and federal agencies as well as private plans supply information to a national data bank which contains reports of "final adverse actions" against physicians and other providers concerning violations of health care fraud abuses. The term *final adverse actions* does not include malpractice claims but does include

- Civil or criminal judgments against physicians related to the delivery of health care
- Formal or official actions by state or federal agencies responsible for licensure, such as revocation of licensure, reprimand, censure, or probation
- Any loss of the right to apply for or renew a license, whether by operation of law, voluntary surrender, nonrenewability, or otherwise
- Any other negative action by federal or state agencies that is publicly available
- Exclusion from participation in state or federal health care programs
- Any other adjudicated action or decisions that DHHS establishes by regulation[6]

"Final adverse actions" are entered into a data bank known as the "Healthcare Integrity and Protection Data Bank" which contains all reportable adverse actions taken since the August 21, 1996, enactment date of HIPAA.[7]

To allow for the implementation of this program, HIPAA allows for the sharing of information by health plans, providers, and others. Immunity from prosecution is granted to those persons or entities who provided information to DHHS or the attorney general unless the information was false or the person providing such information had reason to believe the information was false.

In order to finance this program, HIPAA has established a separate Fraud and Abuse Control Account which is funded from moneys from a variety of sources including civil monetary penalties, criminal assessments, and whatever other damages can be recouped through successful health care fraud actions. The funds in this account can then be used to finance additional investigations into fraud and abuse so that a synergistic relationship exists between moneys recovered and additional investigations.

THE PROBLEM OF MEDICAL NECESSITY

How does one judge medical necessity in psychiatry? The American Psychiatric Association has adopted the AMA's definition of medical necessity piecemeal, possibly in deference to the parity concept that all physicians should be treated equally even though some of us may be more equal than others. Medical necessity is defined as follows:[8]

> Health care products or services that a prudent physician would provide to a patient for the purpose of diagnosing or treating an illness, injury, disease or its symptoms in a manner that is: (1) in accordance with generally accepted standards of medical practice; (2) clinically appropriate type, frequency, level, site and duration; and (3) not primarily for the convenience of the patient, physician, or other health care provider.

It is questionable whether such a definition is useful in the evaluation of psychiatric services insofar as the frequency or length of psychotherapy sessions can be interpreted as something done for the "convenience" of the patient. One patient's necessity may be downgraded to another patient's convenience depending on the opinion of an auditor. I believe the medical necessity of any individual psychiatric service should be regarded as a complex decision reached primarily by the psychiatrist, but subject to independent psychiatric reviews based on the needs of the patient. The determination of psychiatric medical necessity should also involve additional information derived from the patient's family, the patient's legal representatives, other professionals involved in the care of the patient, as well as nonprofessionals involved in a caretaking capacity. The current AMA-APA definition of medical necessity does not acknowledge this. These contributions from external sources are in fact very important because, in psychiatry, unlike other medical specializations, we frequently treat patients who are unreliable historians or even who deny illness entirely. It is conceivable that an auditor might not think that the input of a social worker or nonprofessional caretaker is important in the determination of medical necessity given the current APA-AMA definition when such input may be of crucial importance. I believe the concept of medical necessity should be redefined in accordance with the realities of psychiatric practices.

As a specific example, it may not be clear why a patient who was seen in psychotherapy for fifty minutes and charged for this could not be seen for twenty-five minutes thereby incurring a lesser charge. Psychiatrists who are charged with the offense of offering an unnecessary service may find it difficult to defend themselves if the auditor maintains that the fifty-minute session was prolonged "primarily for the convenience of the patient"—to use the term in the quoted definition of medical necessity. Theoretically and legally, the psychiatrist could incur a severe fine for each fifty-minute service that was rendered unless he or she could prove that what was done in fifty minutes could not have been done in twenty-five minutes.

I will concede that if I were asked to justify every visit I made to every patient in terms of the medical necessity criteria currently accepted by American Psychiatric Association or AMA, I doubt whether I could do it. I admit that there are times when I am influenced by the information provided by other professional personnel or caretakers regarding the necessity of making a visit. I do not always know when a patient decompensates because I am not always on the premises, as are caretakers. Frequently I am not in a position to determine the medical necessity of a visit until after I make the visit and make my own assessment.

That is why it is advisable to allow the input of other professionals and caretakers in the determination of medical necessity—and to alter the officially accepted definition of medical necessity to allow supplementary input—even though it is the physician who has and should have the primary responsibility to determine necessity. In my visits to residential care facilities I have generally followed a routine pattern. Sometimes this pattern is every two weeks or monthly depending on the size of the home or the stability of its inhabitants. In the course of many years the expectation has arisen among patients, administrators, and social workers that I should make these routine visits. Perhaps the mere fact that I have been making these visits for over thirty years has contributed to the expectation that I should continue to make the visits even if I chose not to. Frankly, thirty years ago when I was being paid $6.40 per patient per visit, I didn't think much about whether my visits were absolutely necessary. But the expectations of Medicare beneficiaries and their caretakers can easily create the impression of a necessary obligation on the part of the Medicare provider. In this sense, expectation can be the mother of necessity.

Be that as it may, it has been my experience that routine visits by the Modern Psychiatric Team which are not dependent on crises are invaluable in terms of preventing relapses and rehospitalizations. This is true because the psychiatrist can intervene early in the course of an exacerbation, to prevent its development. Generally speaking, routine visits about every two week seem sufficient to create the tight control analog that consists in diabetes therapy—at least in the early phases of a relationship when the patient is not well-known and later shifting to a monthly frequency when the patient is familiar to the psychiatrist and appears reasonably stable.

Nevertheless, some patients demand or expect weekly "sessions."

Such patients are usually educated middle-class expatriates who have abandoned middle-class psychoneurotic ritualisms for an underclass psychosis. Frequently they have the expectation that they can be adequately treated only with weekly or even daily hour-long sessions focusing on insight. Some of these patients have read books on psychoanalysis or have seen movies on the subject starring Gregory Peck. In a sense these are among the saddest of patients, because many of them are ex-achievers who, once having arrived, have been dragged down in the world by their illness. I think in many ways it is more difficult for people who have been dragged down than it is for those who have never been up. An example of this type of patient's questions and commentary follows:

> Do you have any questions for me? Please ask me some questions. How are you? There are twenty-eight days in February. I smoke in the rain and it makes my cigarettes wet. The Artane is working fine and I feel more together. Will you ask me if I have any more side effects? Sometimes my eyes rolled up, but not anymore. My mother said I should take a bath if my eyes rolled up and my eyes would go away. I might be dystonic to my medication. Cary Grant's eyes used to roll up. I used to live with him. Do you want to ask me any more questions? You are the best doctor I have ever had. Can we have psychotherapy sessions?

It is nice to hear the patient say that I am the best doctor he has ever had, but he is not necessarily a reliable informant. It is generally not productive to provide psychotherapy sessions to some patients who are too cognitively impaired to benefit from such offerings. When I refused his request for formal psychotherapy sessions, the patient did not change his opinion that I was the best doctor that he had ever had—possibly my refusal confirmed his opinion.

REDEFINING MEDICAL NECESSITY FOR PSYCHIATRY

With these factors in mind, it might be well for the psychiatric profession to reconsider its piecemeal acceptance of the one-sock-size-fits-all currently accepted APA-AMA definition of medical necessity. What works for socks may not work for shoes. Like it or not, psychiatry as a specialization has distinctive contours which require a more customized approach, and the following definition was offered by me as an approximation of what such a definition might include:[9]

> The definition of "medical necessity" in psychiatry pertains to health care services that a prudent physician would provide to a patient for the purpose of diagnosing and treating a psychiatric illness in a manner that is in accordance with generally accepted community standards of psychiatric practice and clinically appropriate in terms of type, frequency, level, site, and duration. The medical necessity of any individual service is a complex decision reached primarily by the treating psychiatrist but subject to the review of an independent psychiatrist, while taking into consideration the needs of the patient, and which may involve additional information derived from the patient's family, the patient's legal representatives, other professionals involved in the care of the patient, and nonprofessionals involved in a caretaking capacity.

COMPUTERS AND THE MEDICARE AUDIT

I have a naturally sunny disposition but I quickly become very resentful if anyone attempts to undermine my chronic sunniness. In keeping with this, I do not like to receive any letter which contains even the slightest hint of bad news, nor would I willingly continue to read any correspondence that starts with the word *unless,* unless I have been caught unawares. I realize that this reluctance to confront unpleasantries is uncharacteristic for a psychiatrist, and I have little to say in my defense other than to assert that many of my depressed patients seem strangely exhilarated by my unrelenting cheerfulness. However, on occasion I have been accused of having been immunized against empathy. I really don't mind the accusation because it conceals the essential fragility of my moods and it is important for psychiatrists to project the image of emotional stability.

The reason for somewhat inappropriately offering these intensely personal revelations is that I received this letter from someone I don't know who resided in a numbered box in Chico, California, and which I opened with extreme trepidation, and as it turned out, justifiably so. Mind you, all this was before October 2001, when bioterrorists started to mail anthrax in envelopes. This person—a complete stranger—was requesting my "medical legal" records—as if I were both a lawyer and a doctor. This letter, which significantly affected my professional and emotional life for the next three years, started out as follows:

March 15, 1996
Martin Fleishman, MD, Incorporated
2305 Van Ness, Suite F
San Francisco, California 94109

MEDICARE

Provider Review/Utilization Review
Post Office Box xxxxx
Chico, California 95927-2806

IMPORTANT REQUEST FOR MEDICAL LEGAL RECORDS

We annually audit a percentage of claims for services provided to Medicare beneficiaries (patients) as required under Section 1842 of the Social Security Act (SSA). Some claims for services provided by you to specific beneficiaries are included this year.

The audit will review services paid between July 1, 1995, through December listed on the attached sheet. The inclusive dates of service are listed for each patient. Records should reflect all documentation of services rendered including the following:

History and Physical Examinations
Consultations

Al I Test Reports
Office Visit Progress Notes
Operative/Procedure Reports

If any of the patients on the enclosed list were hospitalized during this
period of time, we also require:

Admission History and Physical
Daily Physician Visit Progress Notes
Physicians Orders
Operative/Procedure Reports
Discharge Summary

   Since the audit will involve examination of the records to determine
medical necessity, appropriateness of services, utilization patterns, et
cetera, it is important that you provide copies of any documentation,
even from outside of the review period, that could affect a determination.
   Please send legible photocopies of all records for the patient listed
on the attached sheet within forty-five (45) days from the date of this
notice.
Etc. etc.

   It is obvious that my initial apprehensions were entirely war-
ranted. It is perhaps fitting that the date of this letter was March 15,
1996 (a day sometimes referred to as the Ides of March—the day Jul-
ius Caesar was warned to "beware of"). This letter was to lead to ongoing correspondence with attorneys, Medicare auditors, Medicare
Hearing Officers, Administrative Law Judges, and magazine editors—as well as personal interviews with most of the above. It was to
interfere with much of my sleep, consume most of my waking hours,
and virtually eliminate recreational television as a nightly release for
the next three years. In short it became an obsession, and the usual
treatments for obsessions—group meetings and psychotherapy with
understanding psychiatrists who are understanding because they are
understandably happy that they are not in your shoes—were unavailable because attorneys advise you not to talk to anybody about your
legal difficulties. It is not surprising then, that this letter definitely undermined my aforementioned and otherwise irrepressible sunniness,
and made me irritable and cranky.
   When one is deprived of the strength afforded by the external val-
idations of one's worth from friends and colleagues, it is like being
in a state of not-quite-solitary confinement—that is to say, your
body is not confined but in a sense your mind is so that strange

things can happen. What I mean by this is that strange thoughts can happen. At times I found myself doubting my own worth—wondering if perhaps I had been guilty of inadvertent oversights or, even worse, fraud. The possibility of fraud arises even when there is no fraudulent intent because fraudulent intent is no longer essential for the allegation of fraud—a point that was made earlier in this chapter in bold print. Under such circumstances, it is easy to question one's own motivations and to construct lugubrious premonitions about spending the rest of one's life in a penal colony. By "one's life," I am actually referring to my life.

I really did not understand the reason for the audit, and wondered whether the audit was instigated by patient complaints or was essentially random in nature, so I forwarded a letter to the auditor requesting clarification about this. He was nice enough to respond and his letter was revelatory: My problem was that my use of medication management codes created an outlier aberrant service code profile compared to the codes generated by other psychiatrists, which in and of itself is sufficient to trigger a computer-based audit. Well, the problem is that on-site psychiatric services to schizophrenic occupants of residential care facilities—which necessarily has a psychopharmacological emphasis—is quite different from office-based practices which have more of a psychotherapeutic focus, so the comparison is inappropriate. Probably, I shall be somewhat repetitive about this point since in all truth I am trying to influence Medicare. However, the computer doesn't know what is appropriate or inappropriate—at least in this area because it was not programmed to recognize this. It was just an ordinary run-of-the-mill computer, not a terribly bright one which (or who?) knew which end was up, like Hal, in *2001—A Space Odyssey*.

Another reason why on-site providers are more subject to audits is because Medicare administrators sometimes cast a jaundiced eye on a single provider servicing multiple patients at the same nonhospital site, such as nursing homes, locked facilities, or the aforementioned residential care facilities. Visits to these facilities are sometimes pejoratively viewed as "gang visits," by "high-volume providers" and may be regarded as essentially abusive. High-volume practices may be abusive but not necessarily.

What looks abusive may actually not be abusive because high-volume providers with specialized foci may be able to work much more rapidly than generalists particularly where the high-volume provider sees the same patients recurrently. Such psychiatrists can work very efficiently if they know the patients, know the problems of the patients, and have taken the time and trouble to organize the patient's drug history on the basis of their own progress notes as well as information contained from hospital summaries (assuming the psychiatrists have taken the additional time and trouble to request those summaries and review them in the privacy of their own offices). The issue of abuse should not be inferred from numbers alone but can be inferred from a number of other factors such as usefulness of the progress notes (a quality not necessarily related to length), patient complaints, co-worker evaluations, house staff evaluations, and under certain circumstances, criminality rates, rehospitalization rates, and suicide rates (approximately 10 percent of the schizophrenic population commit suicide according to some estimates).

In keeping with the imperious demands of my aforementioned sunny disposition, I tried to find something good about this audit letter—looking for the needle of hope in this haystack of offal—and I actually found it. John Doe indicated under his signature that he was representing "Medicare Utilization Review." Why was this good? This was good because of what he was not representing. That is to say if the letter was signed by someone who identified himself or herself as "Special Investigator, Medicare Program Integrity Unit," this would have been much worse. This usually indicates a nonroutine problem in which there is a strong suspicion of fraud or abuse.

The role of carrier representatives, such as the aforementioned special investigator, is described in a book titled *Medicare Carriers Manual* which describes their primary role in identifying cases of fraud or abuse. Following is a quotation from the California Medical Association's *2001 CMA On-Call #0625 "Medicare Audits,"* p. 2. CMA On-Call is the California Medical Association's online library of medicolegal regulatory and reimbursement information that is updated annually and addresses issues affecting the practice of medicine in California. [10]

Medicare carriers play an important role with respect to Medicare program integrity. The Medicare Carriers Manual provides that their primary role in this regard is to identify cases of suspected fraud and abuse and refer them to Office of Investigations field officers for consideration of sanctions. Recent changes in the Medicare Carriers Manual mandate that carriers establish and maintain a Medicare Fraud Investigation Branch led by a Program Integrity Coordinator. When detecting fraud and abuse, a Program Integrity Coordinator must be able to coordinate effectively with all departments of a carrier, but particularly the medical review department. Carriers must have written procedures for personnel to identify fraud and abuse situations and are now required to "carefully evaluate completed billing forms to detect apparent inconsistencies in the coverage and payment of services." Additionally, they must maintain documentation in provider files of the details of telephone or personal contacts involving fraud and abuse issues discussed with providers and their staff; this documentation must be maintained for seven years. Carriers must also establish and maintain a communications network with community providers to keep them informed about fraud and abuse issues and "periodically include inserts with Explanations of Medicare Benefits to educate beneficiaries about the types of fraud and abuse they can identify."

The previously mentioned Program Integrity Coordinator implements policy from the Program Integrity Manual, which reflects the principles, values, and programs for Medicare. According to the manual, the primary principle of program integrity is to pay claims correctly. In order to meet this goal, the manual requires contractors to ensure that they pay the correct amount for covered and correctly coded services. Since 2001 the Centers for Medicare and Medicaid Services (CMS) has made a number of changes in the "program integrity" activities of its fiscal intermediaries and carriers. These changes are incorporated in the *2003 CMA On-Call #0625 "Medicare Audits,"* pp. 2-3, to include the following:

- Preventing fraud through effective enrollment and education of providers and beneficiaries
- Early detection of errors or fraud by medical review and data analysis

- Close coordination with partners, including contractors and law enforcement agencies
- Implementation of fair and firm policies

In addition, CMS is now attempting to make the audit process more fair to physicians. In pursuit of this objective, CMS has consented to the following policy changes advocated by the California Medical Association and the American Medical Association:

- Carrier decisions to conduct medical reviews should be data driven.
- Medical reviews should be no more extensive than necessary.
- Carriers should consider the past history of billing errors.
- Actions imposed by failure to meet Medicare rules should be appropriate to the level of noncompliance.
- Carriers should provide comparative data on how the physician varies from same-specialty physicians in the payment locality.
- Carriers should notify physicians in writing when they are placed on or removed from medical reviews.
- Carriers should notify physicians of specific actions that they must take to resolve problems.
- Physicians should be removed from review as soon as possible when compliance is demonstrated.
- Undercoded claims should be considered in calculating physician error rate.
- Carriers should consider administrative law judge reversal rates when implementing medical review.[11]

Obviously all audit notifications should be taken seriously, whether coming from Medication Utilization Review or from the Special Investigator, and physicians so notified should contact an attorney, preferably one experienced in Medicare law.

The audits can come from either Medicare or Medicaid or both. However, if one is the subject of a federal Medicare audit, it is entirely possible that the state Medicaid people will be joining the posse. It's similar to what happens in cases of tax evasion. First one will get an insulting letter from the Internal Revenue Service. Somewhat later one will receive a letter from some nosy person in state government who has been reading your mail.

Here is an officially documented reason for the Medicare audit as sent to me by John. I started calling him John because we had become real pen pals. Did I already mention that the Medicare auditors I was dealing with were really very conscientious and were dedicated civil servants? Well, they were, and presumably still are, so I repeat, if one is going to cross swords with them, one should do so courteously.

MEDICARE

PROVIDER REVIEW/UTILIZATION REVIEW
POST OFFICE BOX XXXX
Chico, California 95927-2806

Martin Fleishman, MD, Inc.
2305 Van Ness Avenue
San Francisco, California 94109

Dear Dr. Fleishman:

This is in response to your letter dated June 7, 1998, in which you request further information on why you were chosen for audit and the extrapolation process.

As we discussed during a recent telephone conversation, your practice was selected for the Provider Audit List (PAL) for medical review in the Utilization Review (UR) unit in accordance with the guidelines as stated in the Medicare Carriers Manual (MCM) section 7500. The Health Care Financing Administration (HCFA) requires that we conduct postpayment reviews of claims of a specific provider or group of providers in order to evaluate his/her/their/billing patterns over a selected period of time. Your practice was selected because our internal reports indicated the possibility of over-utilization of pharmacologic management visits over that of your peers. This profile aberrancy is illustrated in the graph below. The graph compares your usage of Pharmacologic Management versus that of your peers. Your peers are defined as all other psychiatrists billing for Medicare patients in your locality.

When I received this letter I really did not understand the implications of the term, or possibly I should say allegation, of "profile aberrancy." Acting on impulse, I inspected my physiognomy in the mirror to obtain some clue to determine if my profile was really as aberrant as the Medicare statistical gumshoes claimed. During this time I engaged in imaginary conversations with my adversaries, which is what psychiatrists frequently do to preserve their sanity, but rarely admit.

THEM: We regret to inform you that the National Bell Curve Office of Audits and Investigations has determined that you are charging for services that exceed customary and usual practices and you are two standard deviations above the mean. You therefore have an aberrant profile and we are going to audit you in response to orders personally delivered by the surgeon general of the United States of America with you in mind.

ME [in the menacing manner of Robert De Niro's psychotic antihero in *Taxi Driver* as he postures before a mirror and brandishes a pistol]: Are you talking to me? Are *you* talking to *me?*"

Following this narcissistic soliloquy, I turned away from the mirror even though this was difficult for me, and I looked at the world of reality. The letter included the sentence, "Your practice was selected because our internal reports indicated the possibility of overutilization of pharmacologic management visits over that of your peers."

In other words, I qualified for audit status because I had an atypical billing pattern when I was compared to other psychiatrists and I was perceived as possibly rendering services that violated the dictates of medical necessity.

Of course there were good reasons for my profile aberrancy since my practice was aberrant in the sense that I was doing something most psychiatrists do not do. I was providing on-site services to patients residing in residential care facilities. If I practiced office psychiatry my profile would have been similar to other psychiatrists practicing office psychiatry and I never would have been audited. Nevertheless, an audit was initiated. This started out with an initial assessment that I had been overpaid by the sum of over $52,609.59.

Every psychiatrist who does on-site work in residential care facilities or similar facilities can expect to be audited because this kind of work generally demands psychopharmacological evaluations rather than psychotherapy, as previously stated. The computer will then decide that you as the residential care facility psychiatrist are using psychopharmacological codes more frequently than the average psychiatrist. The average psychiatrist is office based, but never mind. The computer throws every one into the same egalitarian pot. The residential care psychiatrist is then relegated to that worst of all destinies. He or she becomes an outlier. To be an outlier in the statistical sense means that one is not typical of the statistical category to which one has been assigned. If that is unclear let us use *Webster's* definition: "One who or that which has been beyond or has been excluded from the main body." So that is it. The computer decides that I as a psychiatrist was "one who or that which has been beyond or has been excluded from the main body," the main body in this instance being the population of psychiatrists. Being an outlier is bad, because Medicare computers are programmed to target outliers for audits. Outliers are somewhat like outlaws except the spelling is a little different and they are audited instead of incarcerated. Outliers are only incarcerated after an audit.

COMPUTERS AND THE MEDICAID AUDIT

Being an outlier is not only a temptation for the federal Medicare computers, but it also identifies one as a "person of interest" for the state (Medicaid) computers. The difference however is this: Medicare starts its audits with a demand for records. The records are then reviewed followed by a demand for money based on an audit of the records. Medicaid, on the other hand, does not request records; they merely request money. The Medicaid program is the federal-state partnership that provides health care to the poor. It is administered at the federal level by CMS and at the California state level by the Department of Health Services and is called Medi-Cal.

Getting money, either by demand or by request, has an obvious advantage over requesting records because if the money is received, records do not have to be obtained and analyzed. Therefore salaries for auditors do not have to be paid. After all, auditors need to eat also—even if they are auditors. This saves money all the way around with the exception of the physician who is providing the money. The exchange of money is a perfect example of a zero-sum game. When one is audited by Medicare, one can expect the Medi-Cal auditors to be in hot pursuit. Here is how it happened.

Shortly after the grueling examination of my physiognomy, I received yet another unsolicited letter. This was from the local friendly state Medi-Cal dealer at the Department of Health Services in Sacramento. For those of you who do not speak Californian, let me explain that Medi-Cal is Californian for Medicaid. This letter was from the Third Party Liability Branch, Recovery Section-Overpayment Unit, so right away I was a little suspicious, and my first impulse was to relegate it to the round file.

However, I opened it anyway although this was against my better judgment. So this was from Medi-Cal, and it started out with "Dear Provider Number xxxxx." Well, addressing me as a number rather than by name made me a little nervous, possibly because I had recently seen a TV program on concentration camps or possibly because it gave me an intuitive premonition as to what my future might be like. Anyway, the letter started out with words like "The Medical Review Branch of Audits and Investigations, Department of Health Services, has analyzed data from your paid claims for the twelve-month period of" blah-blah to blah-blah or words to that effect. It went on to say that on the basis of this paid data my services for procedure code number 90862 exceeded customary and usual practices and I should remit the sum of $32,641.30 which I could do "without penalty" or else. Okay, they didn't really say "or else," but if you present the option of "without penalty," presumably there is the alternative option of "penalty" even if it isn't explicitly stated.

I know one might think that I am exaggerating so here is a verbatim reproduction of this letter from this uncivil civil servant:

DEPARTMENT OF HEALTH SERVICES

714/ 744 P STREET
P.O. BOX xxxxxxx
SACRAMENTO, CA 94234

Martin Fleishman, MD, Inc.
2305 Van Ness Avenue, Suite F
San Francisco, CA 94109

Dear Provider:

PROVIDER NUMBER xxxxx

The Medical Review Branch of Audits and Investigations, Department of Health Services Department has analyzed data from your Medi-Cal paid claims for the twelve-month period of August 1996 through July 1997.

Our analysis of your paid claim data shows that you are claiming for services which exceed customary and usual practices. The service(s) you claimed and were paid for are as follows:

Pharmacologic Management, including prescription use and review of medication with no more than minimal medical psychotherapy, CPT-4 90862—$32,641.30

Reimbursement for CPT-4 90862 is separately payable by Medi-Cal only when: the service as defined in the CPT-4 is performed by you; is medically indicated; and is not billed with any other psychotherapy or Evaluation and Management service on the same date of service for the same patient. Claims for this service billed with any other psychotherapy and/or Evaluation and Management service are not separately payable.

Please assure that the services you claim meet the above reimbursement requirements. In the event that you have been paid for services that did not meet these requirements, you may, without penalty, refund that amount by making a check payable to the Department of Health Services and mailing it to:

Please attach the enclosed copy of this letter with any refund. Questions regarding repayment arrangements should be directed to the Department's Recovery Section—Overpayment Unit at the above address.

The analysis and identification of the paid claims amount for this service does not limit your liability to the Department of Health Services for this and any other services based on any subsequent audits for this or any other time period.

Please be advised that submission of claims for items or services which were not provided as claimed, are not reimbursable under the Medi-Cal program, or were claimed in violation of an agreement with the State, may subject you to civil money penalties in accordance with Welfare and Institutions Code, Section 14123.2 and Title 22, California Code of Regulations, Section 51485.1.

If you have any questions concerning this matter, please contact Mr. John Doe, at blah, blah, blah.

Sincerely,
John Doe (I'm not the federal John Doe—I'm the state John Doe)

Admittedly, this is not an exact verbatim reproduction of the letter from my unwanted pen pal, but most of the letter is verbatim. The part that is not verbatim is the part of it after "Sincerely" that says "I'm not the federal John Doe—I'm the state John Doe." Also the terminal "blah, blah, blah" is not verbatim. The truth is I am slow to anger and at first I planned to respond by assuring the investigator that I was a good provider. However, after some intensive slow thinking it occurred to me in my nonlawyer's mind that this letter was somewhere between fishing-expeditionland and extortionland.

I was definitely irked by this whole experience. I'm sure other physicians in the United States of America have had similar experiences and were also "irked." I'm sure about this because in February 2001, the *American Medical Association News* indicated that other doctors were also "irked," as was reported under the following headline:[12]

Doctors Irked by States' Tactics on Medicaid Fraud

A growing number of states are using sophisticated computer programs to root out Medicaid fraud and overpayment, but doctors are furious about some approaches.

Medicaid programs nationwide face big shortfalls, and a growing number of states are turning to computers to help them make sure existing money is being spent properly. States say intelligent software helps them recover money, correct honest billing mistakes and detect fraud that would go unnoticed. Physicians, though, are outraged at some states' tactics. They believe it's unfair to go back three to five years to look for fraud when most doctors have only a year to file Medicaid claims. They say the system is tainted when companies are paid a percentage of what they recover.

Doctors also question computer algorithms used to find billing errors. In some cases, the computer program made the error, not the doctor, they say. States using outside contractors incorporate the computer audits' findings into letters sent to doctors that say how much the physicians owe Medicaid. These unexpected letters have angered some physicians. (*American Medical Association News,* February 19, 2001, Vol. 44, p.1. Copyrighted 2001, American Medical Association.)

The fact is "state John Doe" really made me even more "irked" than "federal John Doe," and that was even before I read this article about other doctors being "irked." Now English is a very utilitarian language and it invites all to its table providing whoever comes can make a contribution—somewhat like linguistic potluck. *Chutzpah* is just such a Yiddish newcomer that has acquired country club respectability by virtue of its unique ability to express what Webster defines as "brazen effrontery." However, it does this in one word rather than two, which gives it more of an emotional bang for the buck—I mean more of an impact. The first syllable is ushered from that deep part of the throat that is the pharyngeal site of seething indignation followed by the explosive terminal *pah,* which is really the vocalized form of an exclamation mark. Its sense is best expressed if it is uttered with a guttural rendition of the first syllable in which the back of the tongue approaches the soft palate and in which one's attitude, rather than one's teeth, is gritted. This is not a common sound in English so one must practice to get it right, as one must practice with the Spanish double R to get that right.

The word is singularly applicable in certain types of situations, and best defined by a person who kills his parents and then asks the judge for mercy on the basis that he is an orphan. I mean, here is this presumptuous unwanted pen pal, this official state John Doe—this Californian state John Doe—trying to extort some dough from some John—namely me, a fellow California taxpayer whose taxes help pay for the salary of this state John Doe, and he tries to shake me down simply because he doesn't like my profile. Moreover, he doesn't even demand an audit; he simply demands money and talks about penalties if he doesn't get money. I am trying to convey by this mini-exegesis on *chutzpah* that I was more than "irked." My irrepressible sunniness was undermined and I was seething with indignation.

However, other aspects of his letter were irksome for other reasons and really alienated my etymological sensitivities. I refer to the use of "customary" and "usual" in the same sentence as when he claimed that my "services exceeded usual and customary practices." This really is an unforgivable redundancy and if I were his English teacher I would have underlined the phrase and asked him to see me after class.

The phrase "usual and customary" presumes guilt in that "usual" sounds very sinister when accompanied by "customary" or maybe I should say when aided and abetted by "customary," while "usual" unaccompanied by "customary" sounds pretty usual. In fact, "aided and abetted," which I used in the preceding sentence, is another combinatorial phrase implying evil intent. One never uses "aided and abetted" to describe a kindly act such as helping a blind person cross the street by aiding and abetting this person even if it's done in a usual and customary manner. I will admit, however, that I have never seen a physician help a blind person across the street. As a rule, we are too pressed for time and can't be bothered with such petty annoyances. With respect to these observations, I believe that I have already stated in a previous chapter that I am subject to digressive ramblings which bubble to the surface of consciousness and which must then be registered in this document in the manner of a ship's captain as he enters the important vicissitudes of his journey into a ship's log.

I met this state John Doe at a social function some time after I received his letter and he did not seem like such a bad fellow. He felt a little guilty about hassling me and explained somewhat apologetically that he was bucking for a G-12 promotion, or some kind of a civil service rating similar to that, and he was under pressure to be more productive. He had nothing against doctors personally. He confided, sub-rosa, that his brother-in-law was a doctor and he was having him investigated in accord with his civil service ambitions. He relayed the fact that even his doctor was a doctor, and we both broke into convulsive laughter, only mine was pure simulation.

Before I digressed I indicated that I was accused of receiving $52,609.59 in Medicare overpayments and I rather quickly veered away from explaining this. The reason for going public with my dirty little secret is that after my $52,609.59 comeuppance, I cheerfully told my wife that it could be worse. When she asked me what I meant by this, I responded that we should look for the silver lining. Some of us are so blessed by an overabundance of felicity that the meaning of any noxious event, no matter how degrading or destructive, is twisted like a pretzel so as to allow a foolishly positive interpretation. I will admit membership in this fraternity of "irrational exuberance," a term first offered by Alan Greenspan ostensibly to describe the personalities of stock market investors, but two weeks after this memorable utterance he committed marriage, so God only knows what the man had in mind. As far as I know, I am the only one who has noticed this strange temporal syzygy. A syzygy is not a Japanese blue-plate special, but a term which I use to denote a conjunction in time; perhaps such confluences are only registered through the baleful eye of an admitted psychiatrist. I realize that I have already remarked upon this phenomenon in Chapter 3, but since I am the only one who appears to have made this association, it bears repetition. Also before I did not describe it as a syzygy, and syzygy is a killer word in Scrabble.

When my wife questioned me about the content of the silver lining, I provided her with three silver linings. Silver lining number one: the estimates of the overpayments could have even been greater. Silver lining number two: at least I wasn't being prosecuted for fraud. Silver lining number three: the Medicare audit will afford me an opportunity to become rich and famous because I will write a fantastically hilarious book about my experiences in the audit.

I will write this fictional book about this psychiatrist named Dr. Ecks (instead of Dr. X, get it? Easier to explain in print than orally) who was imprisoned because of clerical errors. Not the clerical errors committed by priests, ministers, and rabbis that make the headlines occasionally—okay, more than occasionally—but clerical errors in his billing practices. This book will have a Horatio Alger-type motif, but with an ingenious twist. It will be about Horatio Alger, MD.

In keeping with the Horatio Alger, MD, theme, this Dr. Ecks would start out as a real loser, a sartorially challenged workaholic who would always need a haircut because he would never have time to go to a barber and lacked sufficient self-esteem to go to a hairstylist where he would have to schedule an appointment. He couldn't make any kind of caretaking appointments because he felt guilty about consuming another person's time. To make matters worse, he would wear the same thin limp brown powerless tie which would hang loosely around a predictably frayed collar with an equally predictable asymmetrical knot. He would wear drip-dry shirts, frequently incompletely dried, and trousers with the barely detectable musk of chronicity, threadbare at the cuff and shiny in the seat, and just a wee bit too tight at the crotch to permit unfettered compliance with a rigorously enforced dress code. Instead of sipping fine wine and simulating an easy familiarity with vintage years, he would prefer to guzzle Coca-Cola, where vintage years are not a challenge. He would get Chinese fortune cookies that contained insulting observations about his personality and predicted a dismal future for him—and correctly so. The slightest whiff of his faintest scent would induce ordinarily playful cocker spaniel lap dogs to leap from their proprietary pelvic habitats and cower in corners with their paws over their noses.

Some wags would once describe his personality as magnetic, but with negativity at both poles. Other wags would have other tales if you will permit the pun. For instance, his relationships with people would be no better than his relationship with dogs. He could never remember people's names even though some of them worked with him on a daily basis. Professionally dedicated social workers would eventually refuse to do social work for him or even socialize with him. His dearest and closest friend was a cybernet e-mail pen pal whom he had actually never met. His own mother would try to unload his bronzed baby shoes at garage sales but nobody wanted them, even at rock-bottom prices. She would describe him as a "nervous child" even after he became an adult, while falsely denying that she was his birth mother and encouraging him to search for his biological roots—this having occurred, mind you, after he became a doctor. He would live with her until he was forty-two, and during much of this time she would prepare his bag lunches with day-old sesame seed pumpernickel bagels, hard as concrete, including the sesame seeds—especially the sesame seeds—wrapped in road maps with triple-A triptych routings to exotic destinations. However, he would never take the hint. He was, as they say, slow on the uptake and even slower on the downtake, if there is such a thing. He was not only a loser but a role model for losers. If there were a program such as *America's Least Wanted,* he would have been a guest star. His destiny was to wander about in his own country as a stranger in a strange land without any intimate relationships involving him and a significant other. And if there were any significant others, they wanted no part of him. Even insignificant others—and there were lots of them—would avoid him like the plague. In a pathetic attempt to create other significant others through political alliances, he would plaster his car with large stickers advocating sadly misdirected humanitarian goals such as "Free New Jersey" or "No War on France." In pursuit of humanitarianism he changed his diet so as to avoid the killing of all vegetables—with the exception of broccoli, which he loved. His best and only friend was someone he met on the Internet—an otherwise friendless hermit named Dave who kept a laptop in his cave. He was uncharitably described by others as a kind of personalized Oakland in which there was no "there" there. He was strictly a third-person personality—always referred to by "he" or more likely "him" or even "that." "That" was used as a substitute for a personal pronoun stripped of any personal reference or involvement, and all this done with a wink and a shrug and a nod and other unflattering dismissive one-syllable posturings because there is little that can actually be said about a person whose name evokes neither warmth nor hatred but fanatical apathy—a third-person entity wandering in the land of third-person people, with no friends, confidants, or admirers. His only contacts would be with mental patients and these not among the rich and famous but scattered among the poor and inconsequential, as the residents of residential care facilities are harshly perceived.

Given all of the above, it is not surprising that Dr. Ecks had enemies especially considering the tenor of the times. When I write about Dr. Ecks, I will place him in the pre-9/11 environment during which time the FBI was starting to focus on dishonest doctors. Prior to Global Terror Initiation Day, Medicare fraud was the number-one criminal problem in the United States, and whistleblowing provisions were included as part of the HIPAA legislation. These provisions allowed the whistleblower to retain as much as one-third of the imposed penalties. That being the case, big money was involved and a lot of mean people became fascinated with the prospect of getting even with dishonest doctors—I mean all kinds of people—not only people such as hostile patients but also the hostile relatives of hostile patients with similar identifying DNA miscalculations. This also included people who are neither hostile patients nor their confrontational relatives, such as tattooed muscle-bound professional bounty hunters with semicriminal backgrounds, or righteous impatient patient's rights activists in active pursuit of their whistleblower's rights, or entrepreneurial case managers trying to manage a federal case from the cases they managed, not to mention infuriated NIMBY neighbors of group homes with primordial vendettas against the medical profession because of the perception that "gang" visits by physicians lowered their property values.

In addition to this bunch, there were the hopeful malcontents in the semiprofessional and professional classes who were more dangerous because they had a more intimate knowledge of the physician's procedure code indiscretions. I am talking about such people as alienated employees with sometimes justifiable grievances about their 401(K) pension plans, and disillusioned home-visiting nurses exasperated by the penny-pinching tactics of their managed care home-visiting employment agencies. Also let's not forget about vindictive physicians thirsting for revenge because of real or imagined injustices inflicted upon them by former associates or competitors. Even more dangerous to psychiatrists were some of their colleagues in the mental health professions including politically correct asocial social workers with antiestablishment agendas who perceived whistleblowing as a form of working for the working classes, and outwardly composed clinical psychologists seething with inner deep-seated envious professional-turf hatreds and contesting their territorial prescription-writing claims with the unbridled postpubertal ferocity of the mammalian rut. These groups consisting of the disenchanted and disaffected, the uncivil and the unraveled, the gruntled and the disgruntled—some of them homeless, all afflicted with the same ophthalmological symptom-complex of having dollar signs in their eyes accompanied by severe whistleblowing aspirations—courtesy of the big-rock-candy-mountain, easy-street, 30 percent piece-of-the-action giveaways promised by the whistleblower provisions of HIPAA.

Given the uncharming personality of Dr. Ecks and the predictable impact of the whistleblower law, it is not surprising that among his encyclopedia of enemies, one of the above if not all of the above, fingered Dr. Ecks. Thus, inevitably, he is apprehended. I believe I have already implied that he was convicted because he billed Medicare patients for psychotherapy codes when he should have been billing for medication management codes. To add insult to injury—or more accurately to add injury to injury, the judge confuses the concept of "gang visits" with "gangland visits" with all its RICO ramifications, and for this reason he imposes the maximum allowable sentence, a fact which only serves to contribute to the book's hilariousness.

I know that in recounting this story I went into one of those comedic convulsive ticlike seizures which I am subject to and which I vaguely described in the introductory chapter. As I said, I cannot suppress these states either orally or in print, as is now evident, lest I precipitate one of those akathisia-like episodes which I shall describe at length later in this book, but clearly I was on a roll. If I were a standup comic, people would be rolling in the aisles. My wife, who was not in the aisles, rolling or otherwise, and who is not only my severest critic but also probably my most destructive (which is a formidable combination), responded that the loser scenario was quite familiar to her and that I was really not very funny or very creative; I was merely being autobiographical. She wondered how I could possibly transform such an inveterate loser into a credible winner in keeping with the Horatio Alger, MD, motif.

Actually this was not much of a problem. The conversion was easy. First he will be remanded to Terminal Island because that is a great name for a place to incarcerate a physician convicted of Medicare malfeasance or misfeasance or other types of feasances, and thereby terminate his professional career. Terminal Island is a federal penitentiary near Los Angeles but there is no corollary Beginning Island although there is a Midway Island somewhere in the middle, but that is neither here nor there as the residents of Midway will readily concur, and as is this entire aside.

Because he has such a miserable personality and nobody can stand him, they immediately place him in solitary confinement, for doing nothing at all, and reputedly for his own good until the prison authorities discovered that he was quite introverted and relished his solitude. Actually the administration caught on to his little game only after he submitted a treatment authorization request in which he demanded that his period of solitary confinement be extended indefinitely, at which point they forcibly enrolled him in a resocialization group, this being a placement that was dictated more by sadism than for compassionate or rehabilitative reasons.

Luckily for him, his resocialization therapist practiced a form of group therapy called influential therapy (called IT by knowledgeable insiders but not pronounced as a single word but with a separate articulation of the letters—as with the I first and then later the T, as in I period and later T period—or more precisely I followed by a period of silence and then T followed by silence—I hope I am making myself clear about this) based on a book by someone called Dale Carnegie. Many of the principles Dr. Ecks found quite useful—as for instance the importance of remembering people's names after being introduced for the first time—or even for the second time—which Dr. Ecks could never do until the time he was enrolled in the course. Thus, following an introduction to someone named, as an example, John Smith, a name which one might not be otherwise able to remember; you ingrain the name in your memory by repeating the name in conversation over and over again, such as "Nice meeting you, John," or "How are you feeling today, John?" or "Yes, I remember you from last time, John. How do you spell your last name again, John?" or "Do you know where the john is, John?"

This experience in therapy made a tremendous impact on him giving him a quasi-religious experience. He then becomes born again even though he was not born once, but not in the Charles Coulson sense (the famous Watergate conspirator who was born again after having indeed been born once, and who subsequently found God after being incarcerated). Not at all—he was converted more in the Dale Carnegie-how-to-win-friends sense than the Charles Coulson soulswinning sense. In keeping with this reawakening, he tries to change his personality and become an extraverted joiner. In the process of reinventing himself as a hail-fellow-well-met, he applies for admission to the Aryan Brotherhood but is rejected by their credentials committee as having qualifications of dubious authenticity. Besides, they took umbrage at his nondiscriminatory joviality and socially awkward attempts at gregariousness by addressing every Aryan by his first name without waiting for the courtesies of formal introductions—but not only that—he addressed them all as "John," which in and of itself was an unpardonable gaucherie—even though he was not eligible for a pardon—and sufficient to raise many a tattooed eyebrow.

However, he refused to be deterred from his ambition to become a joiner and subsequently attempted to affiliate with some of the other tattoed mesomorphic confraternities that dominate the prison system such as the Mexican Mafia, but he was rejected because he failed the entrance exam—which was in Spanish. Also the membership committee felt he was being inappropriately patronizing when he addressed all the Latino prisoners as "Juan."

Undaunted, he then attempted to join the Black Muslems, but sadly was rejected once again, this time because he was neither black, nor Muslem. He then becomes very depressed because one of the reasons why he went to jail was because Medicare accused him of making so-called gang visits to residential care facilities, and now he was rejected by these very gangs—or similar to these very gangs (at least in his eyes)—that he used to visit when he made home visits. How quickly they forget. Try to grasp the irony of the situation. Finally, instead of continuing undaunted, he becomes daunted. Increasingly disconsolate as a result of his failed attempts at socialization, and in desperation, he tries to escape and actually succeeds in his efforts by utilizing the techniques that he learned in his IT (I period of silence and then T period of silence) resocialization group therapy sessions based on *How to Win Friends and Influence People*. He did this by winning over and influencing the prison guards. Basically this psychiatrist simply impersonated a normal friendly person, a stratagem which completely fooled the prison guards. He then manages to escape to an overseas destination and tries to found an organization which he calls the National Fugitives Association, but nobody wanted to join because the Swiss police demanded a membership list. He then changes the name of the organization to the Concerned American Expatriate Physicians for Civic Reform. He gets rich because all the doctors in the United States want to join this organization even though it has an unpronounceable acronym and he charges for admission. He then invests all of his money in globalized bank accounts, offshore foreign trusts, Swiss single premium annuities, Isle of Man insurance policies, gold bullion in Barbados, and similar investments of dubious virtue, and gets even richer. He is on the lam, mind you, but still, if one is on the lam, being on the lam is not necessarily a great hardship if while on this lam one can ski at St. Moritz, sunbathe at St. Tropez, wear Brioni suits and Gucci alligator oxfords, drive Ferrari F355 convertible spiders with dual overhead cams, languish in the secured concierge floors of five-star hotels in the Bahamas, Spain, and Switzerland, or watch the setting sun from the portico of one's own travertine villa on the Amalfi Coast as one slowly sips on one's favorite brand of Courvoisier from one's favorite brandy snifter while smoking a Davidoff cigar.

Maybe the book will not be semi-fictional. Maybe it will only be semi-semi-fictional because a lot if it will be real.

I will become famous because everyone will want to read this fantastically hilarious book about Dr. Ecks. The fact is that people love to read books about doctors being in jail, especially when it involves an egocentric manic-depressive psychiatrist with an active imagination who believed he was a genius in the use of the English language. The book will be even more exciting when I describe in detail the psychiatrist's gang visits to residential care facilities and the subsequent pursuit by a tidal wave of FBI agents, DOJ agents, ATF agents, and others with similarly acrimonious acronymic credentials. In addition to these groups, there was the would-be wanna-be prosecutorial lawyers for whom fame was the goal and zeal its key—prosecutors for whom conviction meant incarceration rather than sincerity of purpose, prosecutors whose Hippocratic-equivalent oath meant "First do some harm."

Psychiatrists will absolutely love the book because of its incomparable brilliance. They will organize special group sessions called focus sessions because they will be focusing on the book with psychiatrists quoting from their favorite passages. Then they will analyze the various aspects of the text including the delicately contrived nuanced nuances, the ingenious double double-entendres, and the diabolically conceived hidden puns. They will ponder the psychodynamic implications of the strange cyber-relationship between Dr. Ecks and the hermit named Dave. They will debate on the diagnostic overtones represented by the author's hilarious digressive ruminations, and the diagnostic undertones suggested by his excessively dependent relationship with a rejecting mother. Between the psychodynamic implications, and the diagnostic overtones and the diagnostic undertones, nothing will be left to chance. Do I make myself clear? It will be like literary Tupperware parties for mental health professionals but without the entrepreneurial housewives making their obligatory pitches for the airtight polyethylene containers. Earl Tupper, the expatriate inventor of the ware that bears his name who emigrated to Costa Rica for reasons best known to himself and the Internal Revenue Service, will be turning over in his Costa Rican grave—assuming that he is dead and the Costa Rican government would allow disinterment to permit substantiation.

My book will become number one on *The New York Times* bestseller list for both the fiction and nonfiction lists simultaneously, an event occurring for the first time in recorded history, because people will not know whether it's fiction or nonfiction, or whether it's real or not real. They won't be able to tell because it will be part novel and part autobiography. It has not escaped my notice—and you can quote me on that—that the two elements of fiction and nonfiction will be inextricably intertwined with each other, like the strands of the double helix.

I feel as if I am standing on the threshold of greatness. The title of my book will be *2001—A Psychiatric Odyssey,*[13] as a kind of sequel to Arthur C. Clarke's book *2001—A Space Odyssey,* only even more people will buy it, and they will make this terrific Omnimax movie about it showing huge black gorillas throwing Rorschach cards up into the air as a way of symbolizing the technological advances of civilization in one sweeping overriding gesture, and all this will be in 3-D, so people in the audience will think that these giant technicolored Rorschach cards will be coming right at them, and I will become famous. I will also become rich because before people can read the book, they will have to buy it, not to mention all the money from the movie rights that I will collect from both the domestic market and the foreign market including India and China, where there are hundreds of millions of moviegoers. They are called moviegoers because that is what they do, they literally go to the movies. They go every day because there is nothing else to do in those countries. And then there's syndication—don't forget about syndication! We will go into syndication. And the residuals—we will also go into residuals, and all those things that they rent at video stores like CVRs or VCRs or whatever—we will get commissions on those. And don't forget about the VD things or whatever they call them—those little disk things that kids buy now with the money that they make from their dot.com cybernet one million gigahertz businesses instead of listening to the 33 rpm records that normal people listen to. And don't forget the patented copyrighted musical score which people won't be able to sing unless they pay me money, and even if they only hum it, they will still have to pay—especially when they hum it. Also, don't forget about all the merchandising that goes along with this, like all the patented copyrighted stuff they are going to sell in gift shops—T-shirts with the Dr. Ecks logos, or those cute little beanie hats with the propellers on top, or the Dr. Ecks dolls, or those cuddly little terry cloth replicas of the giant gorillas holding tiny Rorschach cards using their genetically engineered velcro opposable thumbs.

In fact my exact words to my wife—which I vividly remember to this day—were, "I will become rich—rich I tell you—rich beyond my wildest dreams. And since I will become so rich, I will let you have some money too, because I am basically a generous person and California is a community property state, unless I can somehow get the law changed by hiring lobbyists with all this money I am going to make." I was on Mt. Everest along with Sir Edmund Hillary and Tenzing Norgay, if only for a few seconds. Bear in mind, I said all of this without taking a single breath.

When I was through, my wife said that actually it was unlikely that people in 2004 and 2005 and 2006 would max out their credit cards to buy a futuristic book with a 2001 timeline but that I should nevertheless make this pitch to prospective book publishers because they worked hard and needed a good laugh which they will have—not with me, she assured me, but at me.

At times my wife seems to suffer from this strange syntactical aphasia that is characterized by prepositional translocations in which she confuses "with" with "at," and "at" with "with." This is at best a kind of selective dyslexia for which no cure is known.

Be that as it may, I will be among the first to admit that when I am on the summit of Mt. Everest, everything that I have done at that location, I have done without the assistance of portable oxygen canisters—unlike my buddies, Sir Eddy and Norgy, both of whom needed technological assistance. This includes writing checks I could not cover or writing scientific articles that were not of sterling quality or responded to rejection letters with letters or my own that even lacked the diminished Sterling quality of the originally rejected article. As a matter of fact even this narrative with its alternating current of the serious and the trivial bears some resemblance to my former Everest productions. One of them generated such a devastating editorial response that I withdrew from the world and watched MTV for the next three weeks. Eventually I mustered up enough courage to respond as follows:

> Dear Dr. Anonymous editor:
>
> Thank you for your letter of 8-18-97. In your critique of my manuscript you stated that the paper did not contain any new ideas, did not present old material in new ways, was not clearly presented and contained excessive jargon (although you did not cite specific examples), did not include relevant recent references, was not sufficiently sophisticated for a professional audience, was not clearly defined, did not clearly state its objectives, did not have important results that were clearly presented, and did not have conclusions that were supported by the paper's findings. Also it was too long.
>
> I therefore concluded that you did not like it.
>
> It took me about a year and a half to emerge from this avalanche of criticisms after which I was astonished to discover that not only was I still alive but I had actually summoned the courage to submit the manuscript elsewhere.
>
> For some strange reason, my article seems to have also elicited strong feelings in some of the other peer reviewers as well. Thus one reviewer stated, "It does not contribute any science to the area and is not worthy of publication as a regular article." I would rate that as a vote against this article on the Medicare problems of the private psychiatric practitioner from this obviously salaried academician with an ascetic dedication to science.
>
> One reviewer stated, "This is a remarkable fetching article—folksy and unusually informative on a topic that is rarely discussed." I would rate that as a vote for.

So take your choice: One peer reviewer's "Not worthy of publication" versus the other peer reviewer's "remarkably fetching." Same subject, same article, same author. If it is true that beauty is in the eye of the beholder, so is ugliness. This was the first time that I realized that not all hard-drinking editors are intoxicated by my blend of levity and gravity.

I had, of course, reached the height of Greenspan's previously proclaimed "irrational exuberance" without the benefit of syzygys or concatenations. Now I am not completely without insight about these things and I realize that psychiatrists who read this book and others of similar intelligence may well have concluded that at times I am afflicted by certain flights of fancy, certain whims of the mind, as it were, that are essentially cyclical in their expression, but that are nevertheless responsive to treatment. In the preface I teasingly hinted at the promise of additional explanations of my idiosyncrasies that would be forthcoming in the text. This paragraph constitutes such an explanation and it is about as specific as I wish to be, other than to say that most of this book, present chapter excluded, is written between cycles.

I will now describe my descent from Everest: It is a well-known fact that 25 percent of those who reach the summit of Everest do not return alive. Therefore I will remain forever grateful to my wife who assisted in my descent by saying that it was apparent that I had seen too many 007 movies and that if I continued to prattle on this way, she would file for divorce on the grounds of mental stupidity. If there were such a thing as sublingual lithium with instant efficacy, this was it, and I instantly recouped my former acerbic personality. I responded that by filing for divorce she might be providing me with silver lining number four. She was not amused, but clearly my mind was back to normal.

So much for fantasies. To make this unnecessarily long story short, nobody went to jail and I never got to write the book, either fictional or semi-fictional or semi-semi fictional. The compilers of *The New York Times* best-sellers list—both fiction and nonfiction—never even noticed my absence. They didn't write; they didn't call—it was as if I never existed for them. The audits ended this way: The Medicare initial assessment of $52,609.59 was revised downward to zero, zilch, nada, *bupkis*. *Bupkis* is yet another Yiddish word with a specialized utility but is basically a parvenu compared to its *schlep* and *chutzpah* etymological coreligionists. It means zero, zilch, or nada and sometimes even less than zero, zilch, or nada with the additional implication that the resultant state of nothingness was achieved as a consequence of the implementation of some kind of vindictive process or chicanery— like that endured by the beneficiaries of the pension plans of Enron and Global Crossing. That's what they got—*bupkis*.

The $52,609.59 is not fictional. However the whole process took over three years and interfered with much of my prized recreation television time. Here is an extract from the unapologetic letter I eventually received from Medicare:

> July 22, 1999
> Martin Fleishman MD Inc
> 2305 Van Ness Ste F
> San Francisco, CA 94109
>
> RE: Accounts Receivable Number: xxxxxxxxxx
> Beneficiary's Name: Multiple Patients
> Original Overpayment Amount: $52,609.59
>
> Dear Dr. Fleishman,
>
>   Per the Administrative Law Judge decision on Fair Hearings case number xxxxx, the original overpayment amount was overturned . . .
>   Thank you for your cooperation.
>
> Sincerely,
> Medicare Accounting

So, "the original overpayment amount was overturned." In a single word: *bupkis*. That's how it ended, not with a bang but a *bupkis* whimper. The new bottom line—zero overpayments. This letter, brief, unapologetic, and to the point, was the end of the audit. Over three years of work, compiling documents, writing responses negotiating with typists, consulting with attorneys, not to mention the loss in TV quality time—no MTV or Jerry Springer—all of these sacrifices all preempted by my audit priorities. It was all over. No applause, no crowds, no awards, no presentations, no headlines, no lecture circuit offers, no Hollywood overtures, no Oscars, no Emmies, no Grannies, no green jacket, no Stanley Cup, no Davis Cup, not even a (expletive deleted and no Yiddish equivalent) Little Brown Jug.

The Medi-Cal assessment of $32,641.30 was actually much less of a problem. It was creatively handled by me by not acknowledging receipt of their dunning letter. Apparently the feelings of this aforementioned uncivil civil servant were not hurt, because I never heard from him again. This is also not fictional.

The unwritten take-home lesson in this chapter, which is a long one I grant, but which is no longer unwritten, is this: When confronted with adversities, including "the slings and arrows of outrageous fortune," it is important to retain a sense of humor. This, once again, is not fictional.

AUDITS AND HEALTH CARE FRAUD

Despite my ungracious description of the audit process, audits are necessary because of health care fraud. Unfortunately, the extent of health care fraud is staggering and is believed by some to be as high as 10 percent of the approximately $1 trillion that Americans spend every year on medical treatment.[14] Unfortunately, the impetus for the enactment of the aforementioned punitive HIPAA laws is the widespread existence of health care fraud by physicians, other health care providers, health maintenance organizations, laboratories, and even prestigious university hospitals. Medicare is basically an honor system that is not working optimally because the rules are being dishonored by too many dishonorable people. In short, somebody had to do something. That being the case I will attempt an objective description of the Medicare audit process in the next chapter.

Chapter 13

The Medicare Audit Process

As I have stated, audits are necessary. The sad fact is that some physicians and other providers have developed muscle hypertrophy from pushing envelopes heavily laden with claim forms. As I have said before and will repeat for emphasis, Medicare is basically an honor system that did not work optimally because it was dishonored by too many dishonorable people.

The Medicare program is a federal insurance program established in 1965 by Title 18 of the Social Security Act to provide health care to the elderly. It is administered by the Centers for Medicare and Medicaid Services (formerly called the Health Care Financing Administration) at the direction of the Secretary of the United States Department of Health and Human Services. The name of the Health Care Financing Administration (HCFA) was changed to the Centers for Medicare and Medicaid Services in 2001 and is now referred to by the acronym CMS. As a matter of interest, a brief history of Medicare is included in Appendix G.

Medicare audits are generally initiated by an entity called the "carrier." The carrier is the private insurance company that administers the Medicare program in your state or district. There are roughly twenty-four such Medicare jurisdictions nationwide to administer the Part B (nonhospital) programs and each of the carriers is encouraged to develop its own policies through internal directives formerly known as Local Medical Review Policies and now known as Local Coverage Determinations (LCD).

These policies may differ from district to district. The carrier's responsibility to administer the Medicare Part B program was mandated by Congress. Medicare law requires that the Secretary of Health and Human Services delegate to these private insurance companies a number of responsibilities in administering the Medicare program. These responsibilities include undertaking audits of the records of providers' services to ensure that providers are being appropriately recompensed.

The responsibilities of the Medicare carriers are outlined in a book called the Medicare Carriers Manual. One important function of the carriers is to maintain program integrity. The Medicare Carriers Manual mandates that the carriers establish and maintain a Medicare Fraud Investigation Branch led by a Program Integrity Coordinator whose function it is to coordinate with the medical review department. Carriers must have written procedures for personnel to identify fraud and abuse situations and are required to carefully evaluate submitted claim forms to detect apparent inconsistencies in the coverage and payment for services. Also the carriers must maintain documentation in provider files of the details of telephone contacts and/or personal contacts involving fraud and abuse issues discussed with providers and their staff. These records must be kept for seven years.

In order to comply with their contractual obligations, Medicare carriers must routinely conduct audits of physicians' Medicare billing practices. However, the fact that a physician has been selected for an audit does not necessarily mean that the physician is inadequate or fraudulent.

All Medicare carriers are alerted to apply safeguards against unnecessary utilization of services by physicians and other providers. With this in mind, carriers conduct prepayment and postpayment reviews to identify inappropriate, medically unnecessary, or excessive services, and take action whenever a suspicious practice pattern appears. This process is called focused medical review. The purpose of a focused medical review is to identify "aberrant procedures." Each carrier has a list of the procedures within their administrative geographical region that are most subject to potential abuse or overutilization. This is a proprietary list and not subject to public scrutiny. When a physician's use of procedure codes exceeds those of others in the same specialty, the physician is supposed to receive a letter of inquiry at which time educational or corrective actions will be taken and misunderstandings clarified. Hence physicians may be inappropriately targeted because they were placed in the wrong specialty or because they might have a unique patient load. Under such circumstances a focused medical review may reveal that no impropriety occurred and that special factors characterized a physician's practice that explained his or her aberrant profile.

However, physicians targeted for an audit do not always get letters of inquiry before they are audited. Other reasons besides aberrant patterns may precipitate an audit, such as inappropriate advertising, beneficiary complaints, and whistleblower complaints. In addition, audits may occur on a purely random basis.

Medicare audits fall into two broad categories: Prepayment audits review claims before Medicare pays the physician; postpayment audits analyze claims after Medicare reimburses the physician. In general, physicians should be more concerned with postpayment audits than prepayment audits. Prepayment reviews typically seek only one or two claims from a physician. Prepayment audits are usually not troublesome, but sometimes it is advisable for physicians to review their claims before submission and even send an explanatory cover letter describing relevant information that is not readily apparent from the original claim, as long as the new information is properly dated. Obviously, physicians who are worried about information to be submitted should seek legal counsel before supplying any records. Generally speaking, prepayment audits do not create problems.

However, if a carrier believes that a physician has a systematic billing problem, the carrier may place the physician on prepayment review. This will require the physician to submit documentation for every claim before Medicare will allow reimbursement. If the prepayment review involves documentation of hospital visits, the physician must then obtain the records from the hospital for each visit before submitting the claim. Obviously, this involves additional time and creates administrative headaches.

The first step in the postpayment audit process is the request for medical records. These records will then be analyzed by someone who may or may not have sophistication in the medical specialty of the physician being audited. The results of this analysis will then be mailed to the physician within six months in a document titled "Results of the Preliminary Audit." This document will contain a bottom line with a number that indicates how much the physician is alleged to have overcharged Medicare. The findings can then be protested by letter. The arguments presented in the response to the Results of the Preliminary Audit will then be analyzed, and the physician will receive a second document titled "Results of the Final Audit."

This document bears all the trappings of finality by title and tone, but it is not really final. The findings of the not-so-final audit can be contested by requesting a Fair Hearing. A Fair Hearing is managed by a special Fair Hearing Officer and can be conducted by mail, by telephone, or through personal interview.

If the physician believes that the results of the Fair Hearing are unfair, the physician then has the option of presenting the case to someone called an Administrative Law Judge if the disputed amount is over $500. The physician then has sixty days from the date of the Hearing Officer's decision to appeal to the Administrative Law Judge, but once on the waiting list, it can take more than a year until the case is heard. Administrative Law Judges work for the Social Security Administration and generally receive special training in Medicare Part B appeals.

Most Medicare audits generally are terminated by the decision of the Administrative Law Judge and this was true of my audit. However, if the physician is still dissatisfied with the findings he or she has two other recourses. The physician can go before a Medicare Appeals Council by requesting a hearing within sixty days of the decision of the Administrative Law Judge. The Council can then initiate its own review of the judge's decision. The law has not established any deadlines for either holding hearings or formulating decisions.

When all of the above appeals have been exhausted and if the physician is not exhausted, then he or she can still file a lawsuit in federal court contesting the previous decisions.

In considering all of this and the work and time and legal expenses incurred in this process, the question naturally arises as to whether it is really worth it to fight the allegations. If the amount of money in question is small, it may not be worth the effort. If the amount of money is large, it would definitely be a bad idea to surrender. A surrender without a fight could easily be construed or misconstrued as an admission of guilt. Even if the physician surrenders without a fight, it is a relatively easy matter for a physician to be re-audited at a later date. The double jeopardy limitations which protect the rights of common criminals are not necessarily applicable to the rights of common physicians and do not prevent Medicare from auditing a different sample of patients seen during a different time span. If this is difficult to believe I will defer to the opinion of an attorney experienced in Medicare fraud litigation:[1]

Unfortunately, many physicians mistakenly believe that challenging an overpayment is much riskier than merely paying the original assessment. This fear stems from two misunderstandings. First, many physicians think that challenging a claim will only draw more attention to them. This worry ignores other compelling concerns. Medicare views capitulating to an audit as tantamount to admitting guilt. HCFA [CMS] has instructed Medicare carriers that if they collect an overpayment from a physician, they should closely monitor that physician. This means that if a physician simply repays the overpayment with no appeal, the physician nearly guarantees a future audit. Moreover, succumbing to audits strongly encourages Medicare to perform future reviews because they are an easy revenue source, and they allow HCFA [CMS] to claim that physicians overbill Medicare. In short, simply refunding the money unchallenged invites a return Medicare visit.

Chapter 14

Progress Note Problems

Progress notes are particularly useful for those fortunate few for whom recurrent experiences produce the kind of unblinking fascination that is ordinarily elicited by adolescent first crushes. There are those of us among the community of American physicians for whom the remembrance of things past is a pretty thin book. Unfortunately my remembrance of things past is generally restricted to slim slices of time surrounding the immediate present. I don't know who invented the progress note—whether it was Edison or some other iconoclast from the Midwest—but to those of us who are recollection challenged, it came as a gift from the gods.

Unfortunately the gods are not uniformly charitable in their distributions. I am not a Marcel Proust, and the one time that I was ensconced on a psychoanalytic couch—in keeping with the trend of the times—I was rather silent because I had nothing to say because I could not remember anything about the past, virtually nothing about what my mother and father did or did not do, because I could not remember what they did or did not do to make me the kind of person that I was or was not. Had I the prescience to keep progress notes in the course of growing up, I would not have been in that fix, but on the other hand, I was not that much interested in me.

The fact is that if I can get within a couple days of the current date without looking at the calendar, then I would rate myself as having a pretty good day. One cannot be a charming dinner companion without a good memory. In keeping with this thought, I cannot remember the number of times I have not been reinvited to sit down at sit-down dinner parties because I was unable to remember the names of the hosts. As a member of this unselected group, I have frequently been amazed by the perspicacity and wisdom and brilliance reflected in a past progress note, and it was only after the meticulous elimination of all other possibilities that I was forced to conclude that the writer was me!

For those of us experiencing such golden geriatric moments, progress notes are essential because they provide conclusive proof that we were there, and that we made observations and recommendations consistent with our training. In short, the progress note indicates that we are doing something important. The proof of this importance is that society is willing to pay us money for treating the patient and writing a progress note describing this service. I like to think that we do our work not for the money but for the value that society places on our services that the money symbolically represents. That essentially is what money is for—to pay for goods and services that have intrinsic usefulness. When all works well, the progress note is a service of intrinsic usefulness.

When all does not work well, Medicare will deny or challenge the intrinsic usefulness of a progress note. When Medicare does this it will scrupulously avoid referring to intrinsic usefulness as a concept. Rather Medicare will deny payments using phrases such as service denied because of "using repeated verbatim statements as documentation" or, because there are alleged inconsistencies in "level of service versus documentation." If the money has already been paid, Medicare will request the remittance. "Request" is actually a euphemism for demand. Since Medicare can be rather sticky about progress notes, it is useful to have a general outline of what Medicare considers to be poor documentation. Medicare was nice enough to indicate this in a special bulletin, the contents of which are summarized in Appendix G.[1]

In addition to being good for doctors, progress notes are also good for patients. Progress notes are supposed to indicate progress which happens periodically or lack of progress, which also happens. Despite this, progress notes are always called progress notes, never lack-of-progress notes. Progress notes are important for several reasons. For one thing, they provide indisputable proof to the physician, that he or she has actually been there—and done that. I have already conveyed that thought in a previous paragraph using the word "conclusive" instead of "indisputable." The reason why I am being repetitious is because, believe it or not, an auditor actually tried to deny payments for home visits which I made for the purpose of administering IM decanoate injections because he felt my progress notes were inadequate, but he was willing to pay me for the injections at the rate of $3.92 per shot. It's like the injections were there, but I wasn't there.

I am talking about hundreds of home visits, so that the alleged overpayments amounted to a considerable sum. I contested the auditor's overpayment allegations to the Medicare authorities, and all to some avail, although "avail" is usually preceded by the word "no." The case finally got to an Administrative Law Judge, although it took about three years. In making my presentation to the judge I invoked the concepts of Emmanuel Kant and his formulation of the categorical imperatives that describe the dimensions which must be imposed on experiences to make these experiences meaningful. In contrast to categorical imperatives, mutually exclusive imperatives describe states of nonexperience which describe events that will never be experienced because they can never occur—my concepts, not Kant's, although I didn't say so. Thus an object cannot be hot and cold at the same time. Just as there are mutually exclusive states, in like manner there are mutually exclusive activities, such as playing the piano with boxing gloves, or performing oral sex under water—both examples of mutually exclusive imperatives. One can consider such incompatible activities as the reverse of the Kantian categorical imperatives insofar as they describe that which cannot happen rather than that which can happen.

I then went on to perorate, in my best Supreme Court style, that in the Western world we are still ruled by the rules of law and the rules of logic, both of which dictate that it is possible for a physician to make a home visit and simultaneously not administer an injection to a patient while making this home visit (that which can occur—the Kantian categorical imperative). However, it is not possible for a doctor to administer an injection to a patient who is living in a home without making a visit to the home (that which cannot occur—the Fleishman noncategorical imperative). One would think this would have been learned on *Sesame Street* using those cute little puppets to make the point. Therefore I should be paid for the home visit as well as for the injection. The Administrative Law Judge, a dignified aristocratic-looking woman in her mid-fifties with a patrician pedigree, seemed fascinated by the "compelling nature" (her words) of my visual imagery involving boxing gloves and that "underwater thing" (her words), but she really wasn't very interested in boxing. She then asked me if I was still single (her words). She then went on to cancel all the alleged overpayments.

This illustrates that despite the obvious fact that a service was rendered, compensation can be denied if documentation is inadequate. It is generally acknowledged that documentation is required for payment—or to put it in historical terms, no compensation without documentation. But believe it or not, this policy is subject to legal challenge. Since this appears to be a legally arguable point, I will quote from the attorney who makes the point:[2]

> carriers often apply the improper legal standard when reviewing documentation. Carriers sometimes apply documentation guidelines as laws or rules. When conducting a review, carriers often say, "If it isn't written, it wasn't done." They use the documentation guidelines to downcode the claim to the level supported by the documentation. Legally, this is incorrect. When HCFA first introduced the documentation guidelines, it issued a question and answer sheet that explained that physicians do not have to comply with the guidelines. The first question was, "Are the documentation guidelines required?" The answer: No. The memo proceeded to explain that if Medicare conducts an audit and finds insufficient documentation, then the carrier should request additional information from the physician to determine whether the services were rendered as billed. While carriers generally disregard this instruction, the memo confirms that the level of the service the physician actually provides—not the amount of documentation—determines the code. As a result, if a physician has performed the service that he or she has billed and simply has not fully documented the visit vis-à-vis documentation guidelines, the physician should appeal the overpayment. At the hearing, the physician can testify about the service provided by presenting evidence such as schedules, testimony from nurses or patients, production data, and other material demonstrating that the services were really performed.

Nevertheless, even though the policy of no compensation without documentation can be challenged, documentation is still preferable to argumentation. However, there are other reasons why writing progress notes is important aside from the question of compensation such as legal problems that may arise from inadequate progress notes. Parenthetically, it should be added that progress notes make life a lot easier for the psychiatrist—especially if they are of the psychopharmacological type. Thanks to my unelephantine memory, I cannot always remember the latest change in medication dosages when I am treating multiple patients at the same site. Under such circumstances it is not only necessary to write progress notes, but it is advisable to keep separate progress notes for psychopharmacological interventions for reasons described in Chapter 8. Thus if I make one change in a patient's regimen—either in dosage or adding a drug or removing a drug, and the patient is better on my next visit, I generally acknowledge that in a progress note. If he or she is worse, I acknowledge that also. If there is no change, this is also noted. Admittedly it is not rocket science.

EXAMPLES OF PROGRESS NOTES

The following is an example of an acceptable 98062 progress note:

The purpose of this visit is to observe the pt's clinical status, monitor for drug side effects and/or interactions, and consult with staff re: interim management problems and problems of ongoing care. Pt is a _____ yr. old male currently residing at the _____ residential care home with hx of multiple hosp adm. with Sx of hallucinations, delusions, and depression. Currently pt. has good handshake, erratic eye contact, is clean and coherent, and denies voices or depression. Affect is bland, speech pattern lacks inflections, there is paucity of expressive movement and diminished spontaneity consistent with negative symptoms secondary to meds or chronic core illness. Grooming is untidy and clothing is not functional with untidy arrangement in multiple layers. Good appetite, sleeps well, normal BMs, poor socialization with staff and peers—pathological asociality, but seems to enjoy our conversation. Judgment and insight are lacking. Staff reports no recent interim mgt problems, and pt has relatively good ADLs with no problems assoc. with eating, dressing, bathing, incontinence, toileting, or ambulation. Current meds are _____ with no apparent adverse SE. Pt has a hx of poor response to _____ and _____ as indicated in prior history. Will continue current regimen.

Actually, this progress note contains a bit too much and if psychiatrists were to write such notes on every patient they see in a residential care home, they would spend most of their time writing and very little time interacting. Medicare really does not expect that much from a medication management progress note. A bare-bones 90862 acceptable progress note might include the following:

1. Date, age, diagnosis
2. Current symptoms and problems
3. Problems with medications/side effects if present
4. Description of minimal psychotherapeutic intervention if present
5. Medication changes as needed

Time intervals are finite and the more time one spends writing about patients, the less time is available to interact with patients. Time, in that sense, is a zero-sum game although Einstein never described it that way, nor would he, since this would imply that time was absolute rather than relative. However, the parameters of the game can be partially circumvented if one writes progress notes while the patient is present. Although functioning as a scribe may inhibit interactions, it doesn't necessarily prevent them as is indicated in the following progress note:

The patient states that his target date to leave the facility is August 12, only two weeks away. On that day he will receive official permission from the Navy to move to Treasure Island. He states, "I've been pretty patient about it thus far." He states his medication is working fine and he feels fine and has no symptoms or side effects. He has not had any constipation. He continues on clozapine as 100 mg in the a.m. and 200 mg HS. His WBC one week ago was 6,500. Once he stops seeing me in the house he intends to see me in my office. His instructions as to what he will do when he leaves the house are written in the purple code that the Japanese used to utilize before World War II. These instructions are written in a secret part of his body, which is not evident to the naked eye but only becomes apparent under black light. The instructions only become apparent after the black light penetrates twelve layers of mesothelial cells in that secret part of his body.

The patient then proceeds to tell me where these twelve layers are, but by this time I am getting writer's cramp as well as listener's cramp and I don't want to hear much more, so I say, "I'm down near the bottom of the page." He says "Okay, I'll stop talking." The patient seemed to understand the nature of my discomfort and was willing to accommodate me without any hurt feelings. Also he seemed to appreciate the humorous aspect of my complaint. This would not have happened if I had not been writing the progress note in his presence, nor, for that matter, would you be reading about it.

One of the problems with this type of note is that it does not conveniently fit into the categories of notes created by the Health Insurance Portability and Accountability Act of 1996. These rules mandate two sets of records to be kept separately, one containing medical notes and a separate record containing psychotherapy notes. The purpose of this is to afford additional privacy protection for psychotherapy notes. The regulations are fairly recent, going into effect in April 2003 even though the HIPAA law was passed in 1996.[3]

The regulations define psychotherapy notes as "notes recorded by a healthcare provider who is a mental health provider documenting or analyzing the contents of conversation during a private counseling session that are separated from the rest of the individual's medical record." In addition to sessions with individuals, privacy protection also applies to notes taken by psychotherapists in group, joint, or family counseling sessions.

What does not come under the purview of psychotherapy notes? Not- psychotherapy notes are notes addressing information regarding medications, prescriptions, frequency of treatments, session start and stop times, the results of clinical tests, and any summaries describing diagnosis, symptoms, functional status, treatment plans, symptoms, recent progress to date, and prognosis.

The one clear point about the new regulations is that they are unclear. Is the quoted note a psychotherapy note or a not-psychotherapy note? Obviously the progress note contains elements of both a psychotherapy progress note and a not-psychotherapy progress note, so the question is in which part of the medical record should it be placed? I don't know. In the future I will try to compartmentalize my brain so as to make progress note entries that fit into one genre or the other.

Here is another example of a not-psychotherapy note or possibly a maybe-psychotherapy note—this one involving patient loyalties which may be related to transference. In transference phenomena, the patient reincarnates in the therapist some important figure from his or her childhood or past, and consequently transfers to the therapist the feelings and reactions that were initially directed toward this earlier person. Generally speaking the transference has an ambivalent quality and includes affectionate as well as hostile attitudes toward the therapist. Within the psychopharmacological setting in which psychotherapy is incidental rather than primary, it is at best inappropriate and at worst presumptuous to talk about transference in the conventional sense. Yet patient loyalties occur. Such shamanistic loyalties to the medicine man, which is what I am but hopefully not all that I am, can be very important as is self-evident from the following progress note:

The patient is now much improved after starting clozapine therapy. His grooming and concentration have improved and the staff reports that he is much less hostile and is more direct able and appropriate. The problem now is that he is refusing to take blood tests as is required for clozapine therapy. In talking with him he agrees that the clozapine is helping him, but still doesn't want to take any blood tests. He tells me that I am like his father— always telling him what to do. I tell him that it's not a matter of a father telling him what to do—I am legally compelled to order blood tests and that if he refuses to take these tests, I can be held criminally liable in the eyes of the law. He is quite sympathetic with my plight and agrees to help me out of my dilemma by taking the blood tests.

So far this strategy has worked—with the cooperation of the phlebotomist who understands that if the patient refuses the test, he is to invoke the magic phrase, "You promised Dr. Fleishman." So far the patient has cooperated as a way of helping Dr. Fleishman to avoid incarceration.

In most instances such loyalties have a shamanistic rather than a parental basis insofar as the loyalties that are created are dependent on the perceived efficacy of the shaman's activities. It is true that I am in the business of prescribing medications rather than killing chickens, but many times my efforts are perceived in the context of events that are not fully understood by the recipients. If the therapist, psychopharmaco rather than psycho, is successful, he or she can be regarded as an almost magical figure. Thus, patients who have left the residential care facility for sunnier climes, frequently prefer that I continue to care for them as office patients. This has some advantages for me in that Medicare generally will not question whether I have the right to do what and how and to whom, as long as I do it in my office; whereas visits to so-called custodial facilities are always suspect as bordering on the unnecessary.

Sometimes patients want to know what I am writing about when I enter a progress note. When that happens I read my progress note to the patient and ask him or her for input. Would he or she like me to change it or alter it and if so why? This is actually a very good technique for enhancing patient participation and it makes progress note writing part of the therapeutic process. Also progress note writing is perceived by some patients as a kind of honorific activity, so that if I don't write a note about them, they feel out of the loop, in which case I extend the loop. Sometimes patients will jostle each other about whose turn it is to be next on the progress note list.

I frequently tell patients what is in the progress note even if they don't ask me, especially if I am changing a dose. Typically I might say something like this:

> I am going to increase your medicine and I want you to tell me whether it makes you feel better or worse. If it makes you feel worse we will go back to the old dose and try something different. I will be back in two weeks, but if you cannot wait that long, tell Mrs. Caretaker and she will get in touch with me.

Not only does this make the psychiatrist a nice guy, but it also encourages patient participation in the therapeutic process. Did you notice how I said *"we"* will go back to the old dose? Being a nice guy as a therapist can enhance patient compliance and can have a payoff in a number of different unforeseeable ways.

One irritable paranoid patient whom I see every two weeks to administer IM fluphenazine injections was in a confrontational mood and accused me of not caring for anybody. She said, "You just sit there and write things down in your little book and give shots. What are you writing about now?" My progress note, which I read back to her, was as follows:

Patient somewhat angry at me. She accuses me of just sitting here and writing things down in my little book and just giving shots. She wants to know what I am writing about now even as I am writing this.

Strangely enough we both had a good laugh about this note—yet another psychotherapeutic triumph.

The following is a verbatim extract from a progress note written for a patient who was about to be deprived of free access to her asthma inhalant medication by an overly conscientious administrator who was afraid she might run afoul of licensing regulations.

This patient needs to take her asthma inhalants three times a day to control her symptoms. She is quite capable of self-administration and has no history of substance abuse. However, when she is physically isolated from these medications she becomes very apprehensive, which probably increases her asthma symptoms. I believe she can be benefited if she had direct access to these medications and she will not abuse this privilege.

I told the administrator to photocopy the note and send it to licensing if she thought she might have a problem. This patient will kill for me, this being a request that I will make only under the most extraordinary circumstances.

Since very few medical writers have described the mechanics of progress note writing, it is only fitting that in the interests of an encyclopediacal treatment of this subject I should address the problems of hand fatigue. Hand fatigue is usually a subliminal sensation that is generally excluded from consciousness and which is never mentioned in the psychoanalytic literature as a preconscious or unconscious phenomenon. The reason for this is that psychoanalysis, in its embryonic form, was never adversely affected by Medicare audits or malpractice suits.

Hand fatigue plays a subtle role in progress note writing in that the brain may tell the hand not to write even though more should be written. Some would say that progress note writing is not really very important and that it merely proves documentation of patient care but does not contribute directly to quality patient care. I would disagree with that not only for previously stated reasons, but also because progress notes form the chief line of defense in malpractice suits. Also the good progress note can protect the writer in Medicare audits against allegations of overpayment, or worse. "Worse" in this instance refers to fraud and abuse.

I will now reveal one of the dirty little secrets of writing a good progress note. Frequently when I write progress notes I use double entry bookkeeping. What I mean by this is that I frequently switch pens—sometimes in midstream. I do this to avoid the problem of writer's fatigue. A comfortable pen can help a lot—but what is even better is to have two comfortable pens with different weights and/or different contours. The combination is better because writer's fatigue can exacerbate to writer's cramp if the same pen is used repeatedly to describe the vicissitudes encountered by multiple patients at the same facility. The experienced progress note writer will find that switching pens will relax certain muscles that have been over-stimulated and recruit other muscles that are not fatigued. Progress note writers will then find that they can better resist the tendency to be brief with all the attendant dangers that reside in such a decision. The following progress note example illustrates what can happen if one successfully resists the tendency to be brief. The anonymous "one" in the previous sentence is really me:

Attended court hearing yesterday at San Francisco General Hospital. Conservatorship application approved, but the judge did not approve transfer to a long-term facility. He has improved with Clozaril although his improvement has been very gradual. He is now more coherent but still delusional.

Take a second look at that sentence: "Conservatorship application approved, but the judge did not approve transfer to a long-term facility." That little sentence saved me $9,414 in a Medicare audit.

In this book I do not wish to describe the boring specifics of Medicare audits, but basically this involved Medicare's disputed payments for a prolonged hospitalization which the Medicare auditors felt was medically unwarranted. This one sentence established the fact that the prolonged hospitalization was a product of judicial fiat rather than a medical decision. I didn't decide to keep the patient in the hospital; in effect it was the judge's decision. In other words, the judge was practicing medicine—not that I wished to apprise him of that fact nor did I ask him to show me his license to practice medicine—one of the few times in my life that I was able to suppress comedic propensities without getting nervous or lapsing into akathisia. When I wrote the progress note the day after the judicial hearing, I was not thinking defensively, and entered the progress note as an afterthought. Sometimes afterthoughts are additional gifts from the gods along with good memories.

I know that sometimes penned notes are considered old-fashioned and one should use word processors to construct progress notes. I have nothing against computers and readily admit that the original draft of this book was not written in longhand. However, computerized notes, if offensively repetitive, might convey the impression to a Medicare auditor that the note was primarily the product of a pushed button rather than the documentation of an interpersonal relationship.

Sometimes Medicare auditors will reduce payment for a visit because they do not have a full understanding of Medicare policy. This happened when an auditor reviewed my hospital progress notes and attempted to allow only 62.5 percent of 80 percent of the allowable charge of $53.00. This formula is called the outpatient mental health treatment limitation and is only applicable to expenses incurred in connection with the treatment of an individual who is not an inpatient of a hospital. The correct allowable charge is actually 80 percent of allowed charges. In that case it is generally the responsibility of the audited physician to respond in a courteously didactic manner as is illustrated in the following letter which was sent by me to protest this alleged correction:

> The Medicare Reviewers have changed procedure code 90843 to 90862 for services rendered to hospitalized patients. The question of whether procedure code 90862 adequately represents the standard of care for hospitalized patients will be discussed later. The important point here is that the level of compensation for 90862 was apparently calculated using the formula for outpatients which is 62.5 percent of 80 percent of the allowable charge of $53.00. This formula is called the outpatient mental health treatment limitation and is *only applicable to expenses incurred in connection with the treatment of an individual who is not an inpatient of a hospital* as is stated in the Medicare Carriers Manual.

Generally speaking, patients tend to accept writing progress notes in their presence as a routine matter and will not question the process. Occasionally a paranoid patient might ask me why I am writing the notes, and I generally tell the patient that in the course of time I might forget what he or she has told me and I want to remember what is said because it might be useful for future encounters. If I am then asked to be more specific, I might say that if someone is doing well on medication I would want to continue the medication, but it is hard for me to determine whether someone is improving or not improving if I do not have adequate documentation. If my paranoid patient then asks me to see the progress note, I willfully oblige with the request that he or she check it for errors—a request which is always graciously received by the truly paranoid. I then ask for any suggested corrections or amendment.

When progress note material is used this way it can also facilitate medication compliance. In Chapter 9, I wrote briefly about the use of interviewing techniques to facilitate patient cooperation, but progress note interventions can also be used to facilitate medication compliance. I make sure to tell the patient that when I am changing medications and writing about this, the patient may feel better or worse as a result of these changes. Either way I tell patients that I need their input and if they feel worse they should definitely tell me so that I can change the medication or reduce the dosage.

I have never had a problem because of my progress note preoccupations. I think there is probably an unrealized therapeutic potential in the act of writing about another person in his or her presence and then asking the other person to check for inaccuracies or even suggest additions.

Sometimes patients will object to the word *sick* in describing their conditions. I never argue about whether someone is sick or not sick. Generally my response is that I don't like the word *sick* either, but the problem is that you are not sleeping well or are very nervous or are very irritable or are always fighting with people or that you have had a lot of trouble in life, etc. Strangely enough, patients may argue about whether they are sick or not sick, but they will rarely argue about a description of their symptoms, especially if insomnia is one of their complaints, and, in fact, are usually grateful when this complaint is taken seriously. It is through such communications that patient rapport and trust is gradually facilitated. One can easily see how the ordinarily mundane ritualistic act of writing progress notes can gradually cross over into the arena of psychotherapy.

MEDICARE POLICIES REGARDING PROGRESS NOTES

In the evaluation of progress notes Medicare reviewers will not be interested in notes which reflect the perceptiveness and clinical brilliance of the psychiatrist. They will be more interested in those progress notes which fail the internal Medicare criteria for adequacy. These notes will then be counted and penalties will be levied using this absolute count. Once this is done Medicare is allowed to extrapolate from the audited charts to the physician's entire practice and the penalties will be accordingly increased. The process is similar to assessing the productivity of baseball players by counting their strikeouts instead of their batting averages. It should be obvious that the greater the number of times a player comes to the plate, the greater will be the absolute number of strikeouts. Bottom-line sports entrepreneurs know that there is a better way to evaluate job performance.

It should be similarly obvious that the greater the number of progress notes being audited, the greater will be the absolute number of progress notes found to be deficient. It should not be difficult—and possibly preferable—to develop standards using the batting average approach, in which deficient progress notes are calculated as a percentage of the total progress notes being audited.

While all medical providers will come under increasing surveillance as a result of this legislation, residential care psychiatrists will be particularly vulnerable because of several factors. One fact is that residential care psychiatrists tend to see multiple patients at the same site and tend to use medication management codes in a greater degree of frequency than is true for office-based practitioners. Unfortunately in our computer-driven society the mere fact of procedure code profile aberrancy is sufficient to trigger an audit.

Another problem for the residential care psychiatrist is the relative absence of treatment guidelines. Although such guidelines for patients in nursing homes have been formulated as part of the Omnibus Budget Reconciliation Act of 1987, no such guidelines exist for patients in residential care homes. This relative neglect of patients in residential care homes is attributable to several factors—among them the apparent lack of interest by university affiliated psychiatrists because residential care placements are not customarily included in psychiatric residency rotations. In addition, it has been legislatively ignored because historically residential care patients did not have an effective lobby, as has been true for nursing home patients and the developmentally disabled. Fortunately NAMI (the National Alliance for the Mentally Ill) is now closing the gap. Thus there is now an extremely urgent need to formulate a policy with respect to such questions as appropriateness of care, the necessity of on-site visits, the frequency of on-site visits, and the use of medication codes.

The principal vehicle for determining such important questions as medical necessity and appropriateness of treatment are progress notes. Testimonials from patients, patients' relatives or patient advocates, while good for the psychiatrist's ego, will have little effect on the resolution of these important issues. Yet the Medicare criteria for judging progress notes contain intrinsic inadequacies as applied to psychiatric progress notes. The "stand alone" criterion is a case in point.

Medicare payment policies are based on Section 1833(e) of Title XVIII of the Social Security Act which states that payment may not be made under Medicare unless the person rendering the service provides whatever information the Medicare Part B Carrier deems necessary to assure proper payment.

Each progress note entry describing a service must be able to "stand alone," that is to say must support the fact that the level of service billed was rendered. Related records, e.g., laboratory results, may also be required to support the billed service. In the case of Evaluation and Management services, all required elements for the code billed must be reflected in the notes for that date of service. Billings for Evaluation and Management services should be consistent with the criteria for simple, complex, and comprehensive services. It is not always necessary to repeat information from earlier encounters, e.g., a history and physical, if the service billed does not require that a history and physical be performed.

When frequency of service or levels of care billed by a physician are in question, it is up to that physician to document to the satisfaction of the Medicare Part B Carrier that the service meets the criteria for Medicare payment. The medical records should contain all pertinent and essential information related to the patient's medical status. Such documentation may include operative reports, procedural reports, chart notes, progress notes, history and physical reports as well as written narratives. Additional material may be sunmitted if pertinent, but all documentation should be legible.

It is clear that these policies with their "stand alone" criteria are more applicable to the treatment of acute states rather than chronic conditions. Also these criteria relate more to the work of internists and surgeons. If rigorous enforcement of these provisions were applied to progress notes generated by psychiatrists, then every psychiatrist in the country who bills Medicare for on-site visits will find himself or herself vulnerable to adversarial audits. Psychiatrists as a rule do not write progress notes that "stand alone." A progress note that indicates that a patient is "less delusional" or "more delusional" or "less depressed" or "more depressed" is not a note that stands alone. It has meaning only insofar as it has reference to a previous state recorded by a previous progress note. Also the average progress note does not address the problem as to whether the service rendered was "medically necessary." Moreover, the psychiatrist does not routinely address the problem of physical symptoms unless the patient is a hypochondriac or has somatic delusions. Since time is a finite quality, whatever time is spent writing must by subtracted from time spent doing. It is the doing—doing whatever psychotherapy is indicated and making whatever clinical observations are necessary for the performance of medication management—that is the real determinant of clinical efficacy.

Thus, although regulatory pressure seeks to create long progress notes, clinical effectiveness is dependent on short progress notes in which the patient's current psychiatric status and response to medication is briefly described. In the case of residential care patients such operations should be conducted on the premises. The multiple advantages of on-site visits have been described in other contexts[4], but basically involve exploring how patients behave on their own turf, observing how they maintain their own room and how they interact with their peers, and being able to consult with residential care administrators and encouraging the flow of information from maids and cooks. Psychiatrists are not likely to discover such behavioral inelegances if their contacts are limited to the pristine sanctity of their offices.

I cannot leave the topic of progress note problems without discussing the latest fashions in progress note mandates. In January and February of 2004, many of the manufacturers of atypical antipsychotics in response to directives from the FDA sent Dear Health Care Provider letters (formerly known as Dear Doctor letters) warning doctors about the necessity to monitor for the symptoms of hyperglycemia including polyphagia, polydipsia, polyuria, and weakness. That being the case it is important that in those circumstances psychiatrists approach these issues with their patients—not necessarily in those words, and document accordingly and react accordingly in whatever words they prefer—yet another example of the medicalization of psychiatry.

In this chapter I have discussed general progress note problems that were actually not the focus of attention in the audit, such as the outpatient mental health treatment limitation and the "stand alone" provision. Hopefully I will not continue to stand alone in my opposition to the "stand alone" policy in the evaluation of psychiatric progress notes.

Chapter 15

Special Problems

Board-and-care homes have their own set of problems, and psychiatrists should be prepared to alter their work habits accordingly. Medication directions, for example, require special measures. Whereas in office practice one discusses the directions with the patient, one rarely checks the instructions on the bottle because if there were a discrepancy this would be discussed during the psychotherapy sessions, or so one would hope. However, in board-and-care homes such discrepancies might not be routinely discovered. It is therefore desirable to spot-check the labels on the medication bottles. Also, one must discuss the risks of medication with the residential care facility administrator as well as with the patient. When using concentrates or elixirs it is helpful to have the administering person demonstrate an understanding of the calibrations on the droppers.[1]

I wrote the previous paragraph many years ago. Since then medicine has made great progress even in the area of medication dispensing. It is now no longer the duty of the residential care facility psychiatrist to inspect the medication labels for accuracy because now it is the pharmacist who does this, and, as is well known, pharmacists are more accurate than physicians. If that is not well known, it should be well known, and perhaps it will be well known after this book is published. Also pharmacists have much more legible handwriting, mostly because their handwriting is printed by computers. In the old system, pharmacists would deliver the medications to the residential care facilities. in bottles usually containing a one-month supply, and caregiving staff would take the pills out of the bottles and put them in those little familiar paper cups for patient ingestion. Most of the time they did not make mistakes. Most of the time.

In days of yore when the scratches of screaming little children were anointed with iodine and mercurochrome, this was an acceptable way to deliver medications. Nowadays, the little paper cups should now be relegated to horse-and-buggy status because of the advent of those two great hyphenated medication dispensing inventions—the Medi-sets, and the bubble-pack. I predict that these two inventions will soon become so popular that they will both lose their hyphenated status. The point is that medication dispensing is a professional procedure and should not be left to nonprofessionals. This is particularly true since medication regimens have become more complicated than ever before, as explained in a previous chapter.

The use of psychiatric medications should lead to a closer relationship with the patient's internist, since an internist's prescriptions may affect a patient's psychiatric status, and vice versa. Many medications (levodopa, digitalis, theophylline, reserpine, other antihypertensive agents, etc.) have psychiatric side effects. Ideally, the psychiatrist should be aware of their use and in a position to discuss the options with the internist, should the situation warrant. In the past these interactions have led me to a much closer association with internists than ever existed in my office practice. However this is not as true as it once was since internists, like psychiatrists, are now very busy with the nonmedicine-related problems of medical practice, and have less leftover time for telephone calls. What I mean is that managed-care business-type telephone calls have depleted the available time for medicine-related telephone calls. We have already touched on this problem in the previous discussion of time as a zero-sum game. That being the case, I am now much more dependent on pharmacists in the discussion of nonpsychiatric medications.

This is not the place to dwell on the multiple beneficial effects of lithium even in the nonmanic patient. However, it is the place to mention that lithium does have a particular hazard in a residential care facility practice, where many patients are seen only once a month in that serum levels can gradually approach toxicity between home visits. The greatest hazard occurs in diarrhea and vomiting, where the response to toxicity will not be gradual but rapid.

For this reason, all lithium directions bear the instruction: "Do not give if patient has diarrhea or vomiting." I also like to omit lithium for one day a week, preferably a Saturday, so as to retard the approach to toxic serum levels. Saturdays are best in that serum levels drawn during weekday mornings will not then reflect the omission of lithium on the previous day.

Residential care facilities can be very different from one another. Following are a number of different scenarios which the residential care facility psychiatrist may encounter:

THE POORLY ORGANIZED FACILITY
WITH SUBSTANDARD PROFESSIONAL SERVICES

Here the administrator may or may not be present when the psychiatrist visits. Other caretakers may not be readily available because they are busy doing other things or are pretending to be busy. A diminished value appears to be placed upon the visits of the psychiatrist who gets the feeling that he or she is an intruder. Communications between administrator or other caretakers and the psychiatrist are minimized, and the psychiatrist gets the impression that the staff feels that should improve as a consequence of "doctoring" with little responsibility on the part of the staff to provide information or participate in decision making.

Not all of the visits to residential care facility are conducted under felicitous circumstances. I have plied my wares in kitchens on kitchen tables, in garages incompletely converted into something less than a garage, and while standing on one foot. While it may be true that every cloud does not necessarily have a silver lining, some clouds do. The absence of commodious four-star accommodations has sometimes led to more informal and open encounters with residents, and I have sometimes received gossipy information from some patients about other residents that was clinically useful to me and that I might not have received in more formal settings. Also under such circumstances I was frequently put at ease by cooks who took pity on my plight and sometimes brought me cookies. I love cookies.

One of the unexpected advantages of treating patients in a poorly organized facility is that it allows them the opportunity to approach me spontaneously. Sometimes when this is done in the absence of the administrator, this represents the first sign of improvement in a patient who was otherwise withdrawn and isolated. Sometimes patients will never make that approach. In that case it is incumbent on the psychiatrist to make the approach—even to see the patient in his or her room as an uninvited guest. Also a visit to the room can convey information about the patient's current state of mind that might not otherwise be apparent from an encounter in a designated area. Is the room dirty or disorganized? Are irrational letters or memos posted on the wall? Is there evidence of rat-packing—i.e., collecting street junk such as old clothes or shoes and sequestering them under the bed? Although there are some unforeseen advantages in attending a poorly organized home, the disadvantages far outweigh the advantages insofar as there is no free flow of communication between caretakers and mental health professionals.

What has been happening in this type of facility? There are several possibilities: All of us get old, including residential care facility administrators and residential care facility psychiatrists. When that happens, we can lose our energies and our enthusiasm for work. It's called burnout, and the demands placed on administrators in terms of being on call twenty-four hours a day, seven days a week, and fifty-two weeks per year can take its toll. Administrators can get old even when they are young.

What are the other possibilities? There may have been a previous infelicitous relationship with another psychiatrist who perhaps was inexperienced in this type of work. That would not be unusual insofar as few guidelines describe how a psychiatrist should function in these settings. To my knowledge, I am the only one who has written about the subject.[2] (If other psychiatrists have written how-to-do-it manuals on the subject and I have ignored their efforts, my profound apologies—but I did say "to my knowledge.")

Psychiatrists may make several errors in their interactions with administrators: Thus a psychiatrist may feel free to make unscheduled visits to the home, or schedule his or her visits at the last possible minute on the basis of personal convenience to the psychiatrist but with little regard for the time demands made on the administrator. Such policies may not sit well with an administrator who may then decide not to meet with the psychiatrist.

The psychiatrist may make a fetish out of egalitarianism. The psychiatrist may deliberately not dress in a professional manner so as to stress his or her equality with the patients. Such misplaced egalitarianism is essentially hypocritical. The psychiatrist is an expert in a difficult field which requires years of training and dedication. He or she is part of an elite group, whether he or she likes it or not. As a male professional I have generally found it important to wear a shirt and tie. To me this has been the uniform of productivity. Also this is a sign of respect for the patients, caretakers, and administrators. Some people interpret sartorial sloppiness—rightly or wrongly—as deliberately disrespectful or even insulting. Were I to appear in these settings with a nose ring and backpack, and with a salutation such as "Call me Marty," I would gain little respect and little confidence. Democracy is not applicable in every context.

The previous discussion may be construed as an attack on psychiatrists who make a fetish out of antiestablishmentarianism. Such attitudes may work well in an office practice, because if the patient disapproves of the psychiatrist's social message, the patient may choose not to return. There is a factor of natural selection in office psychiatry in that patients may choose not to select a psychiatrist because of a lack of shared value systems. This is not true in a residential care facility practice where patients do not have that freedom. They are not free to not return because the residential care facility is their home and it is the psychiatrist who does the returning.

Just as a zealous anti-traditional approach may be counterproductive in the residential care facility setting, the same may be said for the psychiatrist who observes standard office procedures in the residential care facility setting. I once encountered a psychiatrist who told me that the administrator had refused to let him come to the house. I did not discover the reason for this until some years later when the administrator asked me to visit the home. When I did this, I interviewed a geriatric schizophrenic patient who spent most of the time talking to hallucinated entities in the bookcase. The administrator told me that she did this most of the day. She also told me that Dr. R., the visiting psychiatrist before me, had been seeing her every two weeks, and would spend about an hour with her, trying to make sense of her "ramblings," as she described them. This did not seem to make much sense to her, nor did it to me, since the problem presented by this patient did not warrant that kind of attention. The administrator also noted that the patient did not seem to be much better after the psychiatrist left, so after a while she did not pay much attention to whether the psychiatrist came or went, but she preferred that he not come. My brief psychopharmacological interludes with this essentially demented patient did not seem to produce much of an improvement either, but at least I was not spending much time with her mak-

ing strained interpretations of her incoherent "ramblings." I won't say
that the administrator was everlastingly grateful for my efforts, but
she never locked me out.

While it is standard practice in office psychiatry to dedicate half-
hour or hourly intervals to individual patients, usually nobody is in
the waiting room to judge whether the patient has improved as a result
of such allocations. This is not necessarily true in residential care facilities, where such an investment of time tends to create the expectation of beneficial results. Periodic one-hour sessions with an individual patient are noted by other patients, by staff personnel, and by
administrators, and where such efforts are not accompanied by visible and palpable improvements in a patient's status, the status of the
psychiatrist suffers accordingly.

So what does one do about the poorly functioning home? Alert the
authorities that this must be done or that must be done? Wrong! This
will accomplish very little, will not increase patient care, and will create lasting enmity between the psychiatrist and the administrator, so
that the complaining residential care facility psychiatrist will no longer be able to work effectively in that home. Nor will he or she be able
to work effectively in other homes. This is because of the invention of
the telephone. Administrators talk to one another, and if the psychiatrist develops a reputation as a snitch or feces disturber, his or her career as a residential care facility psychiatrist is over. Mind you, I am
talking about attitudes rather than serious violations of patients
rights, where it may be the legal obligation of psychiatrists to inform
the authorities.

So what can the psychiatrist do about such a home? I discussed this
briefly in Chapter 7, "The Cast," but the lesson bears some repetition
in this context. First of all, when the staff does not freely come to me
with background patient information, then I go to the staff. This may
mean that I may go to the kitchen to actively seek out the cook to find
out about the patient's eating habits, or I may actively solicit the opinion of the maid to determine how the patient takes care of his or her
room. Also I try to obtain additional information by being nosy in an
informal way. Don't forget the additional information that can be obtained via the miracles of psychoperambulation as described in a previous chapter.

Practically all of the time, when I have done some of this, when I
have encouraged staff to communicate with me, when I have appeared

accessible and not withdrawn or arrogant (despite the apparent intimidation suggested by my shirt and tie), where patients have improved as a result of my efforts, I have been able to improve the atmosphere of the home and the attitude of the administrator and other caretakers.

THE WELL-ORGANIZED FACILITY
WITH REGULAR VISITS BY THE MRCPT

When there are regular prescheduled visits by the Modern Residential Care Psychiatric Team—either weekly, biweekly, or monthly, the administrator will practically always be in attendance. (By biweekly I mean every two weeks. It is one of the idiosyncrasies of the English language that biweekly can also mean twice a week. If you don't believe me, look it up.) This is because the confluence of professional personnel emphasizes the importance of the meeting. Also let's not forget that social workers are an important referral source, and this fact is not lost upon administrators.

The administrator discusses the patient's behavior and notes any problems that the patient may be having in the activities of daily living such as with continence, dressing, eating, bathing, or personal hygiene. The social worker addresses other patient problems relating to personal interactions or financial problems, and I discuss medication issues with the pharmacist. If I decide to adjust dosages or change medications, these decisions are recorded in the progress notes and immediately attended to by the pharmacist. I prefer not to await the contemplative isolation of my office before making such decisions because the imperatives of office life have a way of placing medication issues in distant locations on the backburner. What I'm trying to say and will repeat in mostly one-syllable words is that by the time I get to my office I can forget to do what I should do and I don't like to do that.

Off the cuff and on the spot medication changes can be rather difficult, but I always take my office charts to the residential care facility when I make my visit so I can quickly review the patient's past medication history without even opening the chart by reviewing the entries on the manila cover (see Chapter 8 for a full explanation of this system). The disadvantage of this system is that it discourages patient-psychiatrist privacy but if privacy is really an issue, which it rarely is, I can then see the patient in a private room on the premises, or arrange for an office appointment. By and large the advantages of this system far outweigh the disadvantages.

Weekly visits are generally necessary only in very large homes—more than twenty-five patients—because of the multiplicity or problems that may arise. In moderately sized homes—fifteen to twenty-five patients—biweekly visits are usually appropriate. In smaller homes, monthly visits are usually sufficient. In this kind of a setting, patients are generally evaluated by the Modern Psychiatric Team in the presence of the administrator or other caretakers in a semiformal structured arrangement. Also in quiet attendance are my office charts and the special chart with laboratory information described in Chapter 8.

What is lost by such a practice? Psychiatrist-patient confidentiality is lost. Also whatever additional information that could have been obtained via psychoperambulation is lost. What is gained by such an arrangement? The facilitated flow of information between mental health professionals, administrators, and other caretakers is gained by such an arrangement. This is very important and can provide me with more information than is available from the scraps that I can collect via psychoperambulation, although psychoperambulation will have to do when nothing better is available.

When functioning in such a midsized facility with the Modern Psychiatric Team, I try to evaluate all the patients in the facility for reasons I will explain later. Typically, the patient enters the meeting site individually. I greet the patient with the customary salutation and note whether my ritualistic efforts are appropriately reciprocated. I look for appropriate eye contact. I shake hands dutifully and look for the manual laundry-list of ill health which I touched upon briefly in Chapter 5 such as the following:

- coarse tremor secondary to lithium toxicity;
- the fine tremor that occurs as a result of the extra-pyramidal side effects incident to the administration of conventional anti-psychotic medications;
- the unilateral tremor that is sometimes the accompaniment of idiopathic Parkinsonism;
- the bradykinesia of Parkinsonism—either drug-induced or idiopathic;
- the sweaty palms of acute anxiety;

- the palmer erythema of chronic alcoholism;
- the thenar atrophy of amyotrophic lateral sclerosis;
- the ulner deviation of rheumatoid arthritis;
- the Heberden's nodes of chronic osteoarthritis;
- or the Dupuytren's contractures of diabetes or alcoholism.

I also look for the hand signs of schizophrenia and whether they indicate a worsening of the patient's psychotic status, such as whether the hands reveal the presence of the flaccidity that accompanies the flat affect of negative symptom or deficit schizophrenia. I look for the tobacco-stained fingers that generally accompany the exaggerated inhalation of schizophrenic-style smoking when cigarettes are smoked down to the butt. I look for the dirty fingernails that are secondary to laziness and low self-esteem and the bitten-down fingernails of nonspecific nervousness—a symptom not necessarily associated with schizophrenia.

In addition to this psychiatric symptomatic clues are afforded by changes in baseline handshake behavior such as handshakes formerly nonremarkable but now vigorously acknowledged (possible onset of mania), handshakes now tentatively proffered (possible increase in depression), and handshakes once offered but now refused (resurgence of paranoia). I try to make comparisons with previous impressions: Are the fingernails getting dirtier? Are the tobacco stains getting nastier—that sort of thing. These are not the type of progress notes that meet the "stand alone" criterion described in Chapter 14, nor should they stand alone.

An entire third-party compensable progress note can be generated from the mere shake of a hand. So I have become an admitted and chronic handshaker, but I still draw the line at slapping backs. Besides, third-party payers do not pay for slapping backs—or for that matter, slapping fronts.

After dutifully noting the above and after a short understandable delay, I say something like, "How are you?" and start writing a progress note—sometimes even before the patient can answer. Obviously I have a lot of information in hand, so to speak, even before the patient can tell me how he or she is feeling. If the patient is not doing well and needs medication changes, I am prepared to do this immediately. Don't forget, in addition to the presence of the pharmacist, I have in my possession my office charts complete with the special psychopharmacological notation sites detailing years of medication regimens and without intervening progress notes—all literally at fingertip availability.

Additional problems are presented when the patient whose meds or dosages I am about to change is among those many chronic schizophrenics with concurrent nonpsychiatric chronic illnesses such as hypertension, diabetes, arthritis, or chronic obstructive pulmonary diseases. It is entirely possible that the medications the patient takes for these illnesses may interact with some of the medications I prescribe. Fortunately, the presence of the pharmacist on the Modern Psychiatric Team provides me with additional feedback which may prevent me from making mistakes. Psychiatrists are not pharmacologically omniscient. That may seem like a sad fact, but the truth is that because of the proliferation of medications, no specialist can claim that quality. For that reason, I am always happy to greet the pharmacist at our monthly or biweekly residential care facility meetings, although I do not try to diagnose his handshake.

At midsized homes, one should generally try to see all the patients in the home at these meetings. This cannot always be done but the effort should be made, so that if a patient does not show up, the psychiatrist should ask specifically about that patient, such as "Where is Patient A?" Sometimes this can lead to interesting conversations as follows:

ME: Where is Patient A?

THEM: Pt. A is in the hospital.

ME: What happened?

THEM: He jumped out of a window last week.

ME [somewhat irked]: Thanks for telling me. Why didn't you let me know?

THEM: It was only a first-story window. He just sprained his ankle.

ME: When he returns from the hospital after they make him better, please let me know. He may come back with higher aspirations.

Sometimes queries regarding the absent patient can produce the answer that the patient is refusing to leave his or her room or come to meals. Sometimes what is regarded as unimportant and not worthy of mention by house staff, or is inadvertently omitted from discussion, is revealed only by a rosterlike systematic review of all the patients in the home. Naturally, in very large homes this cannot be done, but in midsized and smaller homes the psychiatrist should develop a roster mentality.

This is because if a visible intent is not made to see all the patients, it may understandably create the impression that it is not important to see all the patients. It is important to see all the patients, because the absent patient may be the most problematic—even though not obviously so. In many homes attention-getting or attention-demanding patients will preempt the psychiatrist's time to the detriment of other patients. The opposite of the attention-getting patient is the invisible patient. This patient may actually need much more attention than the attention-getting patient.

Sometimes it is the chronically absent patient who makes his or her presence known acutely—by hanging himself in the closet. When this happens and there is no recent progress note, it is a tragedy for all concerned, and less important but important nevertheless, it is also an embarrassment for all concerned. That is why a roster mind-set on the part of the psychiatrist is important, and if the patient does not present himself or herself at the meeting of the Modern Psychiatric Team, I will then provide psychiatric room service and visit the patients in their rooms. If the door is locked and the patient is present, we make all necessary attempts to convince the patient to unlock the door. Actually, that rarely happens.

The other type of patient who tends to get lost in the akathisic shuffle of large homes is the inattention-getting patient. This person does not deliberately avoid others, like the invisible patient, but is a pathological noncomplainer. Just as there are inveterate complainers who grab attention, there are also pathological noncomplainers who should be complaining but nobody hears about them because they never complain. Only by the systematic application of the roster method will their complaints be aired. Here is an example of one such encounter:

PATIENT: Doctor, I don't like my roommate.

ME: Why?

PATIENT: He snores and plays the TV set too loud, and sometimes he uses my toothbrush.

ME: How long have you had this problem?

PATIENT: Not too long.

ME: How long?

PATIENT: About five years.

Sometimes the illness impairs the desire to communicate, but sometimes the inability to complain stems from low self-esteem so that the uncomplaining patient feels that he or she is unworthy of the attention that would occur if people were to respond to his or her complaint.

In this type of home where periodic visits by the Modern Residential Care Psychiatric Team has established the tradition of regularity, there develops the expectation that everyone should be seen on a regular basis so that these visitations acquire the inviolacy of hallowed tradition.

Perhaps this expectation by all concerned, by staff, by administrators, and by team members as well as patients, creates the necessity that patients should be seen regularly. In this kind of situation, the expectation has become the mother of necessity. However, in a way that is a good necessity because it avoids tragedies in the long run, even though it might be difficult to defend the necessity of any particular visit in any one individual case. In this type of situation, it is the house itself that is upgraded in terms of its ability to provide adequate care, because nonprofessional caregivers are routinely encouraged to participate with and provide feedback to the mental health professionals.

This can create a problem in an adversarial audit, in which an auditor can approach each visit on a piecemeal basis, and avoid the context in which the visit was made. The allegation can then be made of the provider providing "unnecessary medical services," which can trigger penalties that may be potentially very severe. In such cases, the defendant should describe the social environment in which there is the expectation of routine services, and the previously described advantages in using a roster system in terms of decreasing the incidence of hospitalization for the group. He or she should remind Medicare that the costs saved by a decrease of only one hospitalization in one patient can easily be the equivalent of hundreds of 90862 coded visits.

THE WELL-ORGANIZED FACILITY
WITH NO REGULAR VISITS BY THE MRCPT

The formal visit with the presence of the Modern Residential Care Psychiatric Team represents the ideal mode of follow-up but it can rarely be achieved. A useful variant of this is the individual meeting with the administrator where he or she discusses every patient with me before the patient contact, then remains in the room while I interview the patient, then leaves the room to allow private communications. Such an administrator is very conscientious and can relate much information. Such visits are generally done in the living room with available easy chairs. Along with my office charts I generally take along a clipboard so I can make my progress note entries while comfortably ensconced in the easy chair.

Here the administrator is usually in attendance when the psychiatrist comes, but team meetings have not yet been established. The principal communicators here are the psychiatrist and the administrator. Ideally the administrator will present his or her findings to the psychiatrist in the presence of the patient. They will then discuss what should be done, again in the presence of the patient. After this meeting the administrator will offer to leave the room to encourage whatever private communications may appear to be necessary between patient and doctor. Generally speaking, this offer is rarely accepted by the patient because such tête-à-têtes are seldom indicated.

In this kind of a situation information obtained via psychoperambulation and informal conferences with cooks or maids are not as important as they were in the poorly organized facility because the administrator herself is a good source of information. Administrators who behave this way generally have very good rapport with their patients. Ideally, these homes are best serviced by routine visits of the Modern Psychiatric Team, but this is not always possible. Social workers may have other commitments as do pharmacists, and although their attendance is optimal, it is not always possible. Failing that, a reasonably good job of patient follow-up can be done utilizing this two-person system.

THE NONEMERGENCY EMERGENCY

The nonemergency emergency occasionally occurs and can occur in any kind of home—be it well organized or poorly organized. A typical scenario involves a patient who starts making threats against others but does not do anything. This means the police cannot be called and even if they were called, usually not very much would happen. The administrator can then take the patient to a crisis clinic— providing he or she consents, which may not be the case. Besides, this may occur after hours when no crisis clinic or outreach worker is available, so the psychiatrist is called. Obviously the patient is not doing very well on his or her current medications, say, one of the newer atypical antipsychotics.

Okay, I will stop being hypothetical and admit that it happened to me and the patient was not doing well on his 8 mg dose of risperidone. I reviewed the patient's chart and noted that at some time in the past he was seen in an emergency room and responded well to a combo of haloperidol and lorazepam. However, he was not taking these meds currently and all the local pharmacies were closed. What to do?

Here is one of the hidden advantages of following multiple patients at the same site. I reviewed the charts of the other patients in the house and noted that one of them was taking haloperidol and another was taking lorazepam. I then instructed the administrator to take haloperidol out of patient A's box and give it to patient C, then take lorazepam out of patient B's box and also give that to patient C. I knew patient A and B very well and knew that neither one would be hurt by this temporary change. Problem solved. Crisis averted. Aside from helping the patient, this move helped the administrator. She did not know what to do and I don't blame her. If I were the administrator and didn't have me to refer to, I would not have known what to do either.

THE PROBLEMS THAT OCCUR
WHEN MRCPT MEMBERS DO NOT VISIT REGULARLY

Nonvisits by the Modern Psychiatric Team occur because Medicare generally does not compensate professionals for routine visits to residential care facilities.

Residential care facilities and all its synonyms are governed by the same Medicare policies that pertain to rest homes and domiciliaries. As indicated in the preface, these facilities are described on page 57 in the book titled *CPT 2004 Physicians' Current Procedural Terminology** published by the American Medical Association (AMA) as facilities that provide room, board, and other personal assistance services, generally on a long-term basis, but not including a medical component.[3] The administration of medication, regardless of how complex it might be, is generally not regarded by Medicare as sufficiently medical to be considered a medical component. Medicare regards the occupants of residential care facilities as ambulatory and therefore capable of making visits to psychiatrists' offices. Thus, there is no reason to pay for on-site visits unless the circumstances are unusual. There is thus an economic disincentive for professionals to make such visits.

I have previously described the impact of on-site professional interventions on home administrators and staff personnel, namely that administrators and house staff can grow professionally if they can attend team meetings and participate in the discussions. Also the establishment of this kind of routine can decrease the isolation of administrators, which in itself can be demoralizing and lead to nonproductive policies. This is especially true when administrators are confronted with behavior that is bizarre, confrontational, or destructive and which defies quick or obvious solutions. In my experience the effect of systematic prescheduled consultations or meetings should help to upgrade the home in terms of creating a therapeutic environment.

When such a situation does not exist, any number of bad outcomes can be expected.

Some of these bad outcomes were documented in a series of articles in *The New York Times* drawing upon more than 5,000 pages of annual state inspection reports, 200 interviews with workers, residents, and family members, and dozens of visits to the residential care facilities that were described as "places of misery and neglect, just like the psychiatric institutions before them."[4]

I am not claiming that the tragedies described in the *Times* article would necessarily have been averted had there been on-site visits by the Modern Residential Care Psychiatric Team, but many of the sorrowful situations gradually evolved over a period of time and there would have been ample opportunities for prophylactic intervention had professionals been encouraged to make routine on-site visits. *The New York Times* article is probably only the tip of the iceberg and hints at a national scandal. Abuse in residential care facilities is probably widespread but unrecognized. There is no reason to believe that the abuses in New York are not repeated elsewhere.

No national lobby represents board-and-care patients as a separate constituency. NAMI (National Alliance for the Mentally Ill) is a good organization formed by the relatives of mentally ill patients that defends the interests of all mentally ill patients. However, by the time the chronically mentally ill patient has been placed in a residential care facility he or she has been sick for a long time and is frequently out of touch with relatives or the relatives are deceased. Because of this there is minimal familial involvement and minimal pressure on legislators to address this problem.

Another factor contributing to the neglect of this population has already been remarked upon in the opening chapter: there are no national statistics on this population because of the multiplicity of names for these facilities. Adult homes in New York are known by different names in different states, such as board-and-care homes, group homes, adult foster homes, family care homes, residential care facilities, halfway houses, etc. No national statistics means no readily identifiable constituencies and consequently no lobbies, thus minimal pressure is exerted to effect legislative change. ·

In times past, when we walked in children's shoes, we assumed that the abuses of the total institution existed because of their geographical isolation. The total institution has been defined by Erving Goffman as "A place of residence and work where a large number of like-situated individuals, cut off from the wider society for an appreciable period of time together, lead an enclosed, formally administered round of life."[5] Many of the evils of mental hospitals were described as intrinsic to total institutions and schizophrenia was sometimes interpreted as a naturalistic response to an institutional environment. However, although institutions can contribute to dependency, they do not create schizophrenia. An essential distinction exists between contribution and creation. The idea that institutions created schizophrenia was formulated in the days before it was realized that schizophrenia is a disease of the brain. Thankfully, these regrettable sociological territorial incursions into schizophrenic causality have now been relegated to the dustbins of history along with the tattered remains of the schizophrenogenic mother, the double bind, and the marital skews and schisms of Dr. Lidz (Chapter 7).

In my opinion the standards of treatment in residential care facilities could be enhanced if there were OBRA-type recommendations with respect to visitation frequency and treatment. I understand that there is a natural reluctance to implement treatment guidelines by bureaucrats, yet such guidelines could be devised by physicians and follow the Expert Consensus Guideline Series.[6]

Chapter 16

Suicide

Some subjects do not lend themselves to humor, and suicide is one such subject. Suicide is obviously important because of its tragic effect on patients. It is also important because it accounts for the largest number of malpractice suits filed against psychiatrists.[1] Hence a patient's suicide may have a devastating effect on a psychiatrist's self-esteem and career.

In Chapter 8 I have claimed that the psychiatrist should make routine visits to residential care facilities and not wait until crises occur. Such routine visits are invaluable in terms of preventing relapses and rehospitalizations. This is true because the psychiatrist can intervene early in the course of an exacerbation to prevent its development. I have also said that routine visits do not necessarily stop a schizophrenic patient from committing suicide.

One of the problems with suicides in schizophrenic patients is that the suicides are likely to occur with minimal warning signs—unlike suicides in patients with mood disorders which are generally preceded by increases in depression. But even in depression, psychiatrists cannot predict who will commit suicide.[2]

That is why it is important to establish a baseline clinical impression of the patient's status. Thus even minimal departures from this baseline pattern can alert the physician as to an impending exacerbation. The physician can only obtain this baseline expectation by virtue of routine visits.

The risk of suicide attempts is greatest in the first ten years of illness and tends to occur during a psychotic exacerbation accompanied by depressive symptoms.[3] The incidence of suicide attempts in schizophrenia exceeds that of all other psychiatric diagnoses with the exception of major depression. The annual incidence of successful suicide attempts for schizophrenic patients is 0.4 to 1.1 percent with a lifetime risk for suicide attempts between 25 and 50 percent. The approximate lifetime risk for completing a successful suicide attempt is 10 percent.[4] It is estimated that every year 3,600 patients with schizophrenia commit suicide in the United States.[5]

Suicide attempts are sometimes very difficult to predict, and are sometimes but not always associated with a violent history. Some clues indicating a potential for suicide include a past history of violence toward others, a history of substance abuse, a history of past suicide attempts, social isolation, a history of recent rejection, and noncompliance with medications.[6]

The following are the case histories of two patients, one of whom committed suicide.

Patient A. B.

Pt. A. B. is a thirty-nine-year-old Spanish-speaking man who is bilingual and understands and speaks English fluently. He shows a long history of mental illness and psychiatric hospitalizations since he and his family moved to San Francisco from Cuba just after the revolution in 1959. There is a history of four previous hospitalizations at a state hospital as well as numerous community hospitalizations.

The brother called and stated that patient has been very upset for weeks and on this date he drove his older parents from the house by threats and manhandling them. He seemed very paranoid and upset to officers—talked very fast and incoherently. He was judged to be a danger to others and is gravely disabled.

Upon admission to the community hospital he was very paranoid, delusional, and anxious. He showed increased motor activity with pressured and loud speech. Pt. A. B. was described as angry, hostile, and fearful. Pt. A. B.'s family relates that the precipitating cause of Pt. A. B.'s decompensation was his refusal to take his medication. He is no longer welcomed in the family home.

CURRENT DIAGNOSIS: Schizophrenia, Schizoaffective Type

CURRENT MEDICATION:

Lithium 600 mg BID
Stelazine 20 mg BID
Cogentin 2 mg BID

CURRENT PROBLEMS LISTED:
1. Low impulse control
2. Housing
3. Need for conservatorship

Upon interview patient A. B. exhibits much grandiose speech and with delusional thought content. He states that he is a graduate of West Point and that in 1962 he was drugged by the CIA. He states that former President Eisenhower was his grandfather and that Queen Elizabeth of England is his cousin. He further states that he was crowned Kaiser of Germany in 1955. He states that all of his troubles are due to his poisoning by the CIA. Pt. A. B. states that he left over $500 million in Cuba and that he has money in bank accounts around the world. Pt. A. B. further states that he plans to oppose the conservatorship. He does not want to stay at the board-and-care facility nor does he wish to continue treatment in the _____ Mental Health Day Treatment Program. Pt. A. B. states plans to go to West Germany where he will resume his career as a rear admiral in the West German Navy. He shows little insight into his present need for treatment. He shows poor judgment and is incapable of making a realistic discharge plan for himself.

Pt. has been rendered gravely disabled as a result of his schizoaffective illness. At present he is incapable of providing for his basic needs. In addition, Pt. A. B. has proven unwilling and incapable of accepting needed psychiatric treatment on a voluntary basis. Pt. A. B.'s brother states that he would need constant supervision or he wouldn't take his medications. He would then lock himself in his room and barricade the door. Pt. A. B.'s behavior would then escalate to where the family felt threatened and unable to control him. Reportedly Pt. A. B. did well during the period he was under conservatorship. He apparently had a good working relationship with his conservator and his functioning remained stable during that period.

As stated Pt. A. B. came to San Francisco with his parents after leaving Cuba right after the revolution. Pt. A. B. apparently denies that these are his real parents. He refers to them as his stepmother and stepfather. He also refers to his brother as his stepbrother.

Pt. A. B. also refers to being divorced from his wife in 1962. However, the family says that this is delusional on his part. Pt. A. B. remains delusional about his financial matters and states that he has money in London, Bonn, and in San Jose, Costa Rica.

It is recommended that Pt. A. B. remain in a structured living situation such as his current residential care home. It is also recommended that he continue to participate in an intensive psychiatric treatment at the Mental Health Day Treatment Center.

It is recommended that a conservatorship be appointed for pt. He has been rendered gravely disabled as a result of a mental disorder. At present he is incapable of providing for his basic needs or making any realistic discharge plans for himself. In addition, pt. has proven both incapable and unwilling to accept needed treatment on a voluntary basis. He shows no insight into the severity of his mental illness and he has shown no motivation to participate in treatment. Conservatorship is needed to ensure that he participates in his outpatient psychiatric treatment plan.

Pt. C. D.

This twenty-nine-year-old white male has been treated since 1978 for chronic paranoid schizophrenia. He began having suicidal thoughts on 11/29/82 after he had a midterm examination in which he believed he had failed. He became progressively confused, disoriented, bizarre, and disorganized at his residence. His roommate called and described his extreme anxiety as well as his suicidal ideation. He described a near catatonic state in the patient and the patient was able to speak with me over the phone although he exhibited blocking of thought and confusion. He did report feeling suicidal and did agree to come to the hospital.

Today, he described this incident as feeling as though he were two years old and that any task—even walking—seemed burdensome. He admitted to hearing voices and developing a plan to commit suicide by drowning himself in the ocean (something he has attempted in the past). He is quite frightened about this experience and continues to have suicidal ideation at this time.

PAST PSYCHIATRIC HISTORY: The patient's first psychotic break occurred in 1974 during basic training for the services. He has had numerous hospitalizations since that time at private and state institutions. The past few hospitalizations here and during my care have been protracted ones. In 1978 he was hospitalized eight months out of the year including several months at a state hospital. In 1980 he attempted suicide by walking into the ocean and was hospitalized for a total of five months. During this period, he was extremely delusional and overtly psychotic. He did not respond to medications at that time and was transferred to the state hospital and eventually had a remission of his illness. In October 1981, he attempted suicide by overdose. He appeared to clear fairly quickly from this episode and was discharged only to attempt suicide again within a week by smashing his head through a window and attempting to cut his throat and wrist with glass. He was hospitalized for approximately three weeks on that occasion, once again appearing to clear only to attempt suicide the following day by jumping from a window at a 3/4-way house. He was hospitalized at that point for approximately four months partially at a private hospital and then transferred to a state hospital for ongoing care. In August 1982 he attempted suicide by jumping into a lake at Golden Gate Park but was able to seek care at that time and was again hospitalized briefly.

All of these episodes were secondary to acute psychotic experiences and paranoid delusions, for example of being the anti-Christ, and trying to kill himself as a result to save the world. In the past, he has been treated with a large variety of antipsychotic medications (Moban and Loxitane, Stelazine, Mellaril, Haldol, Prolixin, and Navane, etc.), some in very high doses. He has also been treated with lithium carbonate and antidepressant medication both singularly and in combination. He has never responded acutely to pharmacologic treatment and usually when the episodes become full blown he has ended up with several months of hospitalization before what is likely a natural remission in his illness occurs. Between episodes, he has usually done very well functioning in a volunteer job, being able to establish a residence, and managing his own affairs. Sometimes he has been maintained on very low-dose therapy, for example, Mellaril, 50 to 100 mg at bedtime.

Currently he has been followed by me as an outpatient and maintained on Navane, 10 mg PO in the morning and 30 mg PO at bedtime as well as Cogentin I mg twice a day. He has occasionally had delusional thoughts or ideas of reference; however, we have been able to maintain these by frequent contacts and by titrating his medication upward. It is worthy of note that during the past few months of nonhospitalization, he has not appeared to have cleared as completely as he has during past remissions.

PAST MEDICAL HISTORY: Cerebral palsy, mild

MENTAL STATUS: The mental status examination shows currently the patient is alert and oriented to time, place, person, and situation. His mood is slightly guarded; however, he is pleased to see me. His affect appears inappropriate at times, laughing, and then becoming very serious. Occasionally he glances out in a sideways manner and appears somewhat suspicious. He continues to have suicidal thoughts at this time and fears "losing control" and feeling "disoriented." He describes a near catatonic state that he fears entering once again. He has ideas of Satan controlling him and appears to be mildly hyperreligious.

He reluctantly admits to some auditory hallucinations and "bad thoughts." Currently his associations are intact and his sensorium is clear and his insight is fair. His judgment is deemed to be poor and his intellectual functions are intact.

IMPRESSION: Schizophrenia, paranoid type, acute exacerbation

DISCUSSION: This patient has a very serious and lethal disorder and appears to be having more frequent episodes of greater intensity, because he has attempted suicide so frequently in the past during his psychotic episodes. Great care will be taken to attempt to ensure that he is not discharged prematurely. Despite superficially appearing to clear in the past, he has made attempts at suicide and every effort will be made to forestall that occurrence on this hospitalization. He will be watched closely for suicide ideation and precautions will be taken.

Since the above described hospitalization in 1979, pt. C. D. has made several other suicide attempts involving drug overdoses, slashing his throat with broken glass, walking into the surf and attempting to drown himself, running into traffic, jumping out of a window (sustaining a fractured ankle), and swallowing glass.

It should be obvious that patient C. D. is the suicidal case, but I am not documenting case histories to illustrate the obvious. Patient C. D. was not the one who committed suicide. I have been taking care of him for four years now and he is doing fine—thanks to being on clozapine and thanks to his being monitored for compliance in a residential care facility setting. Some patients have a history of violent and recurrent suicide attempts in response to hallucinations, and when the hallucinations have been controlled, they do much better. These are the patients who are suicidal by history but who are no longer suicide threats.

Patient A. B. ended his life by leaping from the Golden Gate Bridge. Although a 10 percent lifelong incidence of suicide is estimated among schizophrenic patients, the suicide of patient A. B. was unexpected. Increasing depression was not indicated nor was the patient confronting any kind of crisis situation. On the day of the suicide he got dressed in his usual double-breasted suit, put his usual handkerchief in his breast pocket, and walked out never to return. He was obviously an extremely bizarre person and had been so for many years, but his level of irrationality had not changed noticeably. Moreover there was no history of suicide attempts or ideation throughout the course of his long-standing illness.

On the last progress note for patient A. B. written about one week before his successful suicide attempt, I noted that the patient had maintained his baseline status. He denied hearing voices and denied depression. He continued obviously delusional. Staff had not noticed any interim management problems. His activities of daily living continued to be rather good with no impairment in terms of bathing, continence, dressing, or eating. He slept well and had a good appetite. He did not appear under any unusual stress and his medications had not been recently changed.

It appears to be true that with respect to some schizophrenic patients, no amount of increase in visitation frequency is sufficient to abort the suicide because the attempt arises out of a sudden impulse that is not apparently related to externally observable symptoms or events. The schizophrenic patient who commits or attempts suicide does not always provide the prodromal warnings that are evident in depressed patients in which suicidal attempts appear as the logical culmination of an intensification of depressive symptoms.

The most extreme example of a sudden impulse suicide unaccompanied by depression is illustrated by the case of patient E. F. Here is a brief hospital summary of this patient.

Patient E. F.

This thirty-three-year-old Caucasian male was discharged from a community hospital in 1976. He became irrational in a family dispute and hurled furniture and threatened to kill his parents. He is casually dressed, well-behaved. Oriented times three spheres. Good memory. Has had auditory hallucinations in the past. Affect is labile. Denies suicidal feelings. Insight and judgment are impaired. In good physical health.

Provisional Diagnosis: 295.90
Psychiatric: 295.90—Schizophrenia, Chronic Undifferentiated Type
Physical: None
Lab Findings: None

REASON FOR ADMISSION: During a family argument pt. broke the furniture and threatened to kill his parents. During the admission interview he was well-behaved, appeared oriented in three spheres. His memory for past events was good. Affect was labile. He admitted to hallucinations in the past, His insight and judgment were impaired.

Problems:

1. Assaultive and destructive behavior in home of father. Realizes now that his behavior was entirely unacceptable.
2. Auditory hallucinations. No sign of any for approximately four weeks.
3. Impaired daily living activities. Has definitely improved.
4. Independent living skills impairment. Pt. has been working on a work detail for several weeks. As to how he might do in the community, only the future will tell.

MEDICATION AND TREATMENT MODALITIES: Mellaril, 200 mgs., h.s.; work detail; encounter group therapy; one-on-one interviews; family therapy as well.

RECOMMENDATIONS: Discharge, Improved. pt. appears to appreciate that his past behavior has caused nothing but trouble. He is ready to try to settle down and develop a mature affect.

5-18-77 DISCHARGED Improved

A second hospitalization within a year revealed the same pattern of episodic destructiveness directed toward his family, but no suicidal attempts or ideation.

A thirty-three-year-old separated Caucasian male returns to community hospital for the second time within a year. He has led somewhat of a vagabond life in the past, hitchhiking from the San Francisco area to Los Angeles and not engaging in any meaningful employment. Lives on county relief. Recently in Reno where for reasons unknown he was jailed. Following his release he returned to San Francisco where he found that his common-law wife had lived but he could not find her. He contacted his father in Los Angeles and asked him to send him money to return home.

As has occurred in the past, patient and his father eventually had a rather severe altercation which resulted in the patient's breaking a window in his father's house. The police were called and the patient was hospitalized.

Mental status is one of flatness, dullness, and colorless in relation to his environment, depicting a loss of affect and feeling tones. He is facetious and tends to make light of his present situation. He has heard voices in the past but not at present; he cannot give their content. He denies suicidal thoughts but rambles and has rather loose associations. He frequently smiles in an inappropriate manner. He denies he needs help at this time. Feels that he has an allergy to grasses.

Patient appears to be oriented in three spheres. He shows marked thought disorganization. He has no plans for the future. There is much guarding, much suspiciousness, as he furtively looks about the room from one team member to another. Physical examination reveals no significant abnormalities.

Diagnosis: Schizophrenia, Chronic Undifferentiated Type

Patient E. F. was briefly described in an earlier chapter on the importance of making routine visits for patients that do not superficially appear to warrant a visit. What I mean by this is that the patient may not be under acute distress and the parameters of the situation might not fit the definition of "medical necessity" as it is defined by the AMA and Medicare as described in a previous chapter. The case of E. F. is repeated more in detail here to demonstrate the unpredictability of suicide. Patient E. F. had no history of suicide attempts prior to the time I assumed responsibility for his care in October 1981. His adjustment to the residential care facility was nonremarkable. In my last progress note I stated that patient continued to maintain his baseline adjustment, denied hearing voices or feeling depressed, his grooming had deteriorated slightly, and that the staff had not reported any interim management problems. I certainly could not detect any signs of increasing depression or suicidal intent.

Fifteen minutes after I wrote that note, the patient leaped from a third-story window into a garden. It had rained heavily the night before and the patient's fall was cushioned by a thick layer of mud, which bore the foot-deep indentations of both elbows and both knees. The patient, however, was none the worse for wear. Shortly after the attempt, I received an angry call by someone claiming to be his brother demanding to know how long it had been since I had seen the patient. Kindly notice I said "claiming to be his brother" because I had had no prior contact with this person despite years of treating the patient. This patient showed no prior depression, did not admit to suicidal ideation, and had no history of suicide attempts. It is difficult for me to see what I did wrong in this case. The point of all this is that suicides happen in residential care facilities, and they cannot always be anticipated or avoided.

If a suicide is anticipated and therefore avoided, it is not a suicide. It is only the leftover suicide that becomes the statistic. It is possible by scrupulous attention to every detail to avoid one hundred potential suicides and yet miss one. The one hundred aborted suicides are statistical nonevents. The one event that is documented is the successful suicide attempt. If baseball statisticians were to use this method of computation, they would only count strikeouts and ignore hits. Successful suicide attempts have occurred in hospital settings which have more security measures than are possible in a residential care home. Although the frequency of suicides may be reduced, there will always be someone who escapes detection.

The lesson to be learned from this last case is that no degree of increased visitation frequency and no amount of extra caution can prevent this type of event from happening. Had I seen patient E. F. every half-hour around the clock, he still would have had ample time to make his leap between visits. If his suicide attempt had been successful, I would have felt very bad, but not guilty.

Thus, the schizophrenic patient who commits suicide may actually not be a suicidal patient in the generally accepted meaning of the term. Schizophrenic patients who commit suicide may have a history of suicidal ideation and suicide attempts in which case the designation of suicidal appears appropriate. However, as indicated by the previous case histories, some patients who commit or attempt suicide have no prior history of this and may not be considered suicidal in the accepted meaning of the term. Also, other patients may be considered suicidal by their case histories, yet they are no longer suicidal threats.

I am not generally frightened by patients who have a suicide history of drug overdoses. Generally speaking, such patients have not overdosed on dangerous drugs and possibly they were on the wrong medications to begin with. Of course, one can say that under such circumstances I am dealing with the survivors, and not the people who have died as a result of drug overdoses, so that my population of overdosers is not truly random. But I am not interested in random samples of a population of overdosers. After all, it is the living patients that I am trying to treat—and if the overdoses were with psychiatric medications that tend to be relatively safe (unless we are talking about tricyclic antidepressants), I feel that I can control such patients in a residential care home setting.

From these case histories the reader may have deduced that it is not wise for some people to live near the Golden Gate Bridge, but we have no way of knowing whether such suicides could have been prevented by changes of address. Sometimes an attempt is made to understand more about an individual suicide through psychological autopsies. The problem with postmortem wisdom is that it is fairly easy to be wise in retrospect. "Should"—as in you "should" have done this or you "should" have done that—is an easy word to apply when describing the professional obligations of others to control past situations that are now beyond control.

By and large it is the quiet, nonobtrusive, withdrawn patients who tend to receive short shrift in therapeutic visitations. This can be quite dangerous because these patients are more likely to get lost in the akathisic shuffle. A suicide attempt in the absence of a recent progress note is not good news for the attending psychiatrist—even if he or she made a recent visit that was undocumented.

The bottom line is that nobody can prove that residential care facilities diminish suicide. If I am wrong about this I wish somebody would tell me, because I would like to be wrong. The problem with statistical breakdowns of suicide in residential care facilities is that, as previously explained, only the negative events are statistically meaningful. Other would-be events are nonevents.

By nonevents I refer to those patients who would have been suicidal had they lived alone or in nonsupervised dwellings but who never became suicidal because of the care and supervision they received in a residential care home. Such people are not in the statistical universe because they are statistical nonevents. Nobody can prove how many patients are in this category, although patient C. D., the previously described chronic suicide attempter, is one such patient.

Chapter 17

IM Medications—
How to Do It and Why

It is generally acknowledged that the use of antipsychotic medications in chronic schizophrenia is necessary to reduce the risk of relapse. Yet many times patients will resist taking medications or will not comply with treatment plans for a variety of reasons. This tends to be less of a problem in residential care facilities with visiting psychiatrists because caregivers can discuss the problems with the psychiatrist and the psychiatrist in turn can discuss the issues with the patient. Some of the reasons for the lack of compliance are the patient's failure to understand the importance of routinely taking medications as a way of avoiding repeated cycles of decompensation and rehospitalization, mistaken ideas about drug addiction, paranoid thinking, ordinary forgetfulness, a poor relationship with the physician, or the experience of unpleasant side effects. Many times such issues can be resolved by the psychiatrist discussing the problems with the patient. Thus, an issue such as unpleasant side effects can be resolved by several methods, such as changing a medication, lowering the dose, or adding another medication to counteract the side effects. Also during such sessions the patient should actually be encouraged to report unpleasant side effects as a way of helping the psychiatrist help the patient. Patients should be invited to ask questions about their medications. Such interventions can only serve to enhance the therapeutic alliance. I have had patients not tell me about adverse side effects because they did not want to hurt my feelings. Sometimes the therapeutic alliance can be a bit much. Nevertheless, some patients will resist taking medications. Frequently patients who demonstrate a resistance to oral medication will consent to long-acting injectable preparations. It may seem strange that someone will prefer an injection to a pill, but schizophrenic patients are not necessarily noted for their rationality.

Despite the abundant literature on the usefulness of depot medications, very little in the psychiatric literature addresses the issue of how to administer long-acting injectable antipsychotic medications to psychiatric patients. Two such preparations have enjoyed historical use in the United States, fluphenazine decanoate and haloperidol decanoate. Both of these preparations are administered by intramuscular injection using a sesame seed oil-based vehicle. The injected antipsychotic drug is chemically bound to a fatty acid side chain to form a prodrug. At the site of injection, the fatty acid side chain is gradually cleaved and the prodrug becomes active. The esterified biochemical structure of both drugs permits a slow rate of absorption from the injection site. Because of this, the terminal serum half-life of fluphenazine has been extended to eight to fourteen days (the half-life of the oral preparation is fifteen to twenty-four hours). Similarly the half-life of haloperidol was extended to nineteen to twenty-one days (compared to the half-life of eighteen to twenty-four hours for the oral medication). It is sometimes preferable to use injectable long-acting antipsychotics when patients are noncompliant with oral meds. Also occasionally IM meds will work on patients who are refractory to oral meds, possibly because they bypass first-pass effects by the liver. Also such preparations can be used to help stabilize patients initially who may later consent to take oral medications.

In October 2003 the FDA approved the use of long-acting injectable risperidone which combines the advantages of atypical antipsychotic with those of a long-acting antipsychotic. The gradual release mechanism differs from that of the conventional long-acting preparations in that the risperidone is gradually released from microspheres enclosed within a biodegradable polymer shell. Along with the advantages of an atypical antipsychotic, long-acting risperidone also includes the disadvantages, namely cost. A 25 mg dose costs $225 versus $50 for a 100 mg dose of haloperidol.[1] According to the early literature it would seem that 25 mg every two weeks would be an adequate dose for most patients.

Theoretically adverse side effects can last a long time because of the long half-lives of the preparations, and for this reason it is a good idea to start with a low dose, such as 0.25 cc of either of the decanoate preparations. In practice I have rarely encountered side effects that were severe or long-lasting. Another way of avoiding adverse reactions is to administer the oral preparations first if the patient consents, and later decide which IM preparation should be employed—if any.

Long-acting depot medications still have some advantages even when compared to the newer oral medications because of the compliance factor. Data from a large study of patients on oral antipsychotic medications indicated that patients with noncompliance or only partial compliance were more than 2.4 times more likely to be rehospitalized than patients who were medication compliant.[2] In addition, long-acting antipsychotics provide a more consistent delivery system which leads to more stable plasma levels. A more stable and predictable plasma level makes it much easier to evaluate the effect of newer add-on medications—and this is becoming increasingly important because of the growing tendency to employ polypharmacy—rightfully or wrongfully.

Many psychiatrists are reluctant to administer IM injections, preferring to automatically relegate such pedestrian medical procedures to a nurse. This is understandable if the psychiatrist works in a hospital or clinic or other settings where nurses are available. However, nurses are generally not available in the psychiatrist's office or at residential care facilities, although it is true that a psychiatrist can order a home visit by a nurse for the purpose of administering an injection. Under such circumstances the home visit by the nurse will cost much more to Medicare than the visit by the psychiatrist. Also most of the proceeds will go to the home visiting nurse agency rather than to the home visiting nurse. Thus if a psychiatrist learns to administer injections himself or herself, then he or she will save Medicare lots of money. This may not be a sufficient incentive for some psychiatrists to learn to overcome their phobia about administering (or receiving) injections, but in the final analysis, we are all taxpayers. Besides, there are other reasons why psychiatrists who make home visits should learn how to administer injections—which I shall describe shortly.

In the administration of long-acting IM depot medications to deltoid and gluteus, the psychiatrist's nose comes in close proximity to armpit and crotch, and as such it affords an exquisite appreciation of the patient's baseline with respect to grooming and personal hygiene. Nowhere else in psychiatry is this degree of nose-to-crotch immediacy professionally acceptable. This information, along with the subtle changes in mental status that accompany the early phases of an exacerbation, can be utilized by the psychiatrist to titrate dosages. Sometimes the early phases of deterioration in self-care can be inferred from the persistence of a Band-Aid that was applied two weeks earlier. Sometimes the changes are not so subtle, as when the patient offers his or her arm but is too preoccupied to roll up his or her sleeve.

Additional information pertaining to the titration of dosages may sometimes be obtained by consultation with the facility staff persons. Where there is a pattern of responsiveness, such that a given patient may start to deteriorate two or three days before the administration of the next scheduled dose (the therapeutic effect of the long-acting injections may last from one to four weeks), the psychiatrist may then decide to administer a larger dose or to administer it more frequently.

For these reasons, under optimal circumstances, the same person should administer the decanoate preparations, and that person should be a psychiatrist or a psychiatric nurse. In less than optimal circumstances these conditions will not be possible, but in such cases quality of care may be compromised.

The administration of intramuscular decanoate preparations has had some unexpected beneficial side effects—not the least of which is that the use of the syringe contributes to the image of the psychiatrist as being at home with modern medical technology and all that this implies in terms of the epidemiological control of a biological illness. Possibly because of this, a relationship builds up between injector and injectee such that even after patients have left the residential care facility and have achieved independence, they frequently prefer to continue seeing me in my office for ongoing treatment. Aside from image building, I will admit that at times administering an injection has given me a spurious sense of achievement by doing something therapeutic that does not involve talking.

IM decanoate medications are effective as long-term maintenance therapy in chronic schizophrenia and are widely used in Europe and the United Kingdom. In the United States, however, physicians have been reluctant to use them. They assume that depot neuroleptics present an increased risk of major side effects, that patients do not accept or tolerate them as well as oral agents, and that prescribing depot neuroleptics increases the possibility of medicolegal problems. Clinical experience has shown these medications to be very safe and that they present no greater risk than oral antipsychotic medications.[3]

However, if side effects do occur, they can last much longer as compared to the effects of orally administered medications. For this reason it is probably a good idea to first administer fluphenazine or haloperidol orally to determine patient sensitivity, and in any case to start with a relatively low dose such as 6.25 mg of fluphenazine (0.25 cc) or a similar dose of haloperidol. It is possible that with the advent of the newer or so-called atypical antipsychotics, the need for fluphenazine decanoate and haloperidol decanoate will diminish.

THE TECHNIQUE OF IM ADMINISTRATION

Only a few articles in the literature describe how to administer depot neuroleptic injections to psychiatric patients. If one is interested in pursuing primary sources one can find such an article in *The Canadian Nurse*[4] that dissects the procedure into twenty-seven different steps. But I didn't read that article until I was in the midst of writing this book so what I have learned, I have learned by the seat of my shiny pants. Therefore, if you are a psychiatrist planning to administer the decanoate injections, please pay attention. This is important because in some instances the IM decanoates—both of the haloperidol and fluphenazine variety—will work better than any other psychopharmacological preparations including the newer generation atypical antipsychotic preparations. This is true because there will be many instances of patient noncompliance, or simulated compliance—as when a patient cheeks his or her medications before making a quick trip to the bathroom to unload. It is understandable that under such circumstances no oral preparation is going to work.

There can be many reasons for noncompliance including failure to fill a prescription, deliberate attempts at stopping medication, misunderstanding instructions, and inability to follow complicated routines. In many of these instances scheduled periodic injections of long-acting antipsychotic medications can help avert the problems of noncompliance. One of the unheralded good aspects of IM regimens is that noncompliance can be monitored whereas it is more difficult to monitor compliance with oral regimens. This makes it easier to correlate noncompliance with hospitalization rates. In one such study, Curson et al. found that over a seven-year period 50 percent of IM depot-compliant outpatients were admitted to the hospital compared with 100 percent of the noncompliant patients.[5] While this indicates that compliance is very important in preventing rehospitalizations, it also indicates that patients' illnesses can exacerbate even when compliance exists.

Injections to the deltoid are best administered to the posterior aspect of the deltoid where it is least painful. I generally aim for a site that is latitudinally about 1 cm posterior to the deltoid midline and longitudinally about 5 or 6 cm below the acromioclavicular joint. Anatomically I cannot specify why the posterior deltoid is less painful than the anterior deltoid since this is an observation based solely on empirical experience, but if I were pressured into an explanation, I would sound very knowledgeable and say something about the decreased density of nociceptive pain fibers in the skin overlying the posterior deltoid as compared to the anterior deltoid—either I would say that or something equally arcane if only to hide my ignorance.

Ask the patient to fold his or her arm across his or her lap. This position will help to relax the deltoid. To stimulate additional relaxation of the muscle, briefly massage the area of the muscle overlying the injection site. This makes it even less painful. I found that I could not do this without touching the patient, much to the possible consternation of my mentors in academic psychology—my first career. However, I never informed them of my transgressions. In administering these injections, it is generally not necessary to use the Z technique. The Z technique involves retracting the skin and subcutaneous tissue from the injection site, then injecting, then withdrawing the syringe and releasing the pressure on the skin to avoid creating a straight-line needle tract that would allow the ready backflow of injected material. The Z technique is used for IM medications that are not very viscous—such as iron preparations, but it really is unnecessary since both of the decanoate preparations are sufficiently viscous to prevent significant backflow through the injection site, providing the injection is slowly administered. By slow administration, I mean about 30 seconds per cc.

If patients appear unduly apprehensive and lock their eyes on the syringe, talk about some unrelated topic while about to administer the injection—or even about a related topic—anything to remove the eye from the needle. Most of the time the injection will be painless and the patient will think you are a great doctor, which is one of the hitherto unheralded advantages of administering painless injections. It is now heralded. It is not necessary to wear a white coat during this procedure. That's about all there is to it. Oh, yes, I almost forgot. Do not stick yourself with the needle.

If despite all your efforts, the patient complains of discomfort or pain, do not despair. What you do under these circumstances is to knowingly assert, "The reason it hurts so much is that your muscles are too tense." If that doesn't work, say, "The reason it hurts so much is that you were looking at the needle. The next time I give you an injection, focus your eyes elsewhere." Exude an air of confidence when you make these statements. In any event, make sure you blame the patient for feeling the pain. This reinforces the patient's impression that you are a fine doctor, even if you are not. Besides, you may be correct.

One other afterthought that really should be a before-thought. Before you inject, pull back on the plunger to make sure the needle has not entered a blood vessel. Both of the IM preparations of haloperidol and fluphenazine are in sesame oil vehicles. Theoretically speaking, IV administration could cause a fat embolus. Also since the preparations are viscous, it can be very difficult to withdraw fluid through the perforation site if you are withdrawing from a partially evacuated vial in which the remaining fluid is under negative atmospheric pressure. To circumvent this is not a very serious problem; inject air into the vial before withdrawing, but remember—I'm talking about injecting air into the vial, not the patient. If you have trouble understanding the theory, just remember the phrase "accentuate the positive."

The instructions in the *Physicians' Desk Reference* for the administration of IM haloperidol decanoate are to administer it as a deep intramuscular injection using a 21-gauge needle and to administer no more than 3 cc at any one injection site. Contrary to popular belief, it is not necessary to administer fluphenazine decanoate as an IM dose. It can be administered subcutaneously if that is preferred, although I prefer the IM route for doses greater than 1cc. If you don't believe me you can look it up in the *Physicians' Desk Reference (PDR)*. The only problem with this is that you won't find any reference to fluphenazine decanoate or Prolixin decanoate in the *PDR* for 2001, or even for 2000. If you still don't believe me, try looking it up again. You still won't find it. That might come as a surprise to doctors—possibly even a bigger surprise than discovering that instructions to administer a medication "biweekly" can mean either every two weeks or twice a week. You will not find that etymological tidbit in the *PDR* either, but it will be in the dictionary—*Webster's,* not *Dorland's.*

I suspect the manufacturers yanked out the reference because fluphenazine decanoate is now generically produced and use of the decanoate might impede sales of the oral product. Since fluphenazine decanoate can be administered subcutaneously, it is possible to administer it using a 5/8", 22-gauge needle for those patients who have a phobia about long needles.

The haloperidol decanoate preparation comes in two concentration strengths, 50 mg per cc and 100 mg per cc. In my experience, the 50 mg per cc is better tolerated in that some patients complain of a painful sensation at the administration site of the 100 mg per cc preparation. This has never happened with the 50 mg preparation and offhand I cannot see any reason to use the 100 mg preparation unless very large doses are required. Even in that circumstance, it could be an option to still administer the 50 mg preparation but with a greater degree of frequency.

CLINICAL EXAMPLES OF THE USE OF LONG-ACTING IM DEPOT INJECTIONS

Sometimes the therapeutic effects of depot injectables might not be apparent for months.

Patient R. S.

R. S. is a fifty-year-old male with a schizophrenic history dating back to more than thirty years and involving multiple hospitalizations. His pattern in the home was to leave the house every day and go on long walks to the beach where he would systematically count the number of people lying on the beach, the number of surfers, the number of fishermen, and the number of dogs—statistics which he would faithfully convey to me during each of my visits. It was my habit to dutifully log these statistics into a progress note while I was in his presence and he was in my presence so as to emphasize that this was important information which I expected him to convey to me at future appointments—somewhat like an intelligence operation with him as the agent and me as his handler. My not-so-obvious ulterior motive underlying all of this was to encourage his presence and cooperation for future haloperidol decanoate injections, which I assured him made him more alert and able to process information better—not even a lie when it works optimally for the disorganized patient.

In addition to census taking he would also retrieve various items discovered on his daily shoreline constitutionals—such as old clothes, old shoes, and discarded umbrellas, then sequester them under his bed. Periodically, piles of junk had to be extracted from his room. The aforementioned haloperidol injections were needed because he refused oral medications and this was my only option other than complete capitulation. Interestingly enough, he did not object to the injections other than to imply that he really didn't need the injections because he was normal.

However, my efforts did not seem to have any effect on his rat-packing proclivities. If anything, he pursued his passion for collectables with an industriousness that only seemed to increase with the passage of time. As a result the administrator was not particularly impressed by my therapeutic efforts or by me personally, since this was the only patient I was following at the house and my failure rate approximated 100 percent, or so it seemed. In fact, there were times when she would unwittingly (to be gracious about it) lock the office door so that I would be unable to obtain the patient's chart to enter a progress note. I think she was under the impression that I was practicing some kind of a Medicare hustle and ultimately she even had me convinced of that possibility. In fact, I had the premonition that if Medicare were to investigate me for providing unnecessary medical services by administering haloperidol injections, which I did about every month, I would have trouble defending myself other than to stress the importance of keeping *au courant* with the changing demography of shoreline habitats—which admittedly is a bit of a reach even in these days of rabid environmentalism. I eventually told her that I would no longer be routinely visiting the home since the patient did not apparently benefit from my treatment. However, she should call me should anything come amiss.

The amiss came three months after the last injection, which can give one a clue as to how long the therapeutic effects of long-acting depot injections can exist. The administrator telephoned me stating that, earlier in the day, the patient had decided too many cars were parked next to the home and proceeded to smash the windows of five cars that were, as is frequently said about human victims, "in the wrong place at the wrong time." Were the police called? Yes, they were. What did they do? They told the administrator the patient should see his doctor. Very thoughtful of them to make referrals.

Now this is really a case of man bites dog. The fact is that such patients rarely, if ever, inflict injuries on cars. It usually works the other way. Cars inflict injury on them because they don't look where they are going. We all have seen people like this—some of them are officially designated as outpatients and some of them are not designated as patients at all—neither the in-type or the out-type. We have seen them strolling across the pedestrian crosswalks of urban America somehow managing to combine sauntering with a grim determination to get to the other side—eventually and in due course. Frequently their heads are encased in headphones, their eyes unwaveringly focused on a distant object like race horses in a horse race, looking neither to the left, nor to the right for incoming objects, so that they neither see nor hear approaching vehicles because that is not their legal obligation nor is it their problem. It only becomes a problem after a pedestrian injury, in which case it also becomes a problem for drivers and subsequently for the taxpayers who have to pay for courts, attorneys, hospitals, doctor bills, and insurance premiums. Possibly there should be a law requiring pedestrian headphone aficionados to wear motorcycle helmets.

So the pattern of patient damaging car is statistically unrepresentative and, of course, I had to get to the bottom of it. Using guile, indirection, and subtlety as an investigatory technique, I proceeded as follows:

ME: Why did you do it?

HIM: Why did I do what?

ME: Why did you smash the car windows?

HIM: I didn't do nothin.'

ME: I am going to give you an injection. Remember, like the ones I used to give you before?

HIM: Why?

ME: To make you into a normal American fellow.

HIM: I already am a normal American fellow.

ME: I know that you are a normal American fellow, but you are a normal American fellow in your own way. I want you to be a normal American fellow in a different way.

HIM: What kind of normal American fellow do you want me to be?

ME: I want you to be a normal American fellow like the kind of normal American fellow who goes around normally and does not smash car windows of normal American cars—or even normal American Japanese cars. That's why I want to give you the shot.

HIM: All right.

End of dialogue. Now if one reads this colloquy out loud, it will become apparent that this represents the interactions of two psychotics. Diagnostic labels do not bother me. I will readily acknowledge that I am eligible for one of those five-digit diagnostic codes with two decimal places that psychiatrists are required to use when submitting claim forms to Medicare. The important point is that the patient is back on the previously maligned haloperidol decanoate injections every three weeks and the NIMBY neighbors are sleeping more easily, as is the administrator—so far.

The decanoate preparations—also called long-acting depot injections—can be used effectively with more violent patients who might otherwise be sentenced to long prison terms, as is demonstrated by the following brief case descriptions submitted to the Medicaid consultant for continued treatment authorization.

Patient G. H.

Thirty-four-year-old male committed to prison in 1970 on penal code for robbery and carrying concealed weapon. Not guilty by reason of insanity. Transferred to a state hospital in 1972. Discharged in 1973 on biweekly Prolixin decanoate, which I currently continue. Gets confused and hallucinates if he misses an injection. Needs 2 cc every two weeks. No hospitalizations have occurred in the twelve years that I have been following the patient.

I started treating this patient thirty-one years ago and the above authorization request is quoted in an article I wrote seventeen years ago. Since that time the patient had improved to the point where he was able to leave the residential care facility and live independently. However, this did not last. What happened is that he felt so good for so long that he decided he no longer needed the IM injections. That is one of the hazards of a good response to the long-acting depot medications. In a way it is understandable. If one takes an injection and feels good for two weeks, why not try for three or four weeks or longer?

Actually he did reasonably well off meds for two months, but then was admitted to a prestigious university hospital where he received a thorough work-up. The admission note states, "Patient reported decreased sleep since his mother's death and now sleeps only three hours per night. He cried the night before admission but he was unable to determine the duration of his tearfulness. He was angry that some of his relatives did not come to the funeral. He was worried that someone was out to get him and he paid $50 for someone to get him a gun."

The patient subsequently improved and in February 1994 was discharged on the following medications:

1. Lithium 300 mg 2 tabs in a.m., 3 tabs HS
2. Trilafon 16 mg 1 tab in a.m., 1 tab HS
3. Klonopin 0.5 mg 1 tab TID
4. Artane 5 mg 1 tab BID
5. Synthroid 0.125 mg 1 tab daily

It is difficult to say whether this combination was hastily contrived or carefully conceived, but it was grossly inappropriate. No psychiatrist in his or her right mind should expect a disorganized schizophrenic patient who is not in his or her right mind and living alone to follow a regimen requiring him or her to take two different pills twice a day, another pill three times a day, and another pill once a day. In addition to this he must remember to take two lithium tablets in the morning and three at night. Personally speaking, I take one 81 mg aspirin tablet once a day to ward off strokes and heart attacks and I sometimes forget to take it—and I'm not even a schizophrenic. Could we really expect this patient to follow this regimen?

The story has a happy ending. Within a month he was knocking on my door without an appointment after I had not seen him for a year. He complained that he could not keep up with "all those pills." I restarted him on fluphenazine injections and discontinued all of the previously described medications except Artane and Synthroid. I do not give him appointments because he cannot keep appointments, but I have taught him to recognize the signs that his fluphenazine shot is wearing off: he starts sleeping too little and starts talking too much. He is pretty sensitive to these signs and comes in for his shots about every three weeks. He has been doing this for the past nine years and has been able to continue living alone successfully with no additional hospitalizations.

One of the unusual aspects of treatment of this patient is that I do not schedule his appointments. I realize that in standard office procedure (SOP) this informality might not work, but it is the most practical option for this patient. Obviously this would not be possible if my day were filled with twenty-five-minute or fifty-minute dedicated blocks of time to individual patients. What I have done in my office practice is to allow large blocks of time for informal drop-ins, since I have other patients who are also not hindered by temporal constraints. To some people an appointment time is an estimate rather than a commitment and this is an unchangeable aspect of their lifestyle. It is of course, difficult to say whether this weltanschauung has its basis in Kant's categorical imperatives or is more simply an application of the Einsteinian principle of relativity as it relates to time.

Obviously not all psychiatrists should see people like that, and in a sense, all of us choose the kinds of patients we treat. But if a psychiatrist does have such patients much more will be gained by adopting novel ways to cope with unusual situations. Obviously—or not so obviously, this dedication of a block of time to a variable number of patients is one way in which my residential care facility practice has effected my office practice.

The next patient is someone who refused to take oral medications. I used to treat him in a residential care facility setting, but he improved sufficiently so that he was able to return home and live with his mother. However he still refused oral medications but consented to continued treatment with IM fluphenazine decanoate. However he would only come to the office if accompanied by his mother and his dog. In a sense he is the opposite of the previously described patient who comes in voluntarily unaccompanied by a mother and a dog. He is in the habit of locking the door when I am with him because he fears intrusions from alien sources. I make light of this and ask him if he is expecting anybody. He responds with comments like "I'm not if you are not." Such scintillating ripostes has kept our relationship going for the past ten years—a record for a psychiatric relationship for this patient.

The following information was obtained from a hospital admission summary:

Patient J. K. is a twenty-nine-year-old, single, Caucasian male currently living with his family in San Francisco. He is unemployed and has a long psychiatric history.

REFERRAL SOURCE: Patient was brought in by the police involuntarily as a danger to others after an altercation at his home.

CHIEF COMPLAINT: "It's my brother's fault; he pulled a knife on me."

HISTORY OF PRESENT ILLNESS: This current admission is one of several for this patient, who began to decompensate around May 1984. At that time he called the president threatening to "flush him down the toilet," which resulted in hospitalization at a federal prison for a few months. He was discharged home under the care of his parents and had been followed erratically by the Day Treatment Center Team. He had apparently done well in a structured situation but was noncompliant when he was discharged (this is a long and recurrent behavior for him). He was therefore on no medications prior to admission for a period of more than six months. Family reported that during the month prior to admission patient was noted to stare out the window in anticipation of hostile parties; he also spent a great deal of time in the family basement chanting and burning charcoal outside of the fireplace. Mother reported volumes of smoke often billowing out underneath the door. During the entire month of December patient remained inside the house because of a fear of a contract out on his life, and only periodically came up to the kitchen to receive food from his parents. Parents reported that patient never in his life cooked a meal for himself, used the banking system, bought food, or lived alone. This admission followed an altercation with his brother who apparently was threatening him with a knife. Patient threw an organ bench and later threatened to kill his brother. The police were called by mother and patient was brought in on a seventy-two-hour hold as a danger to others and gravely disabled.

PSYCHIATRIC HISTORY: Patient's first psychiatric hospitalization was at a state hospital at the age of twenty for paranoid psychotic decompensation illustrated by his writing threatening letters to a variety of public officials, including the president of the United States and directors of the CIA and FBI. He was then hospitalized at a private hospital for the first time in 1978, when he believed he would be taking over the country by 1980. He was again hospitalized in 1978 after writing threatening letters to public officials, which resulted in the Secret Service showing up with a warrant for his arrest in July 1979. Patient was hospitalized again after writing threatening letters in San Francisco to the director of Mental Health Services, and in each case was treated psychiatrically rather than criminally for these offenses. Federal prosecution was deferred with the understanding that he was to continue taking his medications. In October 1980, patient was told the federal government had no further "hold" on him, after which he promptly stopped taking his medications and showed deterioration in his mental status. In the seven months that followed he worked part-time with his stepfather, but became more withdrawn and isolated. He displayed suspicious and delusional traits that he would be killed and, as noted, was spending a great deal of time at the window peeking through the curtains. He was hospitalized again in 1981, 1982, and twice in 1983 for exacerbation of his chronic psychotic condition. In addition to making threats to various public officials, he stated that he was "Hitler reincarnated."

MEDICAL HISTORY: Medical history is unremarkable.

DEVELOPMENTAL HISTORY: Developmental history is unremarkable.

SOCIAL HISTORY: Patient was born in Santa Monica. His natural father left the family when he was six months old. Mother moved to San Francisco when he was sixteen months old and remarried when he was three. Patient attended Catholic schools through the twelfth grade, graduated, and attended a state university for two years. He claimed to do B-average work.

Mother has been in outpatient treatment for a number of years. Throughout patient's hospitalizations she has been extremely ambivalent about his hospitalizations and in a number of legal hearings has changed her mind about allowing him home. Patient has apparently done fairly well when under enforced treatment.

Obviously this is a very severe illness. The newer atypical antipsychotics are not helpful because he refuses oral medications, but he consents to IM fluphenazine as long as I limit the dose to 2.5 cc, which I administer every two weeks. I am certain about the dose because after he enters the office with the mother and the dog and after he locks the door, he always monitors me when I fill the syringe. Strangely enough, this patient has a very good sense of humor and I am generally able to kid around with him about his secrecy.

In the role model sense I am teaching this patient how to go easy and how to enjoy life just a little bit, and he seems to be learning little at a time. As noted in the previous case history information, he has a history of severe paranoia and was actually incarcerated in a federal prison for writing threatening letters to the president. He no longer writes threatening letters. He consents to the IM fluphenazine decanoate injection every two weeks providing I allow him to monitor me when I fill the syringe. He wants to make certain that the dose continues to be 2.5 cc. I don't mind this since this gives him a sense of participating in his treatment which has its positive aspects. Because he is always monitoring me, I tell him he should get a job as some type of sommelier or quality control manager—more funny stuff. He agrees that this is very funny and I believe he is learning that there is more to life than nursing paranoid grudges, although I am not grandiose in my expectations of a cure.

However, at times he threatens to stop taking injections because, as he consistently points out, he is not sick. I counter by saying that even though he does not need to take the injections, I need to give them. He asks me what I mean by this. I respond by saying that I know from personal experience that when he stops taking injections, he stops laughing at my jokes—which happens to be true. This produces laughter which immediately proves my point and we continue uninterrupted on the injection trajectory.

I might add that his mother worries a lot not only about him but also about me. She worries about my state of health and what will happen to her son when I die. I try to assure her that I am in no hurry and that I plan to live a long life. She asks me how I can be sure about this. I respond by saying I don't really know, but if I die prematurely she can call me a liar. This produces even more merriment but the point is that I have defused a potentially confrontational issue in which the patient's condition would not have permitted a rational discussion of the issues. And all this for what Medicare pays for a brief office visit—quite a cost savings when one considers the cost of incarceration or hospitalization which would be his destiny were it not for the injections.

The third patient also shows a pattern of extreme irrationality and partial responsiveness to fluphenazine decanoate except that his violent fantasies have not been limited to letter writing.

This is the first LPI admission for pt. L.M., thirty-eight-year-old, single, white male educated through high school, on Department of Corrections parole since July 1977 from the state hospital. He was living with his parents at the time of entry. Admission was voluntary.

SUMMARY OF PRESENT DISORDER: The patient was paroled from a state hospital in July 1977 and returned to live with his parents, both of whom are elderly and suffer from chronic cardiac disease. The patient's diagnosis has been schizophrenia, paranoid type; prior to parole he was receiving fluphenazine decanoate, dosage unknown. At the parole outpatient clinic, medication was changed to trifluoperazine 50 mg p.o. q.d.

Initially the parents described little difficulty with their son's returning to the community. Over several months they noticed increasing withdrawal, isolation, and evidence of delusional thinking. The patient's behavior in the neighborhood became of concern to the parents; e.g., he would inexplicably accost strangers in an argumentative critical fashion. There was no evidence of observed aggressive physical activity until shortly prior to admission when he beat up a puppy when he thought the dog was a "monster." On the day of admission the patient was throwing objects around the house. The parents contacted the patient's parole officer, who felt the patient should be placed out of the home and suggested that he be brought to a hospital for evaluation and stabilization.

PAST PSYCHIATRIC DISORDER AND TREATMENT: The patient was convicted of rape eleven years prior to admission and referred for psychiatric evaluation, at which time a diagnosis of paranoid schizophrenia was made.

He was institutionalized, at various prisons until July 1977, treated at times with various antipsychotics. He was paroled in July 1977.

SOCIAL HISTORY: The patient graduated from high school, started college, and then began abuse of amphetamines and LSD, leading to a hospitalization for organic brain syndrome. In 1966 he was convicted of rape as noted previously.

BASELINE PERSONALITY: Throughout his institutionalization the patient has been isolative and at times suspicious. His social contacts for the past several months have centered on the parents to whom he can be alternatively compliant or hostile.

INITIAL MENTAL STATUS: The patient appeared nervous with increased psychomotor activity but under self-control. Speech was fluent. He expressed delusions about a "third eye" of God that followed him. He denied suicidal or homicidal ideation. He denied hallucinations. He was oriented X3.

POSITIVE PHYSICAL AND LABORATORY FINDINGS: Physical examination was within normal limits. CBC, urinalysis, and FBS were within normal limits. VDRL was nonreactive.

PSYCHOLOGICAL TEST FINDINGS: No tests were administered.

TREATMENT AND COURSE: The patient was begun on fluphenazine, initially 20 mg PO q.d. increased to 80 mg PO/day at discharge. Delusional thought content was not evident at discharge. The patient had difficulty in tolerating group activities and would often withdraw to his room where he would pace. He gradually was able to tolerate brief periods in group activities, was socially appropriate, but continued to be agitated.

FINAL TREATMENT PLAN: Referral was made for further inpatient hospitalization. Medication was fluphenazine HC1 40 mg PO BID.

DIAGNOSIS AND FINAL FORMULATION: The patient has a background of antisocial behavior, a conviction on a charge of rape, a history of amphetamine and LSD abuse, and incarceration at various institutions for the criminally insane. Treatment over the past eleven years has been sporadic. A major social/cultural shift came in July 1977 when the patient was paroled. Although he initially tolerated this stress well, he decompensated over the ensuing months to the extent that parents felt unable to manage with the patient at home.

Diagnostic Impression: Schizophrenia, chronic undifferentiated type 295.90.

CONDITION: Unimproved

I have gone into such pedestrian detail in the past two cases to emphasize several points with respect to the administration of IM medications. Pt. J. K. and L. M. are similar in that their lives have been affected by violence. The difference between them is that although patient J. K. threatens violence he has never perpetrated it, while patient L. M. has perpetrated violence but never to our knowledge threatened it. The similarities are that in both instances I have used humor to consolidate my relationships with them. I have already described this with patient J. K., who in fact, was the patient I described in a previous chapter who accused me of believing that he could not adjust his affairs after I completed a conservatorship application form for him.

In the treatment of patient L. M., he was frequently preoccupied with voices when I would visit him in the residential care home, but when directly addressed he would usually respond in a socially appropriate manner. When he failed to do this I would sometimes tell him that he was talking to a doctor, and he should tell his voices to have some respect when the doctor is present. Actually I told him to tell them that they should butt out. He generally could see the humor in my superficially cavalier approach.

However, this breezy approach is not as superficial as it might first appear. I have actually utilized it to adjust his dosage. For years I stabilized him with 3 cc (75 mg) of fluphenazine every week. Previous attempts to use the atypical antipsychotics were not effective. In an attempt to find the minimal effective antipsychotic dose I increased the time interval between injections to every two weeks After several weeks of the decreased injection dose, he was no longer able to kid around. My attempts at humor were met with a cold steely expressionless glare. I then reverted to weekly administrations and he was able to return to his former personality with social smiling and the ability to kid around. Surprisingly, he was able to describe the experience as if someone else had entered his mind and was controlling him. In the case of patient L. M., humor was used as an important clue as to the determination of an optimal dose. (This would not have been possible in the treatment of patient J. K. because he monitored the syringe.)

Those who use fluphenazine decanoate or who read the small print in the crimps that accompany the vials might question the use of fluphenazine on a weekly basis. The preparation is described as a long-lasting medication, the effects of which can last for two or three weeks or longer. This is certainly true in most cases. However, some patients metabolize the medication more rapidly than is the norm. One of the reasons for this is cigarette smoking, which appears to induce a more rapid degradation of the drug, but there are probably other less well-understood reasons for a diminished response.

The ability to respond to humor is not customarily acknowledged as important in the evaluation of mental status. My opinion is that along with anhedonia, avolition, akinesia, and alogia, all of which are used in the assessment of negative symptomatology and/or the deficit state, there should be something called ahumor—meaning the inability to respond to humor. In truth, I understand why it is absent. It's absent because many normal people suffer from ahumor, and hence the trait would not entail pathological specificity. I'm certain that there will be critics of this book who are comedically challenged and suffer from ahumor, but who are perfectly normal in every other respect.

It has been my experience that when an aggressive patient can respond to humor, the problems with aggressiveness diminish. It is as if "kidding around" and violent acting out cannot exist simultaneously within the same mind-set. Perhaps rather than refer to "kidding around" I should relabel this quality as comedic nonresponsiveness thereby obtaining a greater degree of respect for its therapeutic potential. I believe that in some patients lessons in humor would lessen the potentialities for antisocial acting out. The problem is I don't know how to give such lessons other than to provide role-model examples with superficial one-liners. There should be a better way to do this, and the comedic school for traffic violators—which some cities in California have established—may be on to something. If it works, perhaps something should be established for people with violence problems—somewhat like cognitive behavioral therapy, but instead it could be called cognitive comedic therapy.

Be that as it may, my view is that minor changes in personality can be important in the determination of an optimal IM dosing schedule. This will not be evident if different people are administering the injections at different times. It is for this reason, as I stated earlier in this chapter, that I think the same person—be it psychiatric nurse or physician, should be giving the injections.

I want to emphasize other points about IM medications, and for that reason I will have to utilize the valuable services of patient L. M. again. I first assumed responsibility for his care in June 1994. He has never been hospitalized since then, but two months before I started treating him he was in the hospital. Here is what his discharge summary says:

Presenting problem: This fifty-four-year-old male was admitted to the psychiatric unit on a seventy-two-hour hold after he decompensated in the community and could not be managed at the _____ House. He was found to be increasingly threatening and angry toward the other clients of the house and also was threatening to the staff. He believed that others were talking about his mother. He also was posing some hazard as a fire danger due to inattentiveness to smoking.

Significant findings and hospital course: he remained extremely regressed, psychotic, and disorganized throughout much of the hospital stay. As it appeared that he should be unsafe for discharge except through placement in structured community living, there was an extended waiting period for his placement to develop. Despite large doses of Prolixin he continued to manifest evidence of psychosis, including internal preoccupation and inappropriate affect. At the time of discharge he was taking Prolixin 15 mg BID and 40 mg HS, Cogentin 2 mg BID and Klonopin 0.5 mg BID. On discharge he was placed at the _____ diversion unit and was referred for day treatment.

Two additional lessons are to be learned here. The first is that the IM decanoate preparations may be effective even though very large oral doses of the same drug were ineffective. In the case of L. M., he received a very large dose of oral Prolixin—70 mg—in the hospital, which was ineffective, but he responded very well to Prolixin when it was administered IM as the decanoate.

The second lesson to be learned is from second commandment of the Ten Commandments of Residential Care Facility Psychiatry: Thou shalt accumulate as much historical information as thou can from external sources utilizing hospital summaries and/or other sources of information.

I reverted to Prolixin decanoate after his unhappy experience with oral Prolixin because I had background information from a hospitalization that was long ago and a hospital that was far away. By so doing I think I saved the state thousands of dollars in rehospitalization costs—not that the governor has ever thanked me for my efforts.

As previously stated the therapeutic effect of both the IM decanoate preparations can last for many months. This becomes a problem when a decision is made to switch a patient from the IM decanoate injections to one of the newer generation antipsychotic medications. This switch can occur for a variety or reasons, such as the need to avoid side effects such as tremor or to avoid potential problems with tardive dyskinesia. Also there is the increased feeling—and justifiably so—that the newer generation antipsychotics should be considered first-line therapy for schizophrenia.

There is a problem however, in that some patients do better on IM medications and that this may not be apparent because of the long duration of their therapeutic actions. Thus when it is decided to make the switch to oral preparations, a resurgence of psychotic symptoms may not occur for many months and the exacerbation may not be perceived as the consequence of stopping the IM medications. What happens is that the long duration of action has the tendency to obscure the relationship between cause and effect. This can be disconcerting if anyone—lawyers, Medicare auditors, or patients—question whether the injections are really necessary.

Thus I had been seeing a psychotic patient for many years who had the delusion that she had given birth to many children and she would hear voices telling her this. Her symptoms were partially controlled with IM fluphenazine decanoate in the sense that she was not agitated even though she continued to hallucinate. I decided to switch her to one of the newer generation so-called atypical antipsychotic oral agents because of the possible early signs of tardive dyskinesia. She did reasonably well on oral medications for as long as five months, but then became very depressed stating that the voices had accused her of having hundreds of babies—sometimes as many as four or five on a single day. Also when she was in the county jail, the jailers took her out into the field and forced her to have sex with a palomino horse—and the memory of this event was extremely painful. I then restarted her on her IM therapy following which she reverted to her former status of experiencing hallucinations that were not terribly traumatic.

Complications can occur at injection sites although they are rare. Hay[6] has noted the occasional occurrence of subcutaneous lumps and indurations, muscle granulomas, abcess formation, fibrosis, and oozing at the injection site. The study appeared in a Canadian journal and most of the complications appear to have occurred using zuclopenthixol decanoate, a preparation that is not used in the United States.

Clearly there is a place for long-acting depot IM medications in the treatment of schizophrenia, and in some patients the injections would appear to be more effective than oral preparations.

PART IV:
REMEMBRANCES OF THINGS PAST

Chapter 18

School Days

I have already described that part of my past in Chapter 3 which described my entry into the residential care system. This chapter addresses the long past—that part of my life that existed before the residential care past—and how I got into psychiatry in the first place, or more correctly, as we shall see, in the second place.

Being somewhat retarded in my development, I contracted chicken pox at the age of fourteen, and since my mother was simultaneously ill, I was transported to one of the infectious disease wards of Los Angeles County General Hospital. As destiny would have it, the ward was within shouting distance of what was then called the psychopathic unit, and I could hear—without eavesdropping—a variety of obscene, maternally directed, orgiastic imprecations. This had relatively little to do with the course of my chicken pox but did arouse a postpubescent interest in the treatment of the mentally ill. My earlier Rockwellian fantasies about treating sick children would have to wait. I was going to concentrate on curing the mentally ill. One could say that I was changing my major.

This interest persisted throughout my high school years and when I enrolled at UCLA, I did so with a major in psychology. Eventually I was admitted to the graduate school in psychology. In those days practically all PhD programs in psychology were academically oriented and not necessarily focused on clinical issues. In order to qualify for the doctoral degree one had to pass difficult tests in two foreign languages and difficult written and oral exams, and write an original dissertation. The whole project could take between three and seven years, and numerous people fell along the wayside for one reason or another. Some of them simply could not overcome the language barrier. I felt sorry for them because many of them could have made good clinicians. Also they had spent years pursuing their academic objectives and much of that time was wasted. At that time UCLA was producing only a handful of PhDs per year and there appeared to be hundreds of PhD candidates enrolled in the program. I could not determine what happened to most of them and I gradually developed the disquieting premonition that I was participating in a Darwinian scenario. In nonacademic English, it put me into a bad mood.

Also there were deep divisions in the faculty that separated the clinicians from the experimentalists and one could get into trouble simply by socializing with the wrong crowd. Someone once asked Henry Kissinger where the most intense rivalries were—in politics or in academia. Henry stated that it was in academia because the stakes were so small. Henry was dead right.

I have always felt that one could construct a reasonably engrossing TV series focusing on the adventures of a group of students in a clinical psychology graduate program given the current widespread but somewhat morbid fascination with the suffering of others. I refer, of course, to the TV program describing the travails of a group of artificially manufactured survivor-castaways deposited in or on a variety of deserts, jungles, and remote islands—all of them willing to endure incredible hardships for the goal of winning the big money "because it is there," and all done without the help of a laugh track.

Instead of the desert island or jungle we could have the clinical psychology doctoral candidates stranded somewhere in the Gulag Archipelago of Ivy League Land. After listening to their objectives and identifying with their goals, they would then be eliminated one by one—some of them because of inability to climb the aforementioned language barrier, others because of failing the oral exam or the written exams, or because of alienating someone on their PhD committee, or because of consorting with experimental psychologists, or because of generalized social ineptitude, or because of insufficient maturity, or because of no maturity—or even worse, immaturity. Immaturity is actually the worst allegation insofar as it is an offense for which there is no defense. There is no defense because when PhD clinical psychology candidates tried to defend themselves against immaturity, they were accused of being defensive, which was then used to justify the accusation of immaturity. Given the confluence of these adversities, it would not be unreasonable to anticipate that the TV series could achieve high Nielson ratings by significantly penetrating the humiliation market.

In addition to vindictiveness there was the problem of exploitation. Faculty exploitation could occur in a variety of ways. When I was a graduate student in psychology I thought I could supplement my non-existent income by grading student exams, and in fact was paid by the department to do this. The esteemed faculty member for whom I was supposed to be doing this had other ideas. It seems he was working on a book about happiness. He had me running to the university library's card catalog, bird-dogging all the references on happiness. There were no fancy-pants Internet search engines then. Those were the days when milk was packaged in glass, cars were made of iron, and card catalogs were made of wood. We were much closer to the earth in those days, although building the card catalogs slam-dunked a lot of trees. I was one unhappy student. I could have written a rather convincing book on unhappiness, but, had I done so, this publish-or-perish tenure-hungry changeling would have immediately switched sides and taken all the credit for my unhappy thoughts. Actually I never discovered whether he ever completed his happiness book but I know it wasn't *The Joy of Sex.*

Subsequently I learned that the eminent educational psychologist, E. L. Thorndike, published almost 500 books and articles on diverse subjects such as learning to fish, methods of statistical analysis, and the elements of aesthetic quality in urban life. After my own unhappy experiences with faculty Brahmins, I wondered how many unhappy students E. L. had working for him. Come on now, 500 books and articles? It may never be known how many graduate school urchins E. L. Thorndike had working for him in his New England textile mills, but one thing is certain; he did not write 500 books and articles all by his lonesome. Although it is true that Henry Ford called all the cars that rolled off of his assembly line "Fords," Henry, unlike E. L., never claimed to have built them himself.

I also had some personality problems with the animal experiments—one of which involved depriving food to irate pigeons. They were confined to Skinner boxes, so named in honor of B. F. Skinner, the bilious dyspeptic misbehavioral psychologist who spent many years at the University of Minnesota in a region of the country otherwise known for its sensibility, and who made grumpiness a household word, possibly because he had to endure the winters there or possibly because he lived so far from a beach.

I was never really very happy about imposing my educational objectives on those poor benighted pigeons who, with their pitifully
overworked beaks, had to learn how to press all manner of levers in
strange sequences, under the most trying circumstances. I'll never
forget their poor little avian faces. That was all in the days before the
ascent of animal rights activism. In those days no real disagreement
was expressed about who was a person and who was an animal. In
those days academic disputations regarding the appropriateness of biological research were settled in accordance with lifelong hallowed
traditions of genteel civility in which the opinions of opposing colleagues were challenged by the exchange of polysyllabic fusillades
of cleverly contrived invective. Nowadays people use bombs. Times
have changed—or did I already say that?

Times certainly have changed. In those times, as preparation for
my career in treating the mentally ill, I had to spend inordinate
amounts of it (time), reading about grumpy B. F. Skinner and his little
boxes, or Ebbinghaus and his little nonsense syllables, or reading en-
lightening books by the eminent psychologist O. Hobart Mowrer who
later stated in *The Crisis in Psychiatry and Religion* that "psychopathology was a moral problem which has gravitated into medical
hands by default and complacency on the part of the Christian Ministry."[1] Fortunately by the time he issued this moralistic pontification in
1961, I had opted for the psychopharmacological over the psycho-
spiritual. Unfortunately, both orientations cannot be accommodated
simultaneously because only so much room is available in the human
brain. Besides, by then I was too jaded to become one of his acolytes,
and even if I had applied to a Christian divinity school as a way of
saving the mentally ill, I probably would have been rejected as lacking the necessary inspirational qualities for that calling.

If the truth be told, I was never quite enchanted by O. Hobart
Mowrer. It is with understandable reluctance that I will admit that in
my days as a graduate student in psychology I entertained blasphemous thoughts wondering about whether O. Hobart Mowrer's friends
called him Mo, or Ho, or simply O, or whether he had any friends.
And if he did have friends—why did they not tell him to change his
silly first initial. The fact is, O. Hobart Mowrer's name did not sound
like a name at all—it carried an inescapable exclamatory cadence
redolent of what a virginal bride might blurt out on a wedding night

during a climactic epiphany—which, of course, is an even more blasphemous thought.

It was only the utmost discretion that prevented me from revealing these innermost speculations to my graduate adviser. This was not easy for me to do in view of my previously described ticlike tendencies to become agitated when I cannot express comedic material—sometimes to the point of akathisia. Yet this would have been fatal to me at the time. This was because Mo, or Ho, or simply O, as the president of the American Psychological Association, was held in such high esteem that any hint of sacrilegious thoughts regarding this moral critic of the Christian ministry might cause me to be excommunicated from the clinical psychology graduate school. Nevertheless Mo, or Ho, or simply O returned to exact his revenge despite all his holier-than-thou-turn-the-other-cheek kind of stuff, as I shall explain shortly.

Chapter 19

How to Fail in Psychology
Without Really Trying

Despite all the aforementioned obstacles, I emerged from graduate school in almost record time (three years), possibly because I did not make any friends and therefore had no enemies. My first job as a psychologist was at Napa State Hospital as a so-called junior clinical psychologist. When I took the test for the position of senior clinical psychologist, I failed the interview, possibly because I was too nervous or had a bad attitude or did something wrong which I had no inkling about or told a few jokes that bombed. It's all rather vague.

Does that sound rather evasive? It is. I will 'fess up, although it is not easy. During my interview with the three examiners, I had to suppress some utterly irrelevant and irreverent and potentially hilarious comedic thoughts which bubbled up into my mind for no earthly reason—similar but not identical to the O. Hobart Mowrer scenario described in the previous chapter, but generated by geographical origins rather than initials—intrusive fantasies undoubtedly insinuated into my unsuspecting and innocent brain by a depraved incubus from another world with a destructive agenda and with malice on his (or her) mind—a message as it were, from the depraved to the deprived. As it turns out, this examiner with the provocative geographical background was a very attractive woman psychologist who, in the process of name-dropping as a career move designed to enhance her standing with the other examiners, let it be known in her best iron-jawed northeastern finishing school nasal English, that she graduated from Vassar and grew up in Oyster Bay, the exclusive East Coast location best known as the former residence of one Teddy Roosevelt.

Well, that artfully designed reference to her tony riparian digs was enough to set my primitive free-association RPMs (an acronym for revolutions per minute, to the mechanically challenged) brain into overdrive. What happened was that this Oyster Bay reference with all the erotogenic encumbrances that oyster ingestion supposedly creates only added to the aforementioned prurient fantasies triggered by the O. Hobart Mowrer scenario—and all of this was like dynamite to my brain with its pre-radically prostatectomized capabilities and vulnerabilities. All of this flooded my RPM brain with His imagery. The object of the capitalized possessive pronoun in the preceding sentence was not God, but it was Cole Porter—Cole Porter, sly, creative, and impossibly brilliant, in all probability the true identity of the aforementioned incubus rather than a God. Cole Porter tiptoed once again into my mind, this time with the "Let's Do It" lyrical provocations involving Oyster Bay:[1]

> Romantic sponges, they say do it
> Oysters, down in Oyster Bay, do it,
> Let's do it, let's fall in love.
> Cold Cape Cod clams, 'gainst their wish, do it,
> Even lazy jellyfish do it,
> Let's do it, let's fall in love.
> Electric eels, I might add do it.
> Though it shocks 'em I know.
> Why ask if shad do it?
> Waiter bring me shad roe.
> In shallow shoals, English soles do it
> Goldfish in the privacy of bowls do it.

Do you see what I am getting at? All these creatures all preoccupied with copulation and obsessed with the prospect of doing it, doing it, doing it, and all described with the incomparable alliterative elegance that only Cole Porter could have devised and with such extraordinary encyclopediacal fornicational specificity—all these images made me want to, well, if the truth be told, do it, with that examiner. Do you get the picture? Here are these examiners asking me questions about the Rorschach test, or the thematic apperception test, or how to compute the standard deviation from the mean, or the analysis of variance, and I am preoccupied by wanting to fall in love and do it—I mean actually have actual intercourse with one of my interlocutors, a person I didn't know and had just met under the most trying circumstances.

This is obviously some kind of a sickness, possibly an arcane allergy in which just one whiff of Oyster Bay—never mind ingestion,

and frankly I don't believe in this theory involving the aphrodisiac capabilities of oyster ingestion—just one whiff via the olfactory tract
was enough to send my undisciplined attention-deficit brain off to the
races with racing thoughts utterly unrelated to anything that was tran-
spiring in the real world. This included intrusive images of various
kinds of piscatorial dalliances—including but not limited to the
above-referenced "cold Cape Cod Clams"—an upwardly mobile
selfish shellfish seeking opportunistic cohabitation with upper crus-
tacean soul mates in the blue-blooded backwaters of Oyster Bay, or
goldfish now requiring private bowls, possibly in accordance with
new privacy laws as interpreted by animal rights activists, or electric
eels inextricably intertwined with their electrically stunned slowly
slithering paramours, or otherwise lackadaisical jellyfish reduced to
quivering masses of jelly flailing their tentacles in wild anticipation
of extramarital entanglements, and even otherwise gentlemanly English soles intent on rape and pillage in shallow shoals and God only
knows where else. So my mind was off and running and for obvious
reasons I had to pretend that nothing was going on. When all is said
and done, not only did I want to dock in Dr. Oyster's bay, but it was all
I could do to prevent myself from telling her about it in just those
words. I'm sure she would have died laughing at which point I would
have made my move.

Frankly it was all I could do to keep from standing up in front of
this inquisitorial troika and doing standup comedy shtick. (This is another Yiddish word that carries an English passport, identifying it as
"a mannerism or special area of knowledge designed to make one appear distinctive or unique.") In Dr. Fleishman's case this is a tendency
to interrupt formal oral proceedings—as in the examination—or written productions—as with books or articles—with comedic incongru-
ities, either high, low, or somewhere in between—that are so bizarre
as to defy description. I use my hands to illustrate certain points like
standup comedians typically do with a certain degree of pleasant vul-
garity—as might be derived from such additional Cole Porter lead-in
items as:

> The more refined ladybugs do it,
> When a gentleman calls,
> Moths in your rug do it,
> What's the use of moth balls?

Such great rhetorical questions with their winking testicular under-pinnings and ribald concealment of hidden puns would have been just my meat if I could have pulled it off—that is to say, if I could have had the balls to stand up and deliver shtick in front of these three grim-faced serious-minded overeducated academicians. I could use my hands again and parody other Cole Porter–induced visual images that were running through my brain like wild cherry pickers, like seventeen-year cicadas in impatient anticipation of connubial bliss as opposed to katy-dids who already did it. I mean I could have gone on and on, and even more on, with an unending procession of brilliant biblical Ark-like im-ages—describing the whole world as a throbbing kaleidoscopic bio-sphere. I could have been great. I could have been a riot. I could have been—a contender.

With the insight afforded by hindsight, I realize that this labored treatise on ecstasy was little more than the product of a wild hypomanic journey beyond the Cole Porter belt of outer space, al-though at the time—without the visual aids of insight or hindsight—my feeling was that if I had had the guts to perform, I could have been on a roll.

But instead of being on a roll, I was on an ideational roller coaster and by now my compulsive tendency to tell all—this ticlike thing was ticking—ticking like a time bomb in a boiler room with this pressure gauge going up and up so that the boiler would have exploded even if there were no bomb around. I hope I am being clear about this. Because of this idiosyncratic affliction that I suffer from involving the inability to suppress drollery, I became motorically agitated. I was then cata-pulted into an episode of barely controllable akathisia. Akathisia is generally described as a feeling of restlessness accompanied by fidg-ety movements of the legs, rocking from foot to foot, pacing, or the inability to sit still or stand in one place. My episode, I hasten to add, only involved a little of that and was nothing overtly grotesque. I was able to sit down quickly after standing up and shuffling my feet which I did with extreme rapidity so that nobody would notice. This was fol-lowed by some truncal rocking that was barely discernible to the nonmedical naked eye. To make matters even more intolerable, this was accompanied by an intense desire to forcibly extrude my tongue beyond the dental margin and twist it laterally, which I successfully resisted by gritting my teeth. Following this I tried to simulate the fidgety nervousness that a normal person might make during a normal job interview, such as clearing my throat, asking for water, and lighting a cigarette, and looking at my watch and drumming my fingers—all the understandable response to stress of a quintessentially normal person.

Unfortunately this pathetic simulation of normality fell on deaf eyes and only confirmed the worst suspicions of the examiners, namely that I was unfit to engage in the practice of clinical psychology, senior or otherwise. In addition, I noticed that they were looking at one another in uneasy ways as if something were making them uncomfortable. I mean, glancing at one another in strange ways. Nothing obvious mind you, just eye-to-eye type stuff; glances that could be described as fleeting or furtive or darting; Glances Ping-Ponging quickly from medial canthus to lateral canthus and then back again; glances exchanged like strangers in the night only they weren't strangers and it wasn't night. However it was night for me. I blew it and I knew it. The poetry only served to increase the pain, as poems frequently do.

Did I say I had no inkling about what happened? I had inkling aplenty. The important thing is not to lose sleep over something like that, but I didn't know that at the time. I was just a young lad then and I lost a lot of sleep. I was too young to know that an occasional failure was good for a person in that it broadens one—like travel is supposed to do. But I actually got even with whomever it was who failed me. The next time I took the test, I finished first in the state. That was my way of getting even, but the problem was that I didn't know who to get even with, who to taunt, so to speak—which was very frustrating at that time—and still is. Obviously I didn't learn anything from O. Hobart Mowrer, not even to turn the other cheek.

Chapter 20

Life in the Prechlorpromazine Era of Nongeological Time

The historic interview encompassing lessons in how to fail in psychology without really trying occurred almost fifty years ago in what might be archaeologically called the prechlorpromazine era. In those days when patients went into a state hospital it was the equivalent of an internal exile to a distant archipelago where green lawns grow and relatives and friends are never seen. Seven out of ten first admissions to Napa State Hospital never made it back to civilization. State hospital populations expanded every year without the benefit of a birth rate.

In those days I could stand outside a building and easily distinguish the violent ward from the nonviolent on the basis of the grunts, groans, and screams that emanated from within. Also, I could use this system to differentiate the male wards from the female wards, not on the basis of pitch, which would have been too easy, but on the basis of the levels of productivity and obscenity. The women won hands down on both accounts.

In those days straitjackets were still very much in evidence, if not in vogue. Tens of thousands of dollars were spent on psychohydraulic pack paraphernalia—hot packs, cold packs, lukewarm packs, etc., and there existed an action-oriented colloquialism called "necking out," the implications of which are not fully grasped by the younger generation of psychiatrists. Necking out involved tying a towel around the neck of an agitated patient and squeezing until the patient lost consciousness.

In those days psychiatric aids, popularly known as bughousers, responded to obscenity and combativeness with countermeasures similar in character, not because of their inherent brutality, but rather because brutality was employed as a means of control—control over the behav-

ior of others whose behavior was neither understandable nor predictable, and control over one's own fear of being overwhelmed by these
incomprehensible and unpredictable others. I recall entering a ward
where all the patients were in straitjackets. It was a women's ward—
old women. Nobody has captured the essence of this era better than
Frank J. Ayd Jr.[1]

> To appreciate the unprecedented advances since the advent of
> chemopsychiatry, it is necessary to recall what conditions were
> like in the predrug era. There were few outpatient clinics and no
> day and night hospitals and community mental health centers as
> there are now. Despite the prevalence of psychiatrically ill pa-
> tients, more than half of the general hospitals in the United
> States would not admit a known psychiatric patient, one-third
> admitted such patients solely for diagnosis or emergency treat-
> ment, and only one per cent had a psychiatric service primarily
> for short-term treatment. An attitude of pessimism and despair
> toward mental illness was prevalent.
>
> Because of a lack of effective therapies, each year the na-
> tional increment to the mental hospital population rose steadily.
> Within the bare walls of isolated, overcrowded, prison-like
> asylums were housed many screaming, combative individuals
> whose animalistic behavior required restraint and seclusion.
> Catatonic patients stood day after day, rigid as statues, their legs
> swollen and bursting with dependent edema. Their comrades
> idled week after week, lying on hard benches or the floor, deteri-
> orating, aware only of their delusions and hallucinations. Others
> were incessantly restive, pacing back and forth like caged ani-
> mals in a zoo. Periodically the air was pierced by the shouts of a
> raving patient. Suddenly, without notice, like an erupting vol-
> cano, an anergic schizophrenic bursts into frenetic behavior,
> lashing out at others or striking himself with his fists, or running
> wildly and aimlessly about.
>
> Nurses and attendants, ever in danger, spent their time pro-
> tecting patients from harming themselves or others. They
> watched men and women who either refused to eat or gorged
> themselves. They tube-fed to sustain life. Trained to be thera-
> pists, they functioned as guards and custodians in a hellish envi-
> ronment where despair prevailed and surcease by death offered
> the only lasting respite for their suffering charges.

Compounding this ghastly situation was the restricted therapeutic armamentarium of the psychiatrists. How frustrated and
impotent they felt as they watched the number of chronically ill
swell the burgeoning population of long-term resident patients.
They knew from bitter experience that psychotherapy for psychotics was fruitless, that insulin coma and electroshock therapy
offered little or no improvement to schizophrenics continuously
ill for more than two years, and that psychosurgery benefited
only a very small percentage of the chronically ill. For lack of
more effective remedies, they secluded dangerously frenetic individuals behind thick doors in barred rooms stripped of all furniture and lacking toilet facilities. They restrained many others
in cuffs and jackets or chained them to floors and walls. Daily
they sent patients for hydrotherapy, where they were immersed
for long hours in tubs, or were packed in wet sheets until their
disturbed behavior subsided. These measures, barbaric and in-
humane as they appear in retrospect, euphemistically called
therapy, at best offered protection to patient and personnel and a
temporary respite from the most distressing symptoms of psychoses.

This lack of effective antipsychotic therapies accounted for the
bleak outlook for the chronically ill. Unless they were released
within two to three years of admission, they were destined to remain indefinitely, prisoners of psychoses, unresponsive to the existing therapies.

That is the way it was—*in those days*. Not until chlorpromazine
(also known as Thorazine) came to California in 1954 did the situation improve dramatically. However, we knowledgeable and sophisticated psychological insiders in the market of mental illness were immediately prepared to be unimpressed. Previous fabulous claims had
been made before for appendectomies, adrenalectomies, clitoridectomies,
transorbital lobotomies, dental extractions, barbiturates, bromides,
deep sleep therapy, fever therapy, and induced convulsions via insulin, metrazol, or electricity. My colleagues assured me that it was a
sociologically proven fact that patients could improve by being the
focus of extra attention—that improvement could occur simply by
virtue of being in the limelight—being the focus of whatever extra attention exists as a result of being in an experiment. In support of this
argument they invoked the famous Western Electric study by the emi-

nent sociologists, Roethlisberger and Dickson,[2] who initially assumed that worker productivity improved when they worked under colored lights—when in fact, worker productivity really improved because the worker took pride in being studied. The increased productivity had nothing to do with the colored lights. So that was it: Thorazine and the piperazine analog that followed it closely in time—Stelazine, were nothing more than results generated by colored lights augmented by smoke and mirrors—no more, no less. If you want to know what really caused schizophrenia go after the schizophrenogenic mother and the double bind.

I was never quite comfortable with such dismissive explanations. I became increasingly impressed by the progress that some patients made on Thorazine, particularly when one patient told me that for the first time in twenty years, he had stopped hearing voices. At that point I did not think his improvement was "all in his mind" so to speak. Think about it. All my efforts in psychotherapeutic hard time, all my convoluted yet brilliant interpretations of dreams and rituals and obsessions, all my sensitive responses to the nuances of conversation and behavior, to say nothing of my disciplined imperturbability in the presence of the unkempt and the malodorous—in brief all of my professional travails in the face of numerous provocations and annoyances—all drops in a very large bucket in terms of their ultimate effects. Here was this man struggling for years in psychotherapy using words in an attempt to master strange thoughts and threatening voices, with progress measured in millimeters rather than miles—the tiny steps for feet that were not so little but were necessary because they prevented hardworking psychotherapists from becoming completely demoralized because they could feel they were doing something more than nothing at all. Tiny steps were even good for patients but in most instances the steps were not large enough to allow them to walk away from the asylum. All this was accomplished or not accomplished in years of real time, and then this ingrate with virtually no appreciation for the wisdoms I have bestowed upon him by virtue of my intensively contemplative pipesmoking tweedy psychodynamic intrusions into the inner depths of the inner reaches of his unconscious mind—this ingrate, I repeat, for emphasis, this ingrate—plunks a pill in his mouth, swallows it, and then has the temerity to tell me that the voices have stopped—and the world changes. First his world and later my world and later the psychiatric world and even later the whole world—like James Watt and the steam engine. What godgiven right did he have to say that?

This was not a civilized reaction to words—this was not insight. This was more profound, something that penetrates deeply into the primitive recesses of the mammalian brain beyond the levels where fight is measured against flight and which is not subject to the vagaries of words and insights—something as physiologically basic as respiration or peristalsis, variables that insight cannot stop or cannot change. The only insight that was happening was my insight—my insight into the relative impotency of insight when confronting biologically determined dysfunctions. So his world changed—but it was not only his world but my world as well. As early as 1955 I became convinced that medications would play an increasingly important role in the therapy of schizophrenia, and I wanted in.

I had now come to this fabled place that creates so many problems for so many people that we do best to avoid it. That place is called The Fork in the road. Everyone who is anyone knows that it is Yogi, not some superficially impoverished really rich Indian fakir yogi with a small y and big assets; but the non-fakir true Yogi with the big Y—he with the lifetime batting average of 285, and 358 home runs and 1,430 RBIs (acronymic for ribbies) who advised us to take it—take The Fork in the road. It was a difficult decision, and if I took that Fork, it would mean leaving my baronial digs—which I shall describe momentarily, leaving the green lawns and shady trees of the fiefdom, leaving my congenial colleagues in the psychology department, leaving a life of ease and comfort, leaving a salary and a sinecure. To go or not to go—that was the question. Whether 'tis nobler in the mind to live in fat and noble comfort than to suffer the slings and arrows of outrageous medical school—and, forsooth, not to mention the sleepless nights, the daily fights, the quick toboggan when you reach the heights—I'm going back to school again.

So I took The Fork and I ran with it—even though this involved taking some premedical courses. It wasn't easy for a PhD in psychology to take chemistry courses in quantitative analysis and organic chemistry. First, I wasn't used to standing over a hot lab. Second, I had forgotten most of my algebra. I no longer remembered that X stood for the unknown. Third,—well, there were lots and lots of third places. The first thing I did was dump my white shirts and ties and buy one of those sweatshirts that say Alcatraz to show the other students that I was real hip, even though I completed my course work at the University of California at Berkeley, not at Alcatraz. Somehow I survived and was subsequently accepted in 1957 by the University of Southern California Medical School which decided to take a chance on me even though I was over thirty, which was considered over the hill in those days. Later, in the late 1960s, we over-thirty people became untrustworthy. Actually I didn't care—by then I wasn't over thirty anymore; I had become over forty.

Medical school was another experience in survivorship, but I survived. At least nobody bugged me to achieve a mastery in two foreign languages. In a sense medical school was easier than the graduate programs in psychology in that I knew which books I had to read. The courses in medical school are arranged in a pyramidal manner so that the coursework taken at the end of one's training is dependent on the knowledge obtained in earlier courses. Thus, before one can understand pharmacology one must understand biochemistry, pathology, and physiology. In addition, the understanding of each of these subjects is dependent on the understanding of other preparatory subjects. Before one can understand physiology, one must have a background in anatomy and histology. One cannot have a true understanding of pathology without previously acquired preparation in microbiology and neuroanatomy. Biochemistry cannot be understood without a background in organic chemistry—which in itself cannot be understood without preparation in inorganic chemistry. If one can ascend this pyramid, which takes four years, one obtains what is necessary—but not sufficient—for clinical competence. For sufficiency in a specialization, one must trudge the long road through internships and residencies which can take another three to seven years. Many of my classmates decided to take high-intensity prestigious internships where they were on call every other night. I was not that young anymore and I found that after a sleepless night I could no longer assimilate new material. The Southern Pacific Hospital, where I took my internship, had two things going for it. I would only be on call every fifth night and the hospital was in San Francisco. I had always fantasized about working in San Francisco.

Following my internship, I decided to take a residency within the state hospital system. This was considered a low-prestige residency but I had always been stimulated by working with the severely mentally ill, and I had established a certain degree of confidence in treating schizophrenic patients. This occurred partially as a result of my earlier experiences working in a state hospital as a psychologist and partly as a result of interacting with my father's customers in his secondhand clothing store when I was an adolescent. I have never regretted my choice and I believe it helped me considerably in my subsequent career as psychiatrist treating the occupants of residential care facilities. Besides, I never hungered for prestige and still don't— and I suppose that is one reason why I have enjoyed my nonprestigious career in ministering to the severely mentally ill patients of residential care facilities.

Periodically, on my trips involving wine-tasting forays in the Napa Valley, I stop by Napa State Hospital and visit my former place of residence there. For four years I lived in a studio-type room on the third floor with a shared bathroom in a grand old house with two-foot-thick walls to keep out the summer heat. I had never lived so well. I had never lived in such a house. The place was called the Manor House and even though I already mentioned that I was not to-the-manor-born, at least at some point in my life I became to-the-manor-lived-in. To put it in show business terms, I became accustomed to the place. In truth, I was little more than an urban peasant suddenly cast into the habitat of the landed gentry, and not only did I have to learn how to pack my grub, but I also had to learn how to play bridge—real fast.

I loved living there and I loved the psychologists with whom I worked because they were really a grand bunch of people: Gordon and Virginia Riley, and Evalyn Everett and Ernie Belden and Ken Bartolme and Lou Carpenter and Ludwig Lefebre, even though we had some ideological differences as explained previously. When I enter the foyer of the Manor House I can still smell the fragrances and aromas of old wooden paneling and bannisters—aromas that continue to this day because the paneling and oiled bannisters are still there, even after fifty years, all of which vividly revives old memories and old emotions. I then ascend to the third floor in a strange state of semi-exaltation, as if I were on a pilgrimage, not one encompassing vast horizontal distances as an affirmation of faith, but secular in nature and primarily vertical. I go even if I don't have to go—even if the well is dry. Sometimes I do this even if it requires a heroic effort on my part, which may be easy or hard to visualize depending on how one chooses to interpret the preceding phrase. The problem with written language is that it cannot utilize intonation as a way of enhancing nuances. The whole experience is tremendously nostalgic.

I was unable to explain these feelings until, for no apparent reason, I had a flash of insight, even though I am ordinarily against insight—which proves that such prejudices can be limiting. For all of my early life I have lived in apartments in urban areas—not being to-the-manor-born, as already explained, and whenever I have returned to former places of residence, they did not retain their early character—different people, decaying buildings, different neighborhoods—no familiar scents or aromas to reactivate old memories, no residual wainscotted wooden paneling, no oiled bannisters. The Manor House is different. It is still there, still authentic, still unchanged, still singular in that it is the one structure where time passes slowly, if at all, the one structure that lingers from my past and continues to the present.

So there you are. Old memories and fragments of memories triggered by vesicular urgencies proving that the body affects the mind just as the mind affects the body, memories that I didn't even know I had, until I remembered them; the psychologists, Napa State Hospital, and the Manor House, baronial in its manneristic style, under the stately shade trees and out where the green lawns grow, a relic of a bygone era. It resembles a dream from the antebellum South—like Tara in *Gone with the Wind,* only it's not gone—the Manor House at Napa State Hospital, my home, my roots, shallow as they may be—memories that drift in the wind and linger like the soft scent of jasmine.

PART V:
ISSUES IN
PSYCHOPHARMACOSOCIOECONOMICS

Chapter 21

How Antipsychotic Drugs
Have Changed the World

It has now been almost fifty years since I lived in the Manor House and worked as a clinical psychologist in the prechlorpromazine era of nongeological time at Napa State Hospital. Since that time we have witnessed extraordinary changes that, in all probability, could not have occurred in the absence of antipsychotic medications. I will give myself credit in the sense that even as a young person I had the capacity to anticipate the vital role drugs would play in the treatment of schizophrenia. What I did not anticipate—what nobody did anticipate or could have anticipated—was how psychiatric drugs were going to change the world. Even as I retrospectively listed some of these changes originally noted by me in a recent article, titled "Psychopharmacosocioeconomics, and the Global Burden of Disease" (reprinted with permission of the American Psychiatric Publishing, Inc.), the results are amazing.

It could be argued that many of the social changes I list are the result of inevitable social and economic trends that would have occurred even in the absence of antipsychotic medications. We will never truly know, but it is difficult to imagine the emergence of such trends without the antidelusional, antihallucinatory, antiagitation, and decibel-dampening effects of the antipsychotic drugs. The neighbors—those people whom we collectively term the community—would not have tolerated the noise. This fact may be difficult to comprehend by those of us unfortunate to have missed the exhilarating experience of having lived in the B.C. psychiatric era (Before Chlorpromazine). The impact of antipsychotic drugs is generally unappreciated, and is best understood in the context of psychopharmacosocioeconomics—a useful but personally constructed neologism which addresses the subject of how psychiatric drugs have produced profound social, economic, and legal changes. Some of these changes include the following:

1. The migration of most chronic mentally ill patients out of state hospitals
2. The transformation of other state hospitals to exclusive repositories for the criminally insane
3. The return of many chronically mentally ill patients to their families
4. The ability of some chronically mentally ill patients to resume their careers or education
5. The transfer of many other chronically mentally ill patients to special residential facilities in the community (variously known as residential care facilities, board-and-care homes, adult residential facilities, adult foster homes, adult homes, group homes, domiciliary homes, rest homes, personal care homes, and family care homes)
6. The creation of special alternative diversion domiciliary facilities as alternatives to hospitalization which differ from board-and-care homes in the sense that they offer on-site treatment
7. The increased exposure of many mentally ill patients to jails and prisons
8. The transfer of some geriatric mentally ill patients to nursing homes
9. The transformation of some nursing homes into geriatric mini-mental hospitals
10. The proliferation of acute psychiatric treatment facilities in community hospitals
11. The creation of special nonhospital treatment facilities in community mental health centers, in rehabilitation programs, in substance abuse clinics, in psychosocial rehabilitation clubhouses, in shelters for the homeless, and elsewhere
12. The creation of a minivan transportation system to transport people—sometimes called patients, sometimes called clients, consumers, or customers, to physicians' offices, clinics, activity centers, partial hospitalization programs, or other programs
13. The passage of rights-driven legislation based on "the least restrictive alternative" so as to restrict civil commitment even to the manifestly irrational

14. The passage of other laws designed to facilitate the treatment of the mentally ill in the community, such as the Community Mental Health Centers Act

15. The creation of special industries (some cottage and some not-so-cottage) dedicated to the treatment and rehabilitation of the mentally ill

16. The emergence of a homeless mentally ill constituency that is either unwilling or unable to live in specialized mental health community facilities

17. The growth of special neighborhoods peopled by the mentally ill and characterized by urban decay and poverty

18. The rise of the NIMBY movement among the non-mentally ill homeowners wishing to preserve the tradition of their neighborhoods

19. The rise of consumer advocacy groups such as the National Association for Rights Protection and Advocacy, the purpose of which is to fight the use of medications and question the biological basis of mental illness

20. The rise of patient advocacy groups such as the National Alliance for the Mentally Ill created by the families of the mentally ill to defend the rights of the mentally ill and to lobby for increased funding for mental illness treatment and research

21. The decline in psychoanalytically dominated faculties in medical schools

22. The demise of purely psychogenic etiologic theories of schizophrenia involving "schizophrenogenic mothers," "double binds," and "marital skews and schisms"

23. The elimination of parent bashing as a sufficient basis for understanding schizophrenic pathology

24. The rise of legislative militancy as a legitimate means of expanding prescription writing privileges to nonmedical professionals

25. The increased pressure by managed care companies to reduce psychotherapy services

26. The increased incentive to discover other medications for other psychiatric conditions formerly thought to be treatable only by psychotherapy

27. The creation of a vast potential market for antipsychotic drugs for formerly hospitalized patients, and the realization by phar-

maceutical drug houses that the funding for this market could
be extracted from public budgets

28. The creation of a class of patients best described as psycho-
    pharmacosocioeconomic addicts—a class of patients whose
    improvements are dependent on drugs that they cannot afford
    and who are thus perpetuated into a state of economic depend-
    ency

Undoubtedly, antipsychotic drugs have changed the world in other
ways and the list is not presented as necessarily exhaustive. The mo-
mentous changes in society generated by the antipsychotic drugs are
generally not appreciated by the general public as having occurred as
a consequence of the actions of these drugs—possibly because most
of us were born after the chlopromazine revolution and we are unaware of the nature of life as it existed in the era before chlorpromazine. It is difficult to make before-and-after comparisons if there is no
experiential equivalent of the before. I pursue the after in the forthcoming chapters, which focus on the economic impact of psychopharmacosocioeconomics.

Chapter 22

The Cost of the Treatment of Schizophrenia for Society

Much of the contents of this segment appeared as an original article by me in *Psychiatric Services.*[1]

In 1991, the annual cost for the treatment of schizophrenic adults totaled $65 billion. Costs were broken down into their direct and indirect components.[2] Direct costs totaled $19 billion. This consisted of treatment-related expenditures such as those for inpatients and outpatients, as well as nontreatment-related expenditures such as costs generated by the criminal justice system for the incarceration of schizophrenic criminals. Indirect costs, which were $46 billion, included the lost productivity of both wage earners ($24 billion) and homemakers ($4.5 billion). Indirect costs included the lost productivity of individuals who were in institutions ($4.5 billion) or who had committed suicide ($7 billion). Indirect costs also included the cost of caregivers of schizophrenic family members ($7 billion).

These estimates did not include the cost of treatment of schizophrenic children. Also it was acknowledged by the authors that the costs for transitional housing such as halfway houses and "bed-and-board" houses (yet another name for residential care facilities) could only be roughly estimated. For other domiciles, such as shelters, the estimated annual cost for schizophrenics was $410 million. This assumes that the occupancy rate of schizophrenics in shelters was 14.5 percent of the total shelter population. The authors acknowledge that this may be a conservative estimate.

The estimated cost of antipsychotic medication in 1991 was $115 million, but this represents the costs incurred by the nonhospitalized schizophrenic population, which was estimated to be 485,491 at this time. It does not include the cost of medications to the hospitalized population.

Obviously, in 2004 medication costs are many times greater due to the increased costs of the newer and widely used newer generation antipsychotics. The preceding chapter focused on the extent to which psychoactive drugs have produced profound social, economic, and legal changes. One of the reasons for listing these changes is that the changes are not understood as having occurred as a consequence of drug interdictions. If one were transplanted to earth from a distant planet to certain intersections in San Francisco graced by raggedy psychotics pushing their life's belongings in shopping carts, one would assume that this has always been true. Not so. Such pedestrian tragedies were not evident in the prephenothiazine era when shopping cart pushers were confined to state hospitals—for sometimes better or sometimes worse.

One of the listed psychopharmacosocioeconomic changes was the creation of a vast potential market for antipsychotic drugs for formerly hospitalized patients, and the realization by pharmaceutical drug houses that the funding for this market could be extracted from public budgets.

With this last trend in mind, pharmaceutical manufacturers worked hard at developing new drugs that could work more effectively than the conventional antipsychotics and without the troublesome side effects of conventional antipsychotics such as drug-induced Parkinsonism and tardive dyskinesia. The new drugs, in the spirit of NASA, were supposed to work "faster, better, and cheaper" but along the way it eventually became obvious that "cheaper" did not mean cheap.

"Cheaper" meant that because of the new medications, the patient's psychiatric status could improve and recurrent hospitalizations could be avoided, thereby saving society a vast sum of money. Many of us uncritically accepted these macroeconomic justifications for high prices and ignored the microeconomic consequences of price escalations—such as what happens to a consumer when payment has to be made on an out-of-pocket basis.

These new medications are sometimes referred to as "new generation" antipsychotics or "atypical" antipsychotics because they were different from the conventional antipsychotics and worked via different pharmacological mechanisms. However, the new drugs were also atypical because their prices were atypically high. How high is high?

The macroeconomic costs of all psychiatric medications, including the so-called conventional antipsychotic medications, is accelerating rapidly as is evidenced in Table 22.1, published by the Lewin Group, a

TABLE 22.1. Antipsychotic prescription trends in Medicaid, total expenditures, 1995-1998

Year	Cost
1995	$484,000,000
1996	$641,000,000
1997	$894,000,000
1998	$1,264,000,000

health and human services consulting firm, as part of a study, on antipsychotic medications done under contract with NIMH.[3]

Although this table lists the costs for both conventional and atypical antipsychotics, the bulk of the cost is attributable to the atypicals. The Lewin Group offers the following data regarding the interpretation of the $1.264 billion spent in 1998 for antipsychotic medications as represented in Table 22.1.[4]

1. Atypical antipsychotics account for the vast majority of expenditures on antipsychotics: just over $1.1 billion in 1998, or 89 percent of expenditures.
2. In 1998, 51 percent of the 11 million prescriptions for antipsychotics were for atypical antipsychotics. In contrast, atypicals accounted for only 17.5 percent of 9.1 million Medicaid antipsychotic prescriptions in 1995. Only one new generation atypical was available in 1995 (risperidone).
3. The use of atypical antipsychotics in Medicaid has more than doubled since 1995. Concomitantly, the use of typical antipsychotics in Medicaid has dropped by 25 percent since 1995.
4. Olanzepine accounted for the largest share of spending for antipsychotics at $536 million (42 percent). Risperidone ranked second at $395 million (31 percent), followed by clozapine at $172 million (14 percent). Oral haloperidol and phenothiazines accounted for only 2 percent ($12.3 million) and 6 percent ($75.6 million) of expenditures, respectively. Quetiapine accounted for 2 percent of total antipsychotic expenditures ($24 million). The comparatively low use of quetiapine is probably explained by the fact that in 1998 it was a newly marketed drug and most psychiatrists were unfamiliar with it.

But Table 22.1 lists only the costs of psychiatric medications to the mentally ill as inferred from Medicaid data. It does not include the additional cost incurred by Medicare and by other third-party payers. Also it does not include money paid out of pocket by private individuals. How big is this bigger market? In 2003 it was estimated that the total domestic sales for the atypical antipsychotics alone (clozapine, olanzepine, risperidone, quetiapine, ziprasidone, and aripiprazole) exceeded $6 billion.[5] As the song goes in Chapter 7, "Times have changed."

Nor can the blame for the high cost of the treatment of mental illness be laid only at the door of the atypical antipsychotics. The pharmacological treatment of mental illness is now much more complicated and involves other psychiatric medications in addition to atypicals. For many mental patients stabilization is dependent on complicated pharmacological regimens which in addition to atypical antipsychotics may include other antipsychotics, antidepressants, mood stabilizers, anticonvulsants, minor tranquilizers, beta-blockers, anti-Parkinsonian agents, lithium, and stool softeners.

But that's not all. Mental patients are now getting older and they are not immune to the chronic physical illnesses that can afflict the non-mentally ill—such as diabetes, arthritis, asthma, chronic obstructive pulmonary disease, hypertension, or other cardiovascular conditions. In one of the residential care facilities that I visit, a previously described audit of the medications revealed that out of a total population of twenty-seven patients, twenty-three were taking medications for the treatment of accompanying medical illnesses. Aspirin was not included in the audit. The average mental patient is no longer a psychiatric patient in the sense of taking only psychiatric drugs. Perhaps a better word for the average mental patient would be "broad-spectrum patient."

The use of multiple drugs in psychiatry (sometimes disparagingly referred to as polypharmacy), is now more and more common because combinations have frequently been found to be more effective than single drugs. However, this tendency to use more than one drug to treat one illness is not unique to psychiatry. Polypharmacy also characterizes the treatment of other chronic diseases such as hypertension and diabetes, as briefly described in Chapter 8.

Unfortunately the picture is even more complicated in that some of the newer antipsychotic medications may actually induce these chronic diseases, either directly or indirectly be virtue of their tendency to induce the side effect of weight gain. In addition to precipitating diabetes, weight gain can also contribute to hypertension and hyperlipidemia which then must be treated with more drugs and which, if left untreated, can in turn can lead to heart attacks and strokes. Even if the patients did not develop these diseases, practically all of the patients on the newer generation antipsychotics have to be systematically screened for the detection of these diseases. This means periodic blood draws for blood sugars and lipid panels among other tests. One medication (clozapine) mandates weekly blood draws for white blood cell counts for the first six months, and every two weeks thereafter as long as the patient takes the medication.

Since I have criticized the pharmaceutical industry by implication, a bit more should be said. It should be acknowledged that tremendous financial risks are involved for corporations in drug development. Many compounds fail for every compound that is eventually put on the market. Moreover, the fully capitalized cost to develop a new drug, including the cost of post-approval studies as required by the U.S. Food and Drug Administration to determine long-term safety and effectiveness, is estimated to be approximately $803 million.[6] The whole process can take between ten and fifteen years.

Chapter 23

The Costs of the Treatment
of Schizophrenia for the Patient

The atypical antipsychotic medications are not only increasing the costs of mental illness treatment to government and agency budgets, the increased costs are also a burden to the consumer who pays out-of-pocket costs.

The prices in Table 23.1 represent the monthly cost of average therapeutic dosages for uninsured consumers in San Francisco. Uninsured consumers pay more for medications because they do not enjoy the advantages of the lower prices afforded by bulk purchases, although such prices are not spectacularly lower. The following drug prices are based on the average wholesale price as listed in the *Drug Topics Red Book* plus the retail markup of an average chain pharmacy.[1]

The cost of clozapine, which may be regarded as the first of the atypical antipsychotic drugs, is somewhat less—$279 for a 400 mg dose as the generic preparation and $333 for the same dose of the brand preparation (Clozaril), but the savings to the uninsured consumer are more than offset by the increased laboratory costs necessitated by mandatory weekly or biweekly blood counts for clozapine patients. Also the cost of Seroquel may be higher than indicated in the table because the therapeutic range of Seroquel is quite large, ranging up to 800 mg daily, and the cost of the drug increases proportionately.

It is undeniably true that these drugs are an improvement in many respects over the conventional antipsychotics. By way of justifying the high costs of the new generation antipsychotic medications, pharmaceutical manufacturers offered the quid pro quo argument that the high prices are justified (the quid) because they decrease the incidence of hospitalizations and thereby lower the costs of health care to society (the quo). This quid pro quo pricing philosophy does not seem to have proportionately affected the pricing policies of newer

TABLE 23.1. The cost of new generation atypical antipsychotic medications to uninsured consumers

Medications	Cost of thirty-day supply (rounded to nearest dollar)
Aripiprazole (Abilify) at 15 mg tabs 1 daily	$323
Ziprasidone (Geodon) at 60 mg tabs 2 daily	$364
Quetiapine (Seroquel) at 200 mg tabs 2 daily	$370
Risperidone (Risperdal) at 2 mg tabs 2 daily	$370
Olanzepine (Zyprexa) at 15 mg tabs 1 daily	$443

generation medications used to treat other chronic diseases that cause multiple hospitalizations, such as the new oral antidiabetic pharmaceuticals. A month's supply of metformin (Glucophage) at 500 mg 2 tabs daily costs $37, approximately nine times less than most of the listed antipsychotics listed in Table 23.1. It is interesting to speculate on what the cost of antibiotics would have been had the quid pro quo marketing philosophy been used to justify their cost since pricing policies could have reflected the value of preserving life.

However, unlike antibiotics that are administered over the course of several days or weeks, antipsychotics tend to be administered over the course of a lifetime. What is unclear at this point is whether the savings in costs associated with decreased hospitalizations have been offset by the increase in costs associated with the long-term day-to-day use of atypicals when extended over a lifetime. To estimate this cost in macroeconomic terms, one would not only have to consider the lifetime costs of the medication, but also the difference in costs incurred by a lifetime tax-revenue-dependent patient when compared to the revenues created by a lifetime tax revenue.

In a sense, the new generation atypical antipsychotic drugs have created a new type of addiction not amenable to treatment by conventional programs. This occurs in best-case scenarios in patients who have improved enough to resume a working career. However, they have become psychopharmacosocioeconomic addicts—psychopharmaco because they are dependent on the new generation antipsychotic medications for emotional stability; economic because once they have improved enough to live independently, they are unable to afford the drugs that induced the improvement; socio because as a result of the previous factors they are locked into a social class that is dependent on government subsidies. Under such circumstances best-case scenarios have become worst-case scenarios. I know of no good way to estimate the number of patients who are, or will be, in this position, but the probability is that for many patients the high cost of these medications will prevent their conversion from tax-revenue recipients to employable tax-revenue generators.

In addition, other factors contribute to high costs. Hospitals are now under increased pressure to discharge patients rapidly, and sometimes the discharges involve patients who are very disturbed. Sometimes it seems as if the number of medications that a patient is taking on discharge is inversely proportional to the length of the hospitalization. Whatever the reason, patients are now being discharged on very complicated and very expensive drug regimens. The discharge regimen of a patient (Patient A) released from a local hospital and admitted to a board-and-care home on May 9, 2002, is listed in Table 23.2.

Of this list, four medications are for a psychiatric condition (haloperidol, fluoxetine, divalproex, and quetiapine), one is for the side effects produced by the psychiatric medications (benztropine), one is for the side effects of the medication used to treat the side effects of the psychiatric medications (DSS, for constipation), and six are for the treatment of concurrent medical conditions (benazepril for hypertension, metformin and glyburide for diabetes, iproniazid for tuberculosis prophylaxis, calcium carbonate for osteoporosis prophylaxis and aspirin for its preventive effect in cardiovascular diseases).

In Table 23.2 the cost of the nonpsychiatric medications was less than the cost of the psychiatric drugs, but this is not always true as is shown in Table 23.3 for the chronic schizophrenic patient (Patient B) with the accompanying complications of asthma, diabetes, hypertension, glaucoma, and hypercholesterolemia, all of which may have been aggravated by the patient's history of smoking, alcoholism, and street drug abuse.

Granted, this is an extreme example, but it provides an idea as to what frequently occurs to a somewhat lesser degree. Only two medications in the previous list (divalproex and risperidone) can be regarded as purely psychiatric.

TABLE 23.2. Discharge regimen and monthly costs of medications for Patient A

Medications	Cost of thirty-day supply (rounded to nearest dollar)
Psychiatric medications	
1. Benztropine 1 mg 1 tab daily	7
2. Haloperidol 10 mg 1 tab daily	20
3. Divalproex 500 mg 1 tab twice daily	111
4. Fluoxetine (generic Prozac) 60 mg 1 tab daily	197
5. Quetiapine 200 mg 4 tabs daily	639
Nonpsychiatric medications	
6. Aspirin 81 mg 1 tab daily	1
7. Benazepril 5 mg 1 tab daily	31
8. Calcium carbonate 125 mg 1 tab daily	3
9. INH (iproniazid) 300 mg 1 tab daily	6
10. Metformin 500 mg 2 tabs daily	37
11. DSS 250 mg (stool softener)	3
12. Glyburide 5 mg 1 tab daily	20
Total monthly cost of psychiatric meds	974
Total monthly cost of nonpsychiatric meds	101
Total monthly cost of all meds	$1,075

I can easily cite other discharge regimens that are even more costly but the fact is that an average working person with no history of disability is not able to incur the drug expenses listed here. I leave it to my colleagues to speculate about the reasons for this increase in complexity, although some of the possibilities are:

TABLE 23.3. Discharge regimen and monthly costs of medications for Patient B

Medications	Cost of thirty-day supply (rounded to nearest dollar)
Psychiatric medications	
1. Divalproex 500 mg 2 tabs twice daily	195
2. Risperidone 3 mg 2 tabs daily	361
Nonpsychiatric medications	
3. Isosorbide mononitrate 60 mg 1 tabs daily	35
4. Metformin 850 mg 1 tabs three times a day	107
5. Clonidine patches once a week	82
6. Hydrochlorothiazide 25 mg 1 tab daily	4
7. Colace 250 mg twice daily	5
8. Benazepril 20 mg 1 tab daily	31
9. Pravastatin 20 mg 1 tab daily	83
10. Betaxolol eye drops twice daily	98
11. Dorzolamide eye drops twice daily	51
12. Triamcinolone inhalers four puffs twice daily	69
13. Ipratropium inhalers two puffs twice daily	49
14. Aspirin 81 mg tabs one daily	1
15. Oyster shell calcium tabs twice daily	3
16. Multivitamins tabs once daily	3
Total monthly cost for psychiatric meds	556
Total monthly cost for nonpsychiatric meds	621
Total monthly cost for all meds	$1,177

1. The prescribing of medications on a preventive medicine basis—that is, to prevent illnesses that have not yet occurred but which may occur in the future
2. Rapid hospital discharge policies with shotgun treatments

3. Adherence to the dictates of treatment algorithms of ever increasing complexity
4. The increasing acceptability of polypharmacy in the treatment of psychiatric and other chronic medical illnesses or
5. The necessity to treat the unanticipated medical complications created by the new generation atypical antipsychotic medications such as type 2 diabetes, weight gain, dyslipidemia, and, as some claim, osteoporosis.

No doubt other reasons exist, but regardless of the reasons, these regimens are much more expensive than they used to be. Since most of my practice involves the treatment of seriously mentally ill patients residing in residential care facilities many of whom have been recently discharge from hospitals, I am in a good position to identify emerging trends. My impression is that recent discharges from psychiatric hospitals now include drug regimens that are far more complex and far more expensive than the regimens that existed only two years ago. Recent discharges from hospitals to residential care facilities are like canaries in coal mines in that they represent the first signs of an emerging medical trend that will affect all of medicine. The consequent increase in costs will eventually contribute to the economic difficulties of all mental health systems and inevitably to all health care systems. "Eventually" generally refers to an event which will take place in the future, but in a sense the future is already happening.

Chapter 24

How On-Site Services Can Reduce the Costs of Treatment

Since mental health budgets are under increasing scrutiny and pressure, it is important to describe the economic savings involved in the provision of on-site care. However, for those readers who are not interested in the details or mechanics of Medicare coding, this chapter can safely be skipped.

For each visit to a patient in a residential care facility, I now generally charge on the basis of Medicare code 99331 as described briefly in Chapter 9. This is called an Evaluation and Management code (E&M). The use of E&M codes generally requires documentation of the relevant parameters upon which the code choice is supported with respect to history, examination, medical decision making, counseling, coordination of care, nature of the presenting problem, and time. E&M codes for on-site services to residential care facilities are either 99331, 99332, or 99333, depending on the level of service provided. Residential care facilities and all its synonyms are governed by the same Medicare policies that pertain to rest homes and domiciliaries. These facilities are described in the book titled *Physicians' CPT Current Procedural Terminology,* published by the American Medical Association (AMA), as facilities that provide room, board, and other personal assistance services, generally on a long-term basis, but the services do not include a medical component. The code that I routinely use is the simplest code, 99331, and is described in the *Physicians' CPT Current Procedural Terminology* as follows:[1]*

---

*CPT © 2004 American Medical Association. All Rights Reserved.

99331: Domiciliary or rest home visit for the evaluation and management of an established patient, which requires at least two of these three key components:

- a problem-focused interval history;
- a problem-focused examination;
- medical decision making that is straightforward or of low complexity.

Counseling and/or coordination of care with other providers or agencies are provided consistent with the nature of the problem(s) and the patient's and/or family's needs.

Usually the patient is stable, recovering, or improving.

Other E&M codes are described as follows:

99332: Domiciliary or rest home visit for the evaluation and management of an established patient, which requires at least two of these three key components:

- an expanded problem-focused interval history;
- an expanding problem-focused examination;
- medical decision making of moderate complexity.

Counseling and/or coordination of care with other providers or agencies are provided consistent with the nature of the problem(s) and the patient's and/or family's needs.

Usually the patient is responding inadequately to therapy or has developed a minor complication.

99333: Domiciliary or rest home visit for the evaluation and management of an established patient, which requires at least two of these three key components:

- a detailed interval history;
- a detailed examination;
- medical decision making of high complexity.

> Counseling and/or coordination of care with other providers or agencies are provided consistent with the nature of the problem(s) and the patient's and/or family's needs.
>
> Usually the patient is stable, recovering, or improving.[2]

Regardless of which code is used, a carrier may determine that the visit may not be justified or compensable. If so, payment denial may be based on the perception that the visit was not needed or not adequately documented or secondary to some other factor.

Medicare carrier audit practices may vary by geographic area, type of service audited, type of provider audited, carrier budget, and many other factors. As long as the E&M description requirements are met (from CPT), and the service is reasonable and necessary, an audit may not be a problem. The general guidelines all carriers follow when conducting an audit are set forth under Progressive Corrective Action, which can be found at the Medicare Web site, <www.cms.hhs.gov>.

Obviously this book advocates the utility of regularly scheduled periodic visits to psychiatric patients residing in residential care facilities. The advantages of these visits are better psychiatric care and reduced rehospitalization rates, resulting in savings in health care costs. However, an argument can be made against this policy as follows: The routine services to psychiatric patients will not necessarily save money because the costs for providing such care will outweigh the cost savings of recurrent rehospitalizations. On-site visits lend themselves to abuse in which patients can be seen with unnecessary frequency or as members of large groups of patients who reside at the same location—the so-called "gang visit." Many psychiatric patients have reached a level of stability that does not necessarily require monthly visits. Also, most residents of RCFs are ambulatory and can be seen in physicians' offices. If they are too confused to come, the caretaker or some family member should, depending on the facility custom and practice, bear the responsibility of bringing them to the psychiatrist's office.

Arguments in favor of regularly scheduled in-site psychiatric visits are made throughout this book and will not be repeated here. Such visits may be questioned by any one of the Medicare carriers. Part of

---

the carrier's function is to monitor Medicare services and audit those physicians whose services appear to be unusual or outside the scope of usual practice patterns. Under such circumstances the physician may be asked to prove that a specific service was reasonable and necessary. In my opinion, the current guidelines based on medical necessity are not sufficiently specific to allow clear-cut decisions, as described in Chapter 12. "Medical necessity" is a gray area, frequently subject to interpretation, and what may seem medically necessary to the goose might not seem medically necessary to the gander. Since different carriers monitor Medicare on a national basis, carriers may apply inconsistent standards regarding what constitutes a medically necessary visit.

I generally use the simplest code simply because I have a simple mind and simply wish to avoid litigious arguments with auditors regarding issues that have no simple solution, such as how much work was really involved in the performance of a service.

Thus with respect to the taking of histories, there are four levels of complexity—problem focused, expanded problem focused, detailed, and comprehensive. My preference is to bill for the simplest history using code 99331*. The reason for this is that I don't like to sustain upcoding violations with an auditor because the auditor claims that I billed for an expanded problem-focused history when I should have billed for a plain problem-focused history. Also I wouldn't like to encounter the same upcoding problem if I billed for a comprehensive history and the auditor claimed I should have billed for a detailed history—another upcoding violation. Obviously I like to avoid trouble.

The same applies to other dimensions such as the examination. Is the examination problem focused, expanded problem focused, detailed, or comprehensive? I will usually go for problem focused. The same applies to medical decision making. Is it straightforward, low complexity, moderate complexity, or high complexity? I tend to go for low complexity even if it was of high complexity. Can one imagine what a dispute might be like when the auditor says moderate complexity and I say high complexity? I mean, how does the song go—you say to-may-to and I say to-mah-to. I would rather say low complexity and call the whole thing off.

Two other Medicare service codes are commonly used for the pharmacological treatment of mentally ill patients. These codes are distinct from the aforementioned E&M codes because their usage is not dependent on the documentation of interval history, problem-focused examination, and medical decision making. These elements may be part of the service rendered, but they do not need to be documented. They are as follows:

> M0064*: When the medical record indicates that a patient is stable from a psychopharmacologic point of view, but still requires pharmacologic regimen oversight.[3]

> 90862: pharmacological management including prescription, use and review of medication with no more than minimal medical psychotherapy,[4]

The difference between the two codes is that 90862 should involve an in-depth assessment because the drugs that are used are considered potent medications with serious side effects but should not be used to bill for a simple dosage adjustment of long-term medication. On the other hand, M0064 is to be used when the patient is stable but requires routine pharmacological oversight even though the drugs being evaluated are the same as for 90862. This distinction is somewhat confusing but in practice what it means is that 90862 is to be used for difficult problems and M0064 is to be used for problems that are not so difficult. Even this distinction is difficult in psychiatry—so difficult that I found I could not tell the difference. In fact, I spent more time trying to determine whether the service I rendered was difficult or not so difficult than the time I spent rendering the actual service—or so it seemed. For this reason I abandoned both 90862 and M0064 as viable service codes and now use only 99331.

The Medicare allowed charge for 99331 is $41.85 in the San Francisco area in the year 2004 (the rates change every year and are not the same for all areas). Since Medicare pays about 50 percent of allowed charges this means that the compensation to residential care psychiatrists would be about $20.92 per patient visit.

The Medicare allowed charge for a 90862 visit in the San Francisco area in the year 2004 is $60.16 meaning that it pays $30.08 (at the 50 percent reimbursement rate).

The Medicare allowed charge for an M0064* visit in the San Francisco area in the year 2004 is $33.51 with an allowed payout of $22.83 (the reimbursement rates for M-codes are greater than 50 percent).

Were such patients to be followed by psychiatrists in office visit settings using psychotherapy Medicare service codes, the cost per visit would be much greater. Specifically, the Medicare allowed charge for a 90805 visit (twenty to twenty-five minutes of psychotherapy) in the San Francisco area in the year 2004 is $82.85 with an allowed payout of $41.42. The Medicare allowed charge for a 90807 visit (forty-five to fifty minutes of psychotherapy) in the San Francisco area in the year 2004 is $120.11 with an allowed payout of $60.08.

All of these figures are from the Medicare Fee Schedule (Area 05) of the 2004 Enrollment Package of the National Heritage Insurance Company (Area 05 includes San Francisco).

My own experiences suggest that providing services focusing primarily on psychopharmacology with a sprinkling of psychotherapy, as described in this book, but using the 99331 code is a more efficient way to deliver services. Obviously there is a big pay differential between the psychotherapy codes that are primarily office based, and the E&M codes that are rendered on-site. Since we are talking about hundreds of thousands of patients nationwide living in residential care facilities with visits monthly or bimonthly, the use of codes 99331, 90862, or M0064, can save Medicare and other health insurers lots of money. But that is only the tip of the iceberg because of the additional cost savings incurred by the decrease in emergency room visits and hospitalizations caused by the effective implementation of home visits.

I cannot compare the cost of on-site residential care facility visits to outpatient clinic visits since I am not privy to the average costs incurred by the thousands of outpatient clinics across the country, but it is safe to say that it is far in excess of $20.92 per patient visit. However, I am not an economist. The implications of these statements are for another author and another book.

Now that I have clarified all the possible ambiguities inherent in the codes, let me add this disclaimer. It's all a delusion. In a study reported by King, Lipsky, and Sharp[5], 300 certified professional coding specialists were randomly selected from the active membership of the American Health Information Management Association and were sent six hypothetical progress notes of office visits along with a demographic survey. The results of the study showed that the coding specialists agreed on the CPT E&M codes for 57 percent of these six cases. The level of agreement for the individual cases ranged from 50 percent to 71 percent. So the take-home lesson is when running into coding problems, discretion is the better part of valor, this being a policy for which I have created a special acronym—DBV.

Chapter 25

Residential Care Facilities and the Cost Savings Associated with Rehospitalization

As our experience with the chronic schizophrenic patient in the community lengthens, it is becoming increasingly apparent that the course of chronicity is not characterized by a steady downward drift as had been thought in the past; but rather is more frequently characterized by recurrent exacerbations and remissions with a consequent production of repeated acute hospitalizations. Chronic schizophrenia is, therefore, not a cheap disease.

In a sense the residential care facility is to chronic mental illness what the nursing home used to be to nonmental medical illnesses except that now many nursing home beds are occupied by patients who suffer from both mental and nonmental medical illnesses. Both kinds of facilities are the domiciles of people who are sick but not sick enough to be in the hospital. However, people with mental illnesses frequently get worse and once rehospitalized tend to improve and return to the facility after which time the cycle may be repeated. This type of cyclic periodicity is probably less true of patients in nursing homes. Thus, the economic burden to society created by the poorly controlled psychotic patient with an accelerated rehospitalization cycle may actually be greater than that imposed by the chronically institutionalized nursing home patient in which rehospitalization usually occurs as a single terminal spell of illness rather than a recurring cyclical event.

The really big savings in the economics of residential care are created by the reduction of rehospitalizations. With costs of acute hospitalization running around $800 per day and costs of state hospitalization averaging $100,000 per year as I write this in the year 2003 (the costs go up every year), this is easy to understand. In fact, the economic justification for residential care facilities is more easily understood than proved. A rigorous proof would necessitate a follow-up of comparable groups—one being within the system, the other living independently. The problem is that the residential care facility population has a history of geographical instability, severe psychosis, and multiple hospitalizations—all of this before placement in the home. Such a group cannot be followed in an unsupervised setting because its members would quickly be lost to follow-up.

Thus if one were dependent on the use of control groups for validation, it would not be possible to prove that residential care was cost-effective. However, if on-site residential care did nothing more than enhance medication compliance, it would by this deed alone significantly impact upon the rehospitalization rate.

The price of noncompliance is frequently rehospitalization. In a previously cited study, I indicated that 50 percent of patients who relapsed within the first two months of chlorpromazine administration were not taking medication.[1] Also, of those patients who relapsed between two and twelve months, 54.5 percent had not taken medication in the month preceding relapse. A more recent study estimated that the relapse rate for noncompliant patients was as high as 75 percent within one year of discontinuation.[2]

The national annual cost of the rehospitalization of schizophrenic outpatients due to a resurgence of psychotic symptoms is estimated at $2.3 billion, with 60 percent of this occurring because of loss of effectiveness of medications and 40 percent as a result of noncompliance.[3]

One of the great advantages afforded by residential care facilities is that compliance is monitored, and while compliance may not be 100 percent, it is much greater than would exist in unsupervised settings. However, it is also true that relapses can occur in other instances even when noncompliance is not a problem because of the loss of effectiveness of medications that were effective in the past. However, the problems created by the loss of effectiveness of medications are much less if the caregiver has access to a psychiatrist skilled in psychiatric pharmacotherapy. In fact, these two factors act synergistically so that loss of effectiveness facilitates noncompliance and noncompliance can contribute to loss of effectiveness. Because of these factors, substantial cost savings can be attained by offering better pharmacological treatment at an early stage of psychotic decompensation along with treatment strategies to enhance compliance.

Other reasons for relapse include returning to environmental situations that are excessively stressful[4] or returning to families that are overly critical, overly protective, or overly emotionally involved.[5] To the extent that residential care facilities can reduce noncompliance associated with medication, and provide a viable living situation for patients who may otherwise have to return to stressful environmental settings, either with the family or in settings of urbanized isolation, the residential care facility is in a position to significantly impact those factors which produce rehospitalization.

PART VI:
SUMMING UP

Chapter 26

Of Wind and Gravity

So there you are—*The Casebook of a Residential Care Psychiatrist*: a casebook involving clinical cases—meaning people—but also addressing issues related to the administration of on-site services as well as broader issues suggested by the term *psychopharmacosocioeconomics*.

My interest in mental illness has traveled a long and serpentine route from adolescence to incipient senescence. The road winds back to a child looking at pictures of doctors taking care of sick little boys and girls, to my first quasi-psychiatric experiences as an adolescent while hospitalized at the infectious disease ward of Los Angeles County General Hospital, to the semi-psychotic customers in my father's secondhand clothing store. As a young adult I confront the mean streets of the graduate psychology program at UCLA, and later I pursue my first professional career as a clinical psychologist at Napa State Hospital until my chlorpromazine epiphany in 1955. After that I took the fabled fork in the road—back to school again. This time it's medical school at USC and ultimately a second professional career as a psychiatrist—first functioning in the California State Hospital System and later as an independent practitioner working in residential care facilities in San Francisco. Along the way I encounter the Medicare audit system and I emerge triumphant after three years of unrestricted haggling. Still later I receive the Arnold L. Van Ameringen Award in 2001—granted by the American Psychiatric Association. The award is given annually to an institution, organization, or individual that has made an outstanding contribution to the field of psychiatric rehabilitation and care for the chronically mentally ill.

I know this is hard to believe after some of the fictionalized hilarity that preceded this chapter, but it really is true. The plaque is there—it is on the wall—so I know it's there, and I look at it periodically as I shall explain momentarily. So after all my kidding around, did the significance of the wording elude you? It says "To that institution, organization or individual . . ." meaning I was competing against places like Harvard or Yale—me, a little old urban country boy from a small town in California called Los Angeles. Surely this has to be literally the absolute pinnacle of my professional career. After that, it's all downhill—"the big toboggan when you reach the heights"—so aptly phrased by Lorenz Hart who knew all about heights and downward toboggans from personal experience.

Obviously this is not quite a textbook because it has a strong autobiographical component. It is not quite an autobiography, because it also has a manual-type how-to-do-it component. These two elements do not completely describe the book because it has a fictional component fueled by the wildly manic digressions of Dr. Ecks, my fictionalized alter ego who accompanied me through much of my Medicare audit misadventures and gave me the strength to prevail. Perhaps the book can be viewed through the Dr. Ecks lens as semi-semi fiction. To quote Dr. Ecks in Chapter 14, "It has not escaped my notice that the specific pairing I have postulated—that is to say, fiction and nonfiction, will be inextricably intertwined with each other, like the strands of the double helix." You can quote me on that without fear of attribution from either Watson or Crick.[1]

Perhaps the compilers of *The New York Times* best-seller list will have difficulty deciding whether this book should be placed on the best-seller list for nonfiction or for fiction—-like the fictionalized book about Dr. Ecks which I never completed because I never went to a jail. Perhaps they don't really care. Perhaps they will not have an opportunity to care. Perhaps the moon is made out of cheddar cheese instead of bleu cheese. Perhaps I really don't care. Perhaps I have trouble telling who is really realer, Dr. Ecks with his fantastic manic voyages into inner space, or Dr. Fleishman with his aforementioned idiosyncratic "comedic ruminations that create the same kind of cognitive urgency that compel the coprophilic utterances of a patient in the final throes of a Tourette's syndrome."

I have titled the book as a casebook, but the word is used in a generic sense in that the cases referred to are more than the patients— just as the patients are more than cases—but the book also addresses the various events of my life that have contributed to making me the kind of person that I am today—the kind of case I am today. I believe I wrote in the preface that I was one of the cases under discussion. So

there you have it, autobiographical impressions and memories and fragments of memories, and with many digressive ramblings some of which
are brazenly irrelevant, some of which are nostalgic, some of which are
comedic. Memorabilia mixed with triviamobilia, which would have been
the title of this chapter—as in, "Memorabilia Mixed with Triviabilia," but
for the fact that triviabilia is really another non-word. Here are some examples of memorabilia mixed with triviamobilia:

I am a child again. I am home again. I am looking at pictures. I see
him:

> . . . *an aged physician seated by the bedside of a sick child—
> a patient, not a client—with his head cradled in his hands pon-
> dering the course of treatment. I think it was by Norman
> Rockwell. If it wasn't, it should have been.*

> *I thought,* How nice of that man to be worried about the treat-
> ment of that sick child. *I identified with that child because I was
> sick as a child, and in my child's mind where magic and reality
> coalesce, I tried to reach out and touch that man and I still re-
> member the disbelief when I felt gloss instead of garment. I
> thought that some day when I grow up I would like to be like that
> real nice man so that I could do good in the world and help sick
> kids grow up to be big and strong.*

—Chapter 7

A small child with small words and big thoughts.

I am growing—no longer a child, not yet a man—somewhere between in the no man's land of adolescence. I am bedded down at the
infectious disease unit of Los Angeles County General Hospital:

> . . . *the ward was within shouting distance of what was then
> called the psychopathic unit, and I could hear—without eaves-
> dropping—a variety of obscene, maternally directed, orgiastic
> imprecations. This had relatively little to do with the course of
> my chicken pox but did arouse a postpubescent interest in the
> treatment of the mentally ill. My earlier Rockwellian fantasies
> about treating sick children would have to wait. I was going to
> concentrate on curing the mentally ill. One could say that I was
> changing my major.*

—Chapter 18

Did I already say that I did it My Way? Perhaps that is also an illusion. Was it my way in the uncapitalized way of accident, or My Way, capitalized as the brand name of my own special plan—my patent on my destiny. Was it My Way to be exposed to an unknown person at an unknown time to an illness which resulted in a hospitalization—and ambitious fantasies? Was it really My Way, or was I simply subject to the caprice of wind and gravity? Some questions can never be answered. Most of us cannot tolerate such uncertainties. Perhaps that is one of the great limitations of the human brain—the inability to admit that there are unanswerable questions, such as what was there before the Big Bang? Carl Sagan—may he rest in peace in the world beyond the Big Bang—never told me.

I am a little older developmentally but not quite yet out of the no man's land of adolscence, but geographically stuck in skid row land. I am at my father's store—no plaques, no certificates on the walls, but the patients are there anyway, some of them really normal but down on their luck, some of them vagrants and derelicts with a misguided allegiance to alcohol, some of them mental cases even to the naked unprofessional adolescent eye:

FATHER [in Yiddish]: *I would have to go out of business with that price. [Writes another number down.]*

CUSTOMER [in Spanish]: *It's too much. There is no button on the sleeve. [Comes up a little bit from his initial offering.]*

FATHER [in Yiddish]: *I don't charge for the missing buttons. [Comes down a little from the initial offering price.]*

CUSTOMER [in Spanish]: *It is still too much. The collar is bad. It's frayed. [Comes up a little more.]*

FATHER [in Yiddish]: *Okay, I'll lower the price a little more.*

CUSTOMER [in Spanish]: *Okay, it's a deal.*

my father endured a hard life that I could have an easy life and I never had a chance to thank the man, except that I will do it now. "Thanks Dad. I know it's a little late to say it, but thanks anyway. I could never tell you that while you were alive because I was always too busy. Thanks for giving me a good life." I have to go now, typographically speaking, because I hate to see a grown man cry, even if it's me looking at my image in the mirror of life—especially if it's me.

—Chapter 8

The moving finger writes; and having writ, moves on,
Nor all your piety nor wit
Shall lure it back to cancel half a line,
Nor all your tears wash out a word of it.[2]

The moving finger writes and having writ moves on. I am at the Manor House:

For four years I lived in a studio-type room on the third floor with a shared bathroom in a grand old house with two-foot-thick walls to keep out the summer heat. I had never lived so well. I had never lived in such a house. The place was called the Manor House and even though I already mentioned that I was not to-the-manor-born, at least at some point in my life, I became to-the-manor-lived-in. . . . In truth, I was little more than an urban peasant suddenly cast into the habitat of the landed gentry, and not only did I have to learn how to pack my grub, but I also had to learn how to play bridge—real fast.

I loved living there and I loved the psychologists with whom I worked because they were really a grand bunch of people: Gordon and Virginia Riley, and Evalyn Everett and Ernie Belden and Ken Bartolme and Lou Carpenter and Ludwig Lefebre . . . When I enter the foyer of the Manor House I can still smell the fragrances and aromas of old wooden paneling and bannisters—aromas that continue to this day because the paneling and oiled bannisters are still there, even after fifty years, all of which vividly revives old memories and old emotions. I then ascend to the third floor, enter the bathroom, and urinate in the toilet bowl. I go even if I don't have to go—even if nothing comes out. The whole experience is tremendously nostalgic. . . .

. . . Old memories and fragments of memories triggered by vesicular urgencies proving that the body affects the mind just as the mind affects the body, memories that I didn't even know I had, until I remembered them; the psychologists, Napa State Hospital, and The Manor House, baronial in its manneristic style, under the stately shade trees and out where the green lawns grow, a relic of a bygone era. It resembles a dream from the antebellum South—like Tara in Gone with the Wind, *only it's not gone—the Manor House at Napa State Hospital, my home, my roots—memories that drift in the wind and linger like the soft scent of jasmine.*

—Chapter 20

The images fall into place like the harmless multicolored shards in a kaleidoscope. We turn the barrel and the thingamajigs tumble into nowhere only to be replaced by more thingamajigs, which in turn are relegated to obscurity with the next turn. The thingamajigs are memories and the barrel is turned, not by the hand, but by the mind.

The turn of the barrel, the turn of the screw. I am much older—possibly wiser. I have graduated from skid row, from Napa State Hospital, from the USC Medical School, from any institution that I have ever attended, and possibly from correspondence schools that I never even corresponded with. I am a real psychiatric big shot. What better place for a big shot to be in May 1986 but at the annual convention of the American Psychiatric Association, and what better city for the presentation of a very important paper than Washington, DC?

> . . . the only people present were the panelists, the wives of the panelists and myself, plus one colicky infant whose paternity was established only later in the program. The situation was not without its comedic aspects: Following each presentation, the wives clapped enthusiastically and even this uninvited, one-year-old, remarkably accomplished baby could and did applaud on cue while simultaneously shouting "Daddy, Daddy" in response to his ambitious mother's insistent prodding. The one-year-old was still too young to harbor the primordial murderous patricidal hatreds which preoccupy the minds of the Oedipal theorists, but at least the rest of us then knew who his father was. Given the opportunity, any one of us could have done the patricide.
>
> However, since I was single at the time, no wife was applauding for me and no precocious infant egged me on. He couldn't even manage one adventitious clap. I think as a result of his phenomenal precociousness that perceptive little future psychoanalyst sensed that I was not eligible for the adulation that ordinarily accompanies consanguinity, much like an ineligible receiver downfield, as they say in football. Because of these factors, my presentation was greeted with a gimlet-eyed silence. I mean if silence could really be deafening, I would now be wearing bilateral hearing aids. I was mortified by the stony nonresponsiveness of the merry wives of Washington. The situation was all the more galling because I was sandwiched between two layers of adored husbands whose presentations were greeted with

wildly enthusiastic proprietary applause by their spouses who
obviously had entered into a cabal involving a barter system in
which equal units of acclaim would be exchanged—you applaud
for mine and I will applaud for yours—that sort of thing. When I
returned to San Francisco I decided to get married.

—Chapter 3

It is later. The turn of the barrel, the turn of the screw. I know it is later than 1986, because now a lot of medicines in psychiatry are spelled with an X. I am in my office surrounded by the accouterments of professional achievement—the sofa, the matching draperies, a gaggle of plaques and certificates that line the walls in mute testimony to my competence. When I am alone, I frequently look at them for reassurance—including the Arnold L. Van Ameringen Award plaque that I described earlier.

Sometimes I do that even when I am not alone. A new patient, not a client or a consumer or a customer, unaccustomed to my idiosyncrasies, asks me if my mind wanders at times. I explain that when my eyes scan my panoplied wall I am simply looking for reassurance. Besides, I am the only one in the room who has the credentialized authority to make such observations and ask such questions. Somehow the patient feels a lot better after I express such confidence in my own abilities. I proceed with the interview:

ME: What medicines are you taking now?

PATIENT: I am taking Zyprexa, Xanax, Celexa, Loxitane, and amoxetine.

ME: Has it ever occurred to you that all the medicines you are taking are spelled with an x?

—Chapter 5

Why am I writing about all of this? I will concede that this is little more than the geriatric reminiscences of an old man so fascinated by himself that he must write about every aspect of this self no matter how revelatory or bizarre or trivial, yet it must be done. It must be done, "Because," as George Leigh Mallory said about conquering Mt. Everest, "it is there," and by so saying ensured his place in history—before Everest conquered him. Now it is Mallory who "is there"—still there somewhere on Everest eighty years after he perished in 1924. So I write about myself because "it is there," although I have no illusions about historical remembrances. In truth, only some of it "is there." What "is there" now are memories. The rest of it used to be there. I mean the days when social skills were abused in the service of mindless procreational urgencies—those days are no longer "there." They exist in the present in real time only as memories of actual events that were once performed in the past, in the days before real time existed as a real word in the real world.

Memories are like the stuff of New Year's Eve—like those horns and hats and streamers, but especially like the streamers. At midnight we toss them into the air, the tinseled streamers catch the glint of the slanted moonlight, they sparkle and glitter like a thousand dangling iridescent effigies suspended in time for one brief glorious instant before fluttering earthward in the inevitable concession to wind and gravity to await their final destiny—motionless, useless, and lifeless with the pretense of once having lived, they await the ultimate and dismal anonymity of the sweeper's broom. Memories live and die. Even tinseled streamers meet their maker. Our memories will die with us, and the memory of us, will die with our mourners. In a sense we are all subject to the caprice of wind and gravity.

However, enough is enough. It is now time to avoid gloomy epistemological digressions and drift back to earth as yet another concession to wind and gravity and to address the goal of this book, which is merely to change the world.

Chapter 27

Summary and Recommendations

THE EVOLUTION OF PSYCHIATRIC TREATMENT IN RESIDENTIAL CARE FACILITIES

In a series of articles I described the characteristics of psychiatric care as it has been practiced in residential care facilities.[1] During this time, which encompassed over thirty years, many advances in medicine and many changes have added to the complexity of the medication management of patients in these homes (as well as in other settings). Among these changes are the development of new medications, many of which have the capacity to accelerate or inhibit the metabolism of other drugs and the rise of atypical antipsychotics now regarded by many as the first-line treatment for schizophrenia. To make matters even more complicated, there is the increasing necessity to follow drug treatment with laboratory tests, some of which are legally mandated, the increased frequency of FDA boxed warnings for rare and dangerous side effects, and the emergence of more sophisticated treatment algorithms in which polypharmacy is presented as a viable alternative when patients do not respond to single drugs.[2]

Residential care facilities are now under increased pressure to accept more disturbed patients from community hospitals, state hospitals, and other long-term facilities because of the increased costs associated with institutionalization. For many of these patients stabilization is dependent on complicated pharmacological regimens that may include typical antipsychotics, atypical antipsychotics, antidepressants, mood stabilizers, anticonvulsants, minor tranquilizers, beta-blockers, anti-Parkinsonian agents, lithium, and stool softeners. More often than not, these patients are taking additional medications to control concurrent medical illnesses such as diabetes, arthritis, asthma, chronic obstructive pulmonary disease, hypertension, or other cardiovascular conditions. This prevalence of chronic medical diseases among schizophrenics is not surprising in view of the sedentary nicotinic junk food soda-pop lifestyle of many in this population. In one of the homes that I visit, an audit of the medications revealed that out of a total population of twenty-seven patients, twenty-three were taking medications for the treatment of accompanying medical illnesses. Aspirin was not included in the audit.

As stated in the introductory chapter, these combinations may be hastily contrived admixtures necessitated by the pressure of the refusal of third-party payers to fund additional hospitalization days. More often these combinations are thoughtfully arrived at and represent the best possible course of action to maximize the chances for stability. Because of these factors, the medication management of psychiatric patients is increasingly complex and when correctly done is more effective than ever before in terms of facilitating the release of severely disturbed patients into the community.

THE SCOPE OF THE PROBLEM

The scope of the problem is described in more detail in Chapter 2 ("The Problem of the Problem") and is repeated here in summarized form.

Unfortunately, little information is available on how many mentally ill residents are serviced nationwide in residential care facilities. However, the Select Committee on Aging of the U.S. House of Representatives has estimated that approximately 1 million elderly and disabled persons reside in approximately 68,850 licensed and unlicensed facilities.[3] That survey was conducted in 1989 and therefore is somewhat outdated. Undoubtedly the figures are now much higher. Although the committee focused on aging, the statistical reports referred to the "elderly and the disabled." Thus we don't know how much is elderly, how much is disabled, and how much is both.

However, in California the statistics are somewhat clearer in that we have statistics regarding the number of licensed residential care facilities statewide, and a breakdown as to how these homes are divided among the aged, the mentally ill, and the developmentally disabled. In California in 2000, a total of 4,639 licensed nongeriatric residential care facilities had a bed capacity of 39,985.[4] These facilities are categorized as residential care facilities by the Department of Social Services and are occupied by the mentally ill and the developmentally disabled. Of the residential care facility beds, 26,590 (70 percent) were occupied by residents diagnosed as developmentally disabled and 11,395 (30 percent) were occupied by patients with mental illness.

In September 2000 in California the total number of nursing home patients was estimated at 107,084. We already know that the total number of mentally ill residential care facility occupants was 11,395. We now have a residential care facility/nursing home ratio for California (11,395/107,084 or 10.6 percent). If we label the 10.6 percent as the California ratio, it is possible to use this ratio to estimate the nationwide population of residents with mental illness as follows: According to the agency then known as the Health Care Financing Administration, the total number of nursing home beds nationally for this period was 1,490,155.[5] We can now compute an estimate of the nationwide nursing home beds by the California ratio of 10.6 percent. This produces an estimate of 157,959 as a value for the number of residential care facility beds nationally.

This problem is growing in importance because of an increasing number of schizophrenic patients who are attaining geriatric status and who are in danger of statistically disappearing because they are being placed in nursing homes where they become geriatric patients instead of mental patients. This population is increasing because schizophrenic patients being effectively treated for concurrent medical diseases are now living longer. To make matters somewhat more complicated, many geriatric patients who have no prior history of mental illness become psychotic during their stay in the nursing home. Thus, the population of mentally ill patients in nursing homes is increasing because of the increase in patients that are becoming mentally ill only during their senescence and lifetime schizophrenic patients who are becoming geriatric.

When these factors are considered it is highly probable that there are many more than the 157,956 residential care facility beds for the mentally ill than indicated by simplistic extrapolative methods based on the California statistics. Moreover, an additional population of mentally ill residents of unlicensed residential care facilities are statistically stateless because we simply have no statistics for this population. When all of these factors are considered, it is possible that as many as 250,000 patients may be living in licensed and unlicensed residential care facilities for the mentally ill.

GOALS AND RECOMMENDATIONS

I discussed briefly the goals of this book in the Introduction. That was a long time ago. This is a good place to summarize these goals and to make some recommendations, because my goals in the beginning were not completely defined and only emerged more clearly as I progressed with writing the book.

As explained in the Introduction, I originally had four goals in mind: (1) to provide a set of guidelines for on-site residential care services, (2) to change the American Psychiatric Association's definition of "medical necessity," (3) to suggest a method whereby Medicare audit penalties could be more appropriately administered, and finally (4) to suggest certain changes in the Medicare policies regarding the appropriateness of on-site services rendered to residential care facilities. I have already pleaded guilty to the allegation of grandiosity in the formulation of these goals, in the unexpressed hope that this would forestall such charges in book reviews. I still plead guilty to that charge. I still have that hope. If such charges will still be made, let it be written that my admission preceded the accusation.

The other two goals, (5) suggesting legislative changes and (6) recommending university-approved psychiatric rotations in residential care facilities, were not in the original plan of the book. These latter goals slowly emerged as I was in the process of writing the book. As I have said, it was only after I had read what I had written that I developed the courage to make certain additional recommendations. The article in *The New York Times* (Chapter 15) detailing abuses and neglect in the residential care system also contributed to my decision to make recommendations regarding legislation and psychiatric residency programs.

My First Goal

My first goal is to provide a set of guidelines for psychiatrists who do residential care facility work. Very little literature addresses the issues involved in the provision of services in this setting, despite the large population of mentally ill residents of residential care facilities. In pursuit of this objective, Chapter 8 addressed the general problems associated with space and time. Chapter 9 described specific problems regarding frequency of services and special problems relating to the duration of contacts. Chapter 8 also described my own techniques, which I have found useful in the provision of services to residential care facilities. Briefly restated, the Ten Commandments of Residential Care Facility Psychiatry, are as follows:

I. Thou shalt make routine home visits to evaluate patients on the premises and not wait for crises to occur.
II. Thou shalt accumulate as much historical information as you can from external sources utilizing hospital summaries and/or other sources of information and place this information in the office charts.
III. When making a visit to the residential care home, thou shalt schlep the office charts with you.
IV. Thou shalt focus on prodromal signs of relapse.
V. Thou shalt enhance communication with administrators and other caregivers regarding ongoing problems.
VI. Thou shalt enhance communication with social workers and other mental health workers.
VII. Thou shalt segregate psychopharmacological orders into separate progress notes for each patient.
VIII. Thou shalt segregate laboratory test reports into separate folders for each residential care home.
IX. Thou shalt practice psychoperambulation when indicated.
X. Thou shalt involve patients in medication management decisions when indicated.

My Second Goal

The problem of invoking draconian financial penalties as a result of conceptual differences as to what constitutes "medical necessity" leads me to the second goal of this book, that being to convince the American Psychiatric Association to abandon the AMA-approved definition of medical necessity. The current definition is as follows:[6]

Health care products or services that a prudent physician would provide to a patient for the purpose of diagnosing or treating an illness, injury, disease or its symptoms in a manner that is: (1) in accordance with generally accepted standards of medical practice; (2) clinically appropriate type, frequency, level, site and duration; and (3) not primarily for the convenience of the patient, physician, or other health care provider.

This is an unacceptable definition of medical necessity in psychiatric practices for reasons explained in Chapter 12. Adversarial decisions based on this definition of medical necessity can result in severe penalties. The capacity to create a protective change in definitions is not dependent on Medicare, the AMA, or Congress. It can be done by our fellow psychiatrists in the APA. No law prevents us from legally protecting ourselves from the vagaries of prosecutorial interpretations.

The $10,000 per occurrence penalties were originally enacted to punish overtly fraudulent physicians or corporate entities. The understanding in the medical establishment seems to be that such punitive laws will always be implemented in accordance with the intent of the legislators.

Unfortunately history reveals that in the long run, laws with restricted foci tend to become more generalized in their application. A good example of this evolution is demonstrated by the history of the Racketeer Influenced and Corrupt Organizations Act (RICO). Probably a law here can be regarded as an ultra-law because it describes the evolution of other laws—call it the Ultra-Law of Inevitable Generalization that works as follows: A law is passed by Congress with the specific intent of apprehending a certain kind of Mafia criminal, as in the Racketeer Influenced and Corrupt Organizations Act. Eventually, and inevitably, a new legal problem arises for which current laws are inadequate. Then a search occurs to broaden the applicability of whatever laws exist in such a way as to offer remediation to the new problem. Laws with an originally narrow focus tend to become broader when they age. In a certain sense they are like people. It's as if one invents a target pistol that must be aimed and someone else comes along and invents a machine gun that doesn't need to be elegantly aimed but that can be indiscriminately sprayed, thus inflicting a greater number of casualties on the enemy. (One can infer that the Ultra-Law of Inevitable Generalization pertains to guns as well as laws and other phenomena.) So RICO, once a target pistol aimed at the Mafia, eventually mutates into RICO, a machine gun that has broad applicability.

For example, corporations have been sued under the RICO Act for allegedly distributing false advertisements; lawyers, bankers, accountants, and other professionals have been sued under the

RICO Act for allegedly assisting clients in organizing or assisting in the organization of schemes to defraud; spouses have been sued for allegedly concealing the value of marital assets in divorce proceedings; and civil protest groups have been sued for intimidating and extorting the customers of the industries that the protest aimed to disrupt. In the past state medical societies have filed lawsuits against Aetna, United Healthcare, CIGNA, Coventry, Wellpoint, Humana Health Plan, Pacifica Health Systems, and Anthem Blue Cross, alleging violations of the RICO Act, specifically accusing companies of covertly manipulating and exploiting long-standing accepted industrywide practices for financial gain as well as systematically denying and delaying payments due physicians—not exactly the usual Mafia scams.

Although these more unusual applications of the RICO Act may not have been intended by Congress, they can be legitimate uses of this act. Since physicians are now attempting to use the RICO laws against corporate entities, corporate entities will inevitably use them against physicians. What is sauce for the goose is sauce for the gander.

For these reasons, I advise physicians to be ultraconservative in billing for on-site services to residential care facilities. The possibility is that sooner or later average physicians doing average work will be victimized by these laws. This probability is increased by the fact that HIPAA has created unusual programmatic monetary incentives for prosecutors to make recoveries (as described in Chapter 12).

My Third Goal

Despite these problems, I am convinced that it is not the intent of the Medicare policymakers to punish honest physicians. Obviously Medicare can do nothing to repeal the severe penalties since these penalties are legislatively permitted by HIPAA, but what Medicare can do is revamp its audit policies to make the punishment fit the crime. This can be done in many ways. One way is to substitute the current baseball-strikeout statistical system of levying penalties with a batting-average system, as outlined in Chapter 14.

With the current audit system, progress notes are evaluated and penalties are assessed on the basis of how many deficient progress notes are discovered.

These deficient notes will then be counted and penalties will be levied using this absolute count. Once this is done, Medicare is allowed to extrapolate from the audited charts to the physician's entire practice and the penalties will be accordingly increased. The process is similar to assessing the productivity of baseball players by counting their strikeouts instead of their batting averages. It should be obvious that the greater the number of times a player comes to the plate, the greater will be the absolute number of strikeouts. Bottom-line sports entrepreneurs know that there is a better way to evaluate job performance.

It is obvious that the greater the number of progress notes being audited, the greater will be the absolute number of progress notes found to be deficient. It is surprising that such an unsophisticated approach has been accepted by physicians and their defense attorneys. It is patently unfair because the more progress notes are evaluated, the greater will be the number of deficient progress notes. The greater the number of deficient progress notes, the greater will be the assessment of penalties. If an auditor wanted to ratchet up a penalty of say, $100,000, he or she has only to request more progress notes for evaluation.

It should not be difficult, and possibly preferable, to develop standards using a batting average approach, in which deficient progress notes are calculated as a percentage of the total progress notes being audited. It is entirely probable that all physicians generate some progress notes that may be judged to be deficient.

It would be easy to calculate a deficiency index that represents the percentage of deficient progress of the total progress notes generated by the average physician.

When a physician's deficiency index exceeds the average deficiency index generated by other physicians by a certain number of standard deviations, penalties could then be invoked. The size of the penalty would be determined by the extent to which the physician's deficiencies exceeded the average index. In that sense it would make the punishment fit the crime.

If gross differences are found within medical specialties regarding deficient productions, it would not be difficult to calculate deficiency indices for each specialty. This method would be preferable to the current simplistic bean-counting assessment based on absolute numbers. It would have the salutary effect, as previously stated, of making the punishment fit the crime. In addition, it would encourage physicians to improve the quality of their progress notes because their record keeping would be compared to those of their peers.

Physicians are no less competitive than baseball players, and many physicians would be more motivated to strive for excellence if there were some way that excellence could be acknowledged statistically in Medicare audits. Just as a deficiency index greater than average would indicate inferior work compared to the average, a deficiency index of less than average would indicate superior work.

The advantage of having a progress note evaluation method that recognizes superior work, is that such an index could have a ripple effect on medicine that would be both profound and healthful. The effect of the current Medicare audit method is that it focuses on the elimination and penalization of substandard Medicare providers to the exclusion of anything else. A deficiency rating system would still permit this goal, but it would also have a broader effect so as to increase the quality of medical care to Medicare beneficiaries and ultimately to all patients.

My Fourth Goal

My fourth goal is to convince Medicare and other carriers to change their payment policies regarding on-site services rendered to occupants of residential care facilities.

Residential care facilities are considered by Medicare to be in the same category as rest home and domiciliaries. As previously stated in Chapter 15 and the preface, these facilities are described in the book *CPT 2004 Physicians' Current Procedural Terminology* published by the American Medical Association (AMA) as facilities that provide room, board, and other personal assistance services, generally on a long-term basis, but not including a medical component. The administration and supervision of medication that occurs in a residential care facility is not a sufficient reason to merit the designation of "medical facility." Medicare regards the occupants of residential care facilities as ambulatory and in that sense capable of making visits to psychiatrists' offices. Therefore Medicare sees no reason to pay for on-site visits unless the circumstances are unusual.

The problem is that although many patients are ambulatory in the sense that they can walk, many of them are too confused to walk to a destination, or are incapable of keeping appointments, or are too cognitively impaired to utilize transportation systems to get to a doctor's office or a clinic.

The reluctance of Medicare to pay for on-site visits—or even to regard them semi-fraudulently as "gang visits"—comes from an era when the people who lived in residential care facilities were not very sick and were maintained on fairly simple medication regimens that needed minimal medical oversight. This has changed in recent years in that hospitals are now under pressure to discharge very sick patients on complex medical regimens involving multiple drugs with interactive capabilities with patients frequently requiring laboratory tests to determine optimal doses. Moreover some of these medications may precipitate other illnesses as previously described in the text. The possibility is that home visits with appropriate caretaker consultation—an almost totally ignored modality of treatment—may be the most cost-effective way of providing services to this population—cost-effective because consultation with caretakers can enhance patient compliance and facilitate earlier medication interventions in the course of incipient exacerbations. As described in the text, such interventions may involve changing the doses of medications, switching medications, or switching to long-acting IM administrations.

However, no matter how strongly I state my position, psychiatrists will not make on-site visits to residential care facilities as long as Medicare evaluates such interventions through a pejorative "gang visit" lens and as long as certain punitive policies are in effect. These policies follow:

1. The targeting of psychiatrists who provide on-site services for Medicare audits because they generate aberrant procedure code profiles
2. The creation of a two-tier medication management coding system (Medicare codes M0064 and 90862) with ambiguous descriptors so that coding violations may easily be incurred when the codes are confused with each other
3. The currently accepted Medicare practice of assessing penalties on the basis of individual progress note deficits rather than attempting to assess the general quality of all the progress notes
4. The legislative creation of severe penalties per occurrence for the provision of rendering unnecessary services

When push comes to shove, I will admit that, despite all my Medicare procedure-code soul-searching, at times I cannot differentiate the wheat from the chaff. That is to say, I cannot distinguish the compensable from the noncompensable. When this occurs, and it occurs frequently, I have developed certain philosophies based on proverbs. What I mean by this is that certain basic principles govern the behavior of members of organizations and are summarized in slogans. Members of the FBI, for instance, are guided by the motto "Fidelity, Bravery, Integrity," these being words that are obviously based on the FBI acronym.

In like manner, members of the medical profession, when dealing with Medicare, should be guided by the principles embodied by the initials DBV, standing for "Discretion is the better part of valor." When I am torn asunder by the conflict of either submitting a bill for services rendered or not submitting a bill because the service rendered is questionably compensable, I submit to the option of non-submission in accordance with the behavioral standards dictated by DBV.

I do not necessarily advise my on-site colleagues to follow my lead in these philanthropic misadventures and I tell myself that I am doing this temporarily until Medicare provides a clarification of currently described Medicare ambiguities relating to custodial facilities. My billing policies and my problems with Medicare codes have been more fully described in Chapter 14 and I am waiting until the dust settles, but since I am not holding my breath, I am inhaling some of that dust.

This policy may seem incredibly altruistic or self-sacrificing to some, but it is basically self-protective. I prefer not to be paid at all rather than risk the penalties associated with upcoding or rendering services that might be considered medically unnecessary.

Psychiatrists who see multiple patients at the same facility should not be regarded as rendering a service of dubious medical utility. On-site services can increase the quality of patient care and decrease the incidence of rehospitalizations as cited elsewhere (Chapters 8 and 9). Despite this, it appears to be true that psychiatrists who make on-site visits are frequently the focus of Medicare audits because their profiles with respect to medication management and place of service are aberrant when compared with those of office psychiatrists. Psychiatrists who do much residential care facility work *should* have aberrant profiles, for reasons described in this book.

As a result of the economic disincentive created by Medicare payment policies, psychiatrists are very reluctant to accept the responsibility for treating the occupants of residential care facilities. This has a ripple effect in that many residential care administrators are reluctant to accept referrals from hospitals for patients who are not optimally stabilized or have reputations for being difficult placements because the administrators do not have readily available psychiatric backup. As a result of this, patients' hospital stays can become longer than otherwise indicated because of placement problems—resulting in increased hospitalization costs to Medicare.

Even when Medicare decertifies payments for additional hospital days, it frequently occurs only after a period of hospitalization extending beyond the duration of the acute illness. I believe that Medicare would actually save money if routine visits to residential care facilities were allowed—say, on a monthly basis after the OBRA model.

Health care costs would be lowered for several reasons: The average cost per patient for schizophrenic patients treated on-site by psychiatrists using on-site domicile codes (such as 99331*) or medication management codes (such as M0064 or 90862) would be much less than costs generated by office-based psychiatrists because office-based psychiatrists are more likely to employ psychotherapy codes. Psychotherapy administered by psychiatrists is not the cheapest or the most efficient way to treat the chronically mentally ill occupants of residential care facilities—for all of the reasons stated in this book. Generally speaking the allowed charges for psychotherapy codes run about two or three times the allowed charges for medication management codes. The more patients who are followed on-site with medication management codes, the less likely that they would be treated with office-based psychiatrists using psychotherapy codes. It is anticipated that the increase in charges to Medicare generated by the increased provision of on-site services would be more than offset by the decrease in costs occurring as a result of the decreased pressure to treat schizophrenics in the office.

Costs to Medicare (and other third-party payers) would be lowered because on-site services would be more effective in preventing relapses and rehospitalizations for a number of reasons cited in the text, including

---

the opportunity to confer and consult with caretaking personnel. This means I am actually advocating house calls as a means of treating some of the mentally ill as I did in 1984.[7] In Chapter 3 I said that I still like to think of myself as an urban country doctor trudging through the San Francisco snows to do important business despite the hazards involved in generating aberrant computer profiles and the accompanying dangers of incurring Medicare audits. It's still true as in Chapter 12.

I understand that were such visits to be mandated, some physicians might abuse the system by seeing too many patients during one visit. These kinds of abuses, if they occur (as they inevitably will), would only result in a negligible increase in costs to Medicare because of the relatively low rates of payments for the medication management codes. Also abuses could easily be monitored and corrected.

However, I don't think Medicare will effect such changes without legislative mandates, which leads me to my fifth goal.

My Fifth Goal

My fifth goal is to encourage legislation addressing patient care in residential care facilities such that psychiatric on-site visits to these facilities will be mandated. Unfortunately as things stand now, an economic disincentive exists to make such visits, insofar as Medicare considers all residential care facilities as lacking a medical component. Because of this, Medicare will not compensate professionals for on-site oversight services as it does for patients in nursing homes. In nursing homes physicians are required to make routine visits on a monthly basis as part of the OBRA (Omnibus Budget Reconciliation Act of 1987) law. The OBRA guidelines were formulated in response to data which indicated that antipsychotic medications were being used in nursing homes in the absence of clear-cut indications and with inappropriate monitoring.

Since physician visits to nursing homes are now mandated, physicians who make routine monthly visits to nursing homes cannot be accused of making unreasonable or unnecessary visits. However, residential care facilities are not and have never been the recipient of such legislatively dictated treatment obligations. Regrettably, there is no national policy mandating routine oversight for the occupants of residential care facilities as there is for patients in nursing homes.

The OBRA regulations were developed by panels of physicians experienced in the problems of long-term care and were based on reviews of the literature and consultation with colleagues around the country. OBRA eliminated the Medicaid distinction between skilled nursing facilities (SNFs) and intermediate care facilities (ICFs) and combined them into a single level called "nursing facility" under Medicaid. The OBRA regulations can be viewed as creating a national standard of care for pharmacotherapy and documentation in long-term care nursing facilities. This documentation must include a description of target symptoms, the response to medications, and a description of side effects when and if they occur. The regulations also advise planned medication reviews and dosage adjustments if and when indicated by the clinical status of the patient (see Appendix E).

If OBRA-type medication guidelines were applied to residential care facilities, they need not be oppressive and could be based on the Expert Consensus Guideline Series[8] and/or the Texas Medication Algorithm Project.[9] They can be loosely formulated so as to allow the use of combinations of medications in patients who are otherwise intractable to more conventional approaches. The technical problems underlying such recommendations should not be extraordinarily difficult.

Residential care facilities are in need of their own OBRA regulations insofar as residential care facilities are to mental hospitals what nursing homes are to general hospitals. Both types of facilities are for people who are very sick, but not sick enough to be in the hospital. Although it is customary to restrict the term "long-term care facility" to nursing homes, the residential care facility is equally long-term or possibly even longer in the sense that most of the occupants of residential care facilities will spend the rest of their lives at this facility starting at a younger age.

In fact the populations of nursing homes and residential care facilities are converging in the sense that many—if not most of the psychiatric patients in residential care facilities, have accompanying chronic medical disease problems. Many of the occupants of nursing homes have problems requiring psychiatric interventions. The criterion of ambulation that is used to separate the two populations is in many instances more superficial than real in the sense that many supposedly ambulatory schizophrenics may be able to walk but are too confused to walk to a necessary destination—such as a physician's office. It should be acknowledged that Medicare may claim that occupants of residential care facilities are ambulatory, but this is not what is going on in the real world. If Medicare will not allow OBRA-type physician oversights in residential care facilities, then the issue should be pursued in Congress either with respect to creating OBRA-type legislation, or through the enactment of new laws based on recommendations from the American Bar Association.[10] (The American Bar Association developed "A Model Act Regulating Board-and-Care Homes: Guidelines for States" under a grant from the Department of Human and Development Services in 1984.)

The necessity for such legislation is becoming increasingly apparent as is suggested by the recent incidents reported in *The New York Times* article in Chapter 15. However, abuse in the residential care industry is nothing new. In 1989 the General Accounting Office (GAO) conducted an investigation into residential care facilities in six states (California, Florida, New Jersey, Ohio, Texas, Virginia, and alas, not New York) in response to the request of a joint congressional committee on aging in which a wide variety of problems was identified.[11]

These problems ranged from very serious violations in which patients had been subjected to physical and sexual abuse, to problems involving persistent unsanitary conditions, such as improperly stored food and trash. Instances were documented in which patients had been denied heat, were suffering from dehydration, were denied adequate medical care, or had food withheld if they did not work. Situations also occurred that may have contributed to the death of some of the residents. Somewhat astonishingly, since none of the six states audited had aggregated inspection data, the magnitude of the problems was unknown. Moreover, since the examinations were limited to licensed homes, there was absolutely no data regarding possible violations in unlicensed homes, although it can safely be presumed that the violations there occurred with an even greater degree of frequency. As previously stated and as repeated here for emphasis, what is happening in New York may be just the tip of a national iceberg.

Mandated routine on-site services by psychiatrists and other professionals by the Modern Psychiatric Team (i.e., the psychiatrist, social worker, and clinical pharmacist—as described in Chapter 7) would end the isolation of residential care facilities and the potential of abuse that occurs as a result of occupancy within total institutions as described in the article in *The New York Times*. We now know that such institutions, total or subtotal, can exist within the confines of the community without the barriers created by geographical isolation. These island states are able to exist as a domestic Gulag archipelago with their own insular cultures because no national lobby exists militating for change, no routine professional oversight to prevent patient abuses, and not even basic national statistics to estimate the prevalence of the tragedies reported in the *Times* article. Unfortunately, moral scarcity can flourish in the environment of urban abundance.

On the basis of their findings, the GAO recommended that Congress direct the Department of Health and Human Services (HHS) to conduct a comprehensive assessment of states' oversight activities for their board-and-care populations. It was recommended that the assessment target the adequacy of licensing and regulatory requirements and the resources committed to their enforcement. It was also recommended that these assessments should include efforts to identify whether residents' needs are being met. In addition, it was recommended that Congress take subsequent measures to ensure the protection of board-and-care residents.

The Keys Amendment [Section 1616(e)of the Social Security Act] was passed in 1976 to prevent abuses in residential care facilities. It required states to establish, maintain, and enforce standards for a number of different kinds of institutions. These institutions included various types of group living arrangements in which a significant number of Supplemental Security Income (SSI) recipients reside or are likely to reside and to make these standards available for public review. The Keys Amendment also required the states to certify annually to the HHS that they are in compliance with the Amendment's requirements. However, the problem with the Keys Amendment is that it reduced the SSI benefits to the recipients living in substandard homes—so there is little incentive to report violations—neither on the part of the state, the home, or the resident. Thus far GAO recommendations to revise the Keys Amendment have never been acted upon.

My Sixth Goal

My sixth goal, for all the reasons already described in this book, is to encourage university-based psychiatric residency programs to develop rotations within the residential care facility system to encourage their graduates to gain experience in this type of patient care. With this in mind, I have described the aforementioned guidelines for work in residential care facilities. These guidelines are not based on evidenced-based experimental data because such data does not exist. To the extent that these guidelines are based on personal experiences, they may be regarded as merely anecdotal. As such, the information conveyed may be regarded by some as not sufficiently rigorous for the construction of guidelines. If my thoughts about guidelines were demoted to suggestions, I would not mind. Suggestions can still be helpful.

In describing my goals, I have already admitted to the charge of grandiosity. Be that as it may, grandiosity in the service of good intentions is no vice. I believe it was the late Senator Barry Goldwater who did not say that. If I have succeeded in any one of these goals, then I have done enough.

PART VII:
APPENDIXES

Appendix A

The Problem of Competing Acronyms

The plethora of synonyms describing the long-term facilities for the nongeriatric mentally ill has made it very difficult to accumulate statistics about this population. It also has made it difficult to conceptualize the functions of the various types of outpatient facilities that provide services to this population.

Adult residential facilities (ARFs), residential care facilities (RCFs), and residential care facilities for the elderly (RCFEs) are terms and acronyms used in California. Other states have other terminologies and other acronyms. For reasons unknown to me, the original term *board-and-care homes* acquired pejorative status and was subsequently changed to *residential care facilities* and still later to *adult residential facilities.*

Adult residential facilities (ARFs) are facilities of any capacity that provide twenty-four-hour nonmedical care for adults ages eighteen through fifty-nine, who are unable to provide for their own daily needs. Adults may be physically handicapped, developmentally disabled, and/or mentally disabled.

Residential care facilities for the elderly (RCFEs) provide care, supervision, and assistance with activities of daily living, such as bathing and grooming. They may also provide incidental medical services under special care plans. The facilities provide services to persons sixty years of age and over and persons under sixty with compatible needs. RCFEs may also be known as assisted-living facilities, retirement homes, and board-and-care homes. The facilities can range in size from six beds or less to more than 100 beds. The residents in these facilities require varying levels of personal care and protective supervision. Because of the wide range of services offered by RCFEs, consumers should look closely at the programs of each facility to see if the services will meet their needs.

Residential care facilities for the chronically ill (RCFCs) are facilities with a maximum licensed capacity of twenty-five. Care and supervision is provided to adults who have acquired immune deficiency syndrome (AIDS) or the human immunodeficiency virus (HIV). These facilities have not been discussed in this book.

RCFs, RCFEs, and RCFCs come under the guidance of Community Care Licensing, which is part of the California Department of Social Services. Their rules and regulations are contained in Title 22 of the California Code Of Regulations as explained in Appendix D.

The acronymic similarity that exists between RCFs and RCFEs makes for statistical and terminological confusion. To avoid the confusion the authorities in Sacramento, where the statewide statistics are computed, deemed it advisable to change the title of residential care facilities (RCFs) to adult residential facilities (ARFs). I still defer to the term *residential care facility* and that is the term I have used in this book, if only for the reason so stated in the last paragraph of this appendix. If I am misguided about this, so be it. This is not one of the great hotbutton issues of our time.

To summarize, what once was called a board-and-care home (no acronym), then became a residential care facility (RCF) and still later evolved into an adult residential facility (ARF). Board-and-care homes for the elderly (no acronym) later were renamed residential care facilities for the elderly (RCFEs) and the name and acronym are currently in use.

The remaining source of confusion is to clarify the difference between ARFs and ALFs.

I haven't discussed ALFs yet. ALF is the acronym for an assisted living facility. ALFs maximize independence by providing apartment-style living with services designed for senior citizens.

ALFs differ from RCFEs and ARFs in a number of ways. RCFEs and ARFs are state licensed whereas ALFs are not. ALFs typically have apartment units, whereas RCFEs and ARFs offer only rooms. RCFEs and ARFs are subject to regulations for admission agreements, theft and loss policies and eviction procedures as well as periodic inspections by licensing agencies. Generally, admissions to ARFs are arranged by social workers whereas this is not necessary in ALFs. The residents of ARFs are either chronically mentally ill or developmentally disabled. In contrast, one does not need a qualifying mental illness to be eligible for an ALF, and, in fact, a mental illness might render one ineligible. ALFs are generally marketed as "upscale living" although no standard definition exists for assisted living and ALFs are unlicensed. ALFs tend to be expensive and generally provide twenty-four-hour security, emergency call systems for each resident's unit, housekeeping and laundry services, transportation, medication management, social and recreational facilities, and personal care assistance with bathing, grooming, and dressing if indicated. Generally speaking, ALFs fall into three categories:

> The hospitality class of ALFs provides hotellike services such as meals, housekeeping services, and laundry services. ALFs of this type are appropriate for healthy persons with minimal service needs.

The personal care model of ALFs provides personal care assistance for persons in frail health or in situations in which the well spouse and the impaired spouse wish to continue living together with on-site support services.

The aging-in place ALF offers on-site care for chronic conditions. Usually these facilities are equipped to provide some skilled nursing services and can accommodate the changing needs of residents. In California any facility which offers lifelong care must have a "continuing care contract" which is certified by the state.

Generally speaking, ALFs typically provide:

Housekeeping and laundry services
Twenty-four-hour security
Emergency call systems for each resident's unit
Transportation
Personal care assistance with bathing, grooming, dressing, and toileting
Medication management
Social and recreational activities

Unlike the residents of ALFs, the occupants of RCFEs and ARFs are not accustomed to such luxuries. Obviously, given a choice in the matter, it is much better to be a resident of an ALF than a resident of an ARF.

The proposed use of the term *adult residential facility* instead of *residential care facility* or *board-and-care home* has created other potential problems. What about those adults who are not sick and who are residents of dwellings other than their own homes such as, say, hotels? Could it not be inferred that they are living in a variety of adult residential facilities? It is my understanding that there are many people like this. I think the term *residential care facility* avoids this problem and that is why I have used it as the generic term for the domiciles of the nongeriatric mentally ill.

Appendix B

A List of Psychiatric Medications

Here is a list of current psychiatric medications used in the United States and Canada as copied from an Internet source[1] although it has been revised and updated by me. However, do not be misled by the word "current." The changes are occurring so rapidly that by the time this book is published, the list will be obsolete. I am familiar with about 90 percent of the medications on this list, although some of the Canadian names are unfamiliar to me. I don't speak Canadian. Many but not all of the medications are listed alphabetically by both generic names and brand names. Many generic drugs have multiple brand names which may not be listed. The list is not meant to be exhaustive. If nothing else, this indicates why psychopharmacology increases in complexity with each passing year.

Abilify (aripiprazole)
Adapin (doxepin)
alprazolam (Xanax)
amantadine (Symmetrel)
Ambien (zolpidem)
amitriptyline (Elavil)
amoxapine (Asendin)
Anafranil (clomipramine)
Antabuse (disulfiram)
aripiprazole (Abilify)
Asendin (amoxapine)
Ativan (lorazepam)
Aventyl (nortriptyline)
Benadryl (diphenhydramine)
benztropine (Cogentin)
bupropion (Wellbutrin)
BuSpar (buspirone)
Calan (verapamil)
Calcium carbimide
carbamazepine (Tegretol)
Carbolith (lithium)

Celexa (citalopram)
chlordiazepoxide (Librium)
chlorpromazine (Thorazine)
Cibalith-S (lithium)
citalopram (Celexa)
clomipramine (Anafranil)
clonazepam (Klonopin)
clozapine (Clozaril)
Clozaril (clozapine)
Cogentin (benztropine)
Cylert (pemoline)
Dalmane (flurazepam)
Depakene (valproic acid)
desipramine (Norpramin)
Desyrel (trazodone)
Dexedrine (dextroamphetamine)
dextroamphetamine (Dexadrine)
diazapam (Valium)
Dilantin (phenytoin)
diphenhydramine (Benadryl)
disulfiram (Antabuse)
doxepin (Sinequan)
Duralith (lithium)
Effexor (venlafaxine)
Elavil (amitriptyline)
Endep (amitriptyline)
Epitol (carbamezapine)
Eskalith (lithium)
ethosuximide (Zarontin)
Etrafon (perphenazine)
Fluanxol (flupenthixol)
fluoxetine (Prozac)
flupenthixol (Fluaxol)
fluphenazine (Prolixin)
flurazepam (Dalmane)
fluvoxamine (Luvox)
Gabitril (tiagabine)
gabapentin (Neurontin)
Geodon (ziprasidone)
Halcion (triazolam)
Haldol (haloperidol)
haloperidol (Haldol)
imipramine (Tofranil)

Imovane (zopiclone)
Inderal (propranolol)
Isoptin (verapamil)
Janimine (imipramine)
Klonopin (clonazepam)
Lamotrigene (Lamictal)
Libritabs (chlordiazepoxide)
Librium (chlordiazepoxide)
Lithane (lithium)
lithium
Lithizine (lithium)
Lithobid (lithium)
Lithonate (lithium)
Lithotabs (lithium)
lorazepam (Ativan)
Loxapac (loxapine)
loxapine (Loxitane)
Loxitane (loxapine)
Ludiomil (maprotiline)
Luvox (fluvoxamine)
Manerix (moclobemide)
maprotiline (Ludiomil)
Mellaril (thioridazine)
mirtazepine (Remeron)
mesoridazine (Serentil)
methylphenidate (Ritalin)
moclobemide (Manerix)
Modecate (fluphenazine)
Mysoline (primidone)
Nardil (phenelzine)
Navane (thiothixene)
Neurontin (gabapentin)
nefazodone (Serzone)
Norpramin (desipramine)
nortriptyline (Aventyl)
Nozinan (methotrimeprazine)
olanzepine (Zyprexa)
Orap (pimozide)
oxazepam (Serax)
Oxcarbazepine (Trileptal)
Pamelor (nortriptyline)
Parnate (tranylcypromine)
paroxetine (Paxil)

Paxil (paroxetine)
pemoline (Cylert)
Permitil (fluphenazine)
perphenazine (Trilafon)
Pertofrane (desipramine)
phenelzine (Nardil)
Piportil (pipotiazine)
pipotiazine (Piportil)
Primidone (Mysoline)
Prolixin (fluphenazine)
propranolol (Inderal)
protriptyline (Vivactil)
Prozac (fluoxetine)
quetiapine (Seroquel)
Remeron (Mirtazepine)
Restoril (temazepam)
Rhotrimine (trimipramine)
Risperdal (risperidone)
risperidone (Risperdal)
Ritalin (methylphenidate)
Rivotril (clonazepam)
Sabril (vigabatrin)
Serax (oxazepam)
Serentil (mesoridazine)
Seroquel (quetiapine)
sertraline (Zoloft)
Serzone (nefazodone)
Sinequan (doxepin)
Sonata (zaleplon)
Stelazine (trifluoperazine)
sulpiride (Sulpitil)
Surmontil (trimipramine)
Symmetrel (amantadine)
T-Quil (diazapam)
Tegretol (carbamezapine)
temazepam (Restoril)
Temposil (calcium carbimide)
Tiagabine (Gabitril)
thioridazine (Mellaril)
thiothixene (Navane)
Thorazine (chlorpromazine)
Tofranil (imipramine)
Topamax (topiramate)

trazodone (Desyrel)
triazolam (Halcion)
trifluoperazine (Stelazine)
trihexyphenidyl (Artane)
Trilafon (perphenazine)
Trileptal (oxcarbazepine)
trimipramine (Surmontil)
Triptil (protriptyline)
Valium (diazapam)
Valium Injection (diazapam)
valproate injectable (Depacon)
valproic acid (Depakote)
Valrelease (valproate)
venlafaxine (Effexor)
verapamil (Calan)
Vivactil (protriptyline)
vigabatrin (Sabril)
Wellbutrin (bupropion)
Xanax (alprazolam)
zaleplon (Sonata)
Zarontin (ethosuximide)
ziprasidone (Geodon)
Zoloft (sertraline)
zolpidem (Ambien)
zopliclone (Zimovane)
Zyprexa (olanzepine)

As explained, the list is not exhaustive and not exactly up to date and does not include the latest isomers of currently used medications. The problem with any textbook list is that it quickly becomes obsolete. However, it should be noted that if this list were compiled in 1955, it would look like this:

chlorpromazine (Thorazine)
reserpine (Serpasil)
Serpasil (reserpine)
Thorazine (chlorpromazine)

Appendix C

Metabolic Monitoring Recommendations

The following recommendations appeared as an appendix to an article titled "A Retrospective Comparison of Weight, Lipid, and Glucose Changes Between Risperidone- and Olanzapine-Treated Inpatients: Metabolic Outcomes After One Year" by J. M. Meyer in the *Journal of Clinical Psychiatry*.[1] The issues are well described by Dr. Meyer but this is a new area, as Dr. Meyer points out, and there are a lot of issues that are not yet addressed.

There is presently a lack of consensus among psychiatrists on the issue of metabolic monitoring during atypical antipsychotic therapy, but the concern over severe adverse metabolic outcomes (diabetic ketoacidosis and severe hyper-triglyceridemia) necessitates some initiatives in this area. The following suggested program is derived from consultation with psychiatrists in multiple treatment settings and input from endocrinologists. These recommendations can be applied to all adults aged 15 and over, particularly glucose monitoring, as new-onset type 2 diabetes associated with antipsychotic therapy has been seen at Oregon State Hospital, Salem, in individuals as young as 18 years old. This protocol should be considered a first approximation, which hopefully will be refined as the literature in this area continues to grow:

1. **Weight:** Baseline and monthly weights for all patients should be taken, and nutritional and behavioral intervention for obese individuals or those who experience significant weight gain during treatment should be provided.

2. **Lipids:** Given the updated recommendations for hyperlipidemia treatment and the fact that patients with schizophrenia typically possess multiple cardiovascular risk factors, a full lipid panel with fractionation of cholesterol should be performed annually as part of routine health monitoring for inpatients and outpatients. Quarterly fasting total triglycerides and cholesterol should be considered during the first year of atypical antipsychotic therapy. This frequency may be decreased depending on the results obtained and the agent used.

3. **Glucose:** Screening for family and personal history of diabetes should be considered for all patients with schizophrenia, particularly those with high risk due to obesity or ethnicity. Education about the symptoms of diabetes (fatigue, thirst, polyuria) should be performed for those who will be started on higher risk agents or who possess risk factors, particularly those in high risk ethnic groups.

The American Diabetes Association has established the following values for fasting glucose:

Normal < 110 mg/dL
Impaired 110-125 mg/dL
Diabetic range >126 mg/dL for fasting or
> 200 mg/dL (for non-fasting random glucose)

Cases of provisional diabetes should have values confirmed on a subsequent day and must also manifest clinical symptoms if only the random glucose threshold is used.

A baseline and quarterly fasting glucose during the first year of therapy for patients with schizophrenia should be obtained in those receiving atypical antipsychotics and may be decreased to semiannually if no changes in fasting glucose are noted and if the individual lacks other risk factors (e.g., obesity, ethnicity). In general, symptoms of diabetes should be inquired about at each clinical visit. Monthly examination for the first 3 months and a consideration of glucose tolerance testing or postprandial glucose testing may be indicated in those who are at high risk for the development of diabetes due to ethnicity, agent used, family history, or obesity or who manifest abnormal fasting glucose measurements. A high index of suspicion for ketoacidosis should be maintained in these individuals.

Glycosylated hemoglobin (Hgb A1c) values reflect changes in glycemic control over a period of 120 days and thus will lag several months behind abnormalities in fasting and postprandial glucose. It is best used as a monitoring tool for those with established impairments in glucose control, but not as a routine method of screening for diabetes.

I will add parenthetically that it is much easier to obtain fasting glucose values for hospitalized patients than it is for patients living in unregulated environments. Many schizophrenic patients would not honor instructions to fast for eight hours, and some of them may misunderstand the instructions so as to exclude food but not soft drinks. The point is that fasting values are a lot easier said than done for many patients who are not inpatients. For this reason one should not underestimate the value of glycosylated hemoglobin tests as screening tests for schizophrenic populations, even with the afore-mentioned lag-time limitations, insofar as the results of these tests are not dependent on fasting values. It is possible that the most reliable monitoring results might be obtained by combining the results of HgbA1c draws with nonfasting random glucose tests. The HgbA1c would yield a small amount of false negatives most of which would be discovered by the non-fasting serum glucose tests, which are not subject to the vagaries of cooperation demanded by fasting tests. The two tests could be easily administered as a mass preliminary screening device. Fasting glucose tests would only be necessary as confirmatory tests in the event that either one of the preliminary tests were positive.

Psychiatric texts regarding laboratory monitoring rarely address such sordid problems as money. Since this is not a typical psychiatric text—and I am a patient as well as a psychiatrist—I will descend into venality. Differing labs have differing charges, so the prices quoted are rough ballpark estimates of 2004 charges by a lab worker who prefers to remain anonymous—similar to what occurs when reporters quote "authoritative sources in the state department. . . ." etc., etc. A random blood glucose should cost around $26.00. Fasting blood glucoses should cost the same. Tests for HgbA1c are more expensive and should cost about $64.00. White blood counts should cost around $37.00 and complete blood counts around $65.00. Liver function tests—sometimes ordered for patients on atypical antipsychotics—should cost around $54.00.

Other authorities recommend monitoring patients for waist size insofar as waist sizes above forty inches for men and thirty-five inches for women are supposed to indicate vulnerability to type 2 diabetes. I can assure the reader that most psychiatrists are not going to be encircling their male and female patients with tape measures, offering lame excuses about monitoring for type 2 diabetes.

Appendix D

Qualifications and Duties
of the Residential Care Administrator

The following information regarding the qualifications and duties, certifications, and recertifications of the administrators of RCFs is available on the Internet <http://www.dss.cahwnet.gov/ord/CCRTitle22_715.htm> in the document titled Manual of Policies and Procedures, Community Care Licensing Division, Adult Residential Facilities, Title 22, Division 6, Chapter 6, published by the State of California, Health and Human Services Agency, Department of Social Services.

80064 ADMINISTRATOR-QUALIFICATIONS AND DUTIES 80064

(a) The administrator shall have the following qualifications:
    (1) Attainment of at least 18 years of age.
    (2) Knowledge of the requirements for providing the type of care and supervision needed by clients including ability to communicate with such clients.
    (3) Knowledge of and ability to comply with applicable law and regulation.
    (4) Ability to maintain or supervise the maintenance of financial and other records.
    (5) Ability to direct the work of others, when applicable.
    (6) Ability to establish the facility's policy, program and budget.
    (7) Ability to recruit, employ, train, and evaluate qualified staff, and to terminate employment of staff, if applicable to the facility.
(b) Each licensee shall make provision for continuing operation and carrying out of the administrator's responsibilities during any absence of the administrator.
(c) The licensee, if an individual, or any member of the governing board of the licensed corporation or association, shall be permitted to be the administrator provided that he/she meets the qualifications specified in this section, and in applicable regulations in Chapters 2 through 7.

85064 ADMINISTRATOR QUALIFICATIONS AND DUTIES 85064

(a) In addition to Section 80064, the following shall apply.

(b) All adult residential facilities shall have a certified administrator.

(c) The administrator shall be at least 21 years of age.

(d) Have a high school diploma or pass a general education development test (GED).

    (1) Administrators employed prior to July 1, 1996, are exempt from this requirement.

(e) The administrator shall be on the premises the number of hours necessary to manage and administer the facility in compliance with applicable law and regulation.

(f) When the administrator is absent from the facility there shall be coverage by a designated substitute, who meets the qualifications of Section 80065, who shall be capable of, and responsible and accountable for, management and administration of the facility in compliance with applicable law and regulation.

(g) The administrator of a facility for seven to 15 clients shall have one year of work experience in residential care.

(h) The administrator of a facility for 16 to 49 clients shall have graduated from high school, or possess a GED, and shall have one of the following prior to employment:

    (1) Completion, with a passing grade, of 15 college or continuing education semester or equivalent quarter units, three of which shall be in nutrition, human behavior, administration, or staff relations.

    (2) One year of work experience in residential care.

(i) The administrator of a facility for 50 or more clients shall have graduated from high school, or possess a GED, and shall have one of the following prior to employment.

    (1) Completion, with a passing grade, of 60 college or continuing education semester or equivalent quarter units, six of which shall be in administration or staff relations.

    (2) Three years work experience in residential care, one year of which shall have been providing direct care to clients or assisting in facility administration.

(j) The administrator shall perform the following duties:

    (1) Where applicable, advise the licensee on the operation of the facility and advise the licensee on developments in the field of care and supervision.

(2) Development of an administrative plan and procedures to define lines of responsibility, workloads, and staff supervision.

(3) Recruitment, employment and training of qualified staff, and termination of staff.

(4) Provision of, or insurance of the provision of, services to the clients, individual needs and services plans.

(A) The licensing agency shall have authority to approve the use of a centralized service facility to provide any required services to two or more licensed facilities. Prior approval shall be obtained in writing.

(B) Examples of such centralized service facilities are a centralized laundry, dining room or kitchen serving two or more facilities.

(5) Arrangement for special provisions for the care and supervision and safety and guidance of clients with disabilities including visual or auditory deficiencies.

(A) Such provisions may include additional staff, safety and emergency information printed in braille, and lights to alert the deaf to emergency sounds.

(6) Arrangements for the clients to attend available community programs, when clients have needs, identified in the needs and services plan, which cannot be met by the facility but can be met by community programs.

(A) Such arrangements shall include, but not be limited to, arranging for transportation.

(k) Within six months of becoming an administrator, the individual shall receive training on HIV and TB required by Health and Safety Code Section 1562.5. Thereafter, the administrator shall receive updated training every two years.

(l) Administrators employed prior to July 1, 1996 shall be exempt from the requirements of Sections 85064(d), (h), and (i) above, provided that they have no break in employment as an adult residential facility administrator exceeding three (3) consecutive years.

(m) In those cases where the individual is both the licensee and the administrator of an adult residential facility, the individual shall comply with all of the licensee and certified administrator requirements.

(n) The Department may revoke the license of an adult residential facility for failure to comply with all requirements regarding certified administrators.

(o) Unless otherwise provided, a certified administrator may administer more than one licensed adult residential facility.

85064.2 ADMINISTRATOR CERTIFICATION REQUIREMENTS
85064.2

(a) An individual shall be a certificate holder prior to being employed as an administrator.
(b) To receive his/her certificate an applicant shall:
  (1) Successfully complete a Department approved initial Certification Training Program.
  (2) Pass a written test administered by the Department within sixty (60) days of completion of an Initial Certification Training Program.
  (3) Submit an application form to the Department's certification section within thirty (30) days of being notified of having passed the test. The application shall contain the following:
    (A) Proof that the applicant has successfully completed a Department approved Initial Certification Training Program.
    (B) A statement certifying that the applicant is at least twenty-one (21) years of age.
    (C) Fingerprint cards, or evidence that the applicant has submitted fingerprints to the Department of Justice at a live-scan facility, or a statement that the applicant has a current criminal record clearance on file with the Department.
    (D) A one hundred dollar ($100) processing fee.
(c) The Department shall not issue a certificate until it receives notification from the Department of Justice that the applicant has a criminal record clearance pursuant to Health and Safety Code Section 1522 or is able to transfer a current criminal record clearance pursuant to Health and Safety Code Section 1522(h)(1).
(d) It shall be unlawful for any person not certified under this Section to misrepresent himself or herself as a certified administrator. Any person willfully making any false representation as being a certified adult residential facility administrator is guilty of a misdemeanor.
(e) Certificates issued under this Section shall be renewed every two (2) years provided the certificate holder has complied with all renewal requirements.
(f) Certificates shall be valid for a period of two (2) years and expire on either the anniversary date of initial issuance or on the individual's birthday during the second calendar year following certification.
  (1) The certificate holder shall make an irrevocable election to have his or her recertification date for any subsequent recertification either on the date two years from the date of issuance of the cer-

tificate or on the individual's birthday during the second calendar year following certification.
(g) Time deadlines specified in Section 85064.2(b)(2) and (3) above may be extended for good cause as determined by the Department. Any request for extension of time shall be in writing and shall contain a statement of all facts the applicant believes constitute good cause to extend time.

85064.3 ADMINISTRATOR RECERTIFICATION REQUIREMENTS
85064.3

(a) Administrators shall complete at least forty (40) classroom hours of continuing education during the two-year certification period. Continuing education hours must relate to the Core of Knowledge and be completed through any combination of the following:
  (1) Courses provided by vendors approved by the Department, or
  (2) Accredited educational institutions offering courses that are consistent with the requirements of this Section, or
    (A) Examples of accredited educational institutions are Community and State colleges.
  (3) Courses offered by vendors approved by other California State agencies provided that:
    (A) The approval and enforcement procedure of that State agency are comparable to the approval and enforcement procedures of the Department, and
    (B) The course relates to the Core of Knowledge as specified in Section 85090(h)(1)(A) through (I).
    (C) Prior to taking a course from one of the entities specified in Section 85064.3(a)(2) or (3) above, the certificate holder should study the course description carefully to ensure that it fits within the Core of Knowledge as specified in Section 85090(h)(1)(A) through (I). If the course does not fit within the Core of Knowledge, it may not be credited toward the recertification requirement.
    (D) Examples of other California State agencies that meet the Department of Rehabilitation, the Board of Behavioral Science Examiners and the Board of Psychology.
  (4) Certified administrators required to complete continuing education hours required by regulations of the Department of Development Services, and approved by the Regional Center, may

have up to twenty-four (24) of the required continuing education course hours credited toward the forty (40) hour continuing
education requirement.

(A) Community college course hours approved by the Regional Center shall be accepted by the Department for
recertification.

(B) Any continuing education course hours in excess of
twenty-four (24) hours offered by the Department of Developmental Services and approved by the Regional Center
may be credited toward the forty(40) hour requirement provided the courses are not duplicative and relate to the core
of knowledge as specified in Sections 85090(h)(1)(A)
through (I).

(5) Continuing education hours must enhance the core of knowledge. Continuing education credit will not be provided for any
Initial Certification Training Program course.

(b) Courses approved for continuing education credit shall require the physical presence of the certificate holder in a classroom setting except that:

(1) The Department may approve courses where technology permits the simultaneous and interactive participation of the certificate holder, provided such participation is verifiable.

(c) To apply for recertification prior to the expiration date of the certificate,
the certificate holder shall submit:

(1) A written request to recertify postmarked on or before the certificate expiration date.

(2) Evidence of completion of forty (40) continuing education
hours as specified in Section 85064.3(a) above.

(3) Payment of one hundred dollar ($100) processing fee.

(d) To apply for recertification after the expiration date of the certificate,
but within four (4) years of the certificate expiration date, the certificate
holder shall submit:

(1) A written request to recertify.

(2) Evidence of completion of the required continuing education
hours as specified in Section 85064.3(a) above. The total number of hours required for recertification shall be determined by
computing the number of continuing education hours the certificate holder would have been required to complete if he/she had
remained certified. The date of computation shall be the date the
written request for recertification is received by the Department.

(3) Payment of a delinquency fee equal to three times the renewal
fee, or three hundred dollars ($300).

(e) Certificates not renewed within four (4) years of their expiration date shall not be renewed, restored, reissued or reinstated.

    (1) Holders of certificates not renewed within four (4) years of their expiration date shall complete an Initial Certification Training Program as specified in Section 85064.2(b).

(f) Certificate holders, as a condition of recertification, shall have a current criminal record clearance.

(g) A processing fee of twenty-five dollars ($25) shall be paid for the replacement of a lost certificate.

(h) A certificate holder shall report any change of mailing address within thirty (30) days to the Department's administrator certification section.

(i) Whenever a certified administrator assumes or relinquishes responsibility for administering an adult residential facility, he or she shall provide written notice within thirty (30) days to:

    (1) The licensing District Office(s) responsible for receiving information regarding personnel changes at the licenced facilities with whom the certificate holder is or was associated, and

    (2) The Department's administrator certification section.

Appendix E

The Federal Nursing Home Reform Act (OBRA)

In 1987, President Ronald Reagan signed into law the first major revision of the federal standards for nursing home care since the 1965 creation of both Medicare and Medicaid. The legislation created federal standards for long-term care facilities, meaning nursing homes, so that each resident could "attain and maintain his highest practicable physical, mental, and psycho-social well-being." Failure to conform to these standards could result in exclusion of the facility from Medicare and Medicaid funding. This law, titled the Federal Nursing Home Reform Act or better known as OBRA (Omnibus Budget Reconciliation Act), created a set of minimum standards of care and rights for people living in certified nursing facilities.[1]

Part of the law addressed the use of psychotropic medications since mental illness is present in a large percentage of nursing home patients. At the time of the passage of the law, it was felt that antipsychotics and benzodiazepines had been used excessively (and without appropriate diagnosis or monitoring for side effects) and often solely for the convenience of staff, while antidepressants had been underutilized because depression was often overlooked as a cause of behavioral disturbances.

The intent of the regulations was to prevent the misuse of psychotropic medications with their accompanying adverse side effects. One of the objectives of the OBRA-1987 law was to protect residents of long-term care facilities from medically unnecessary physical or chemical restraints imposed for purposes of discipline or convenience.

The Centers for Medicare and Medicaid Services (formerly The Health Care Financing Administration) is responsible for regulating nursing homes participating in the Medicare and Medicaid programs. As such, the agency developed interpretive guidelines for fulfilling OBRA requirements. These guidelines were implemented nationally in 1990 and remain in force. The guidelines were updated in July 1999.

The guidelines addressed the issues involved in the use of long-acting benzodiazepines, anxiolytics/sedatives, sleep medications, and antipsychotics, and required clinical justification for their initial and continued use. In addition, it was recommended that nonpharmacologic measures

412   THE CASEBOOK OF A RESIDENTIAL CARE PSYCHIATRIST

should be tried to address behavioral, psychosocial, and mental disorders. Some of the pharmacological guidelines were as follows:

- Psychoactive medications are regarded as chemical restraints and must be used to treat medical conditions. Psychoactive medications should not be employed to control behavior, nor should they be used for discipline or convenience.
- An attempt must be made to gradually reduce psychoactive medications with the eventual goal being complete discontinuation, unless there are clinical contradictions.
- Psychoactive drugs should be used only to treat specific medical symptoms or conditions. These conditions should be diagnosed and documented in the clinical record. A treatment plan should be developed that addresses the specific objectives of treatment and should also document negative reactions to the medications, should this occur.
- Antipsychotic drugs may be used in the patient with delirum or dementia only if there are psychotic or agitated features resulting in danger to the patient or to others. Such reactions may include screaming, shouting, excessive pacing, continuous crying, or other types of severe distress or functional impairment. Preventable causes of agitation must be diagnosed and excluded if possible. The nature and frequency of such behaviors should be documented.
- Mild agitation, restlessness, aimless wandering, memory deficiencies, and insomnia are deemed insufficient to justify the use of antipsychotic medication.
- Some of the medication abuses noted were:
  Inadequate monitoring of medications;
  Inadequate indications of medications;
  Inadequate documentation of adverse consequences;
  Duplication of medications;
  Excessive dosing of medications; and
  Excessive duration of medications.

Even though the OBRA laws were passed as recently as 1987, they are now probably obsolete. This is because the second generation atypical antipsychotics (SGAs) have less adverse side effects and frequently can be used advantageously to control mild agitation, restlessness, wandering, and can sometimes even increase cognitive functioning. So somebody should do something about OBRA because the regulations are unnecessarily restrictive with respect to the use of the new generation antipsychotics. That being said, I will add this idea as the seventh official goal of this book. The reason that this goal does not appear in the chapter on summary and recommendations (Chapter 27) is that I only thought of it when I was completing the appendixes, and the appendixes came after the final chapter, which is written in stone and cannot be changed. So just as DNA has impacted criminal law, SGA will impact OBRA law. Yet another example of how acronyms have changed our lives.

Although it was clearly stated that the intent of the OBRA regulations was to prevent the misuse of psychotropic medications with their accompanying adverse side effects, there were also other considerations. Thus some felt that the states were using federal money to pay for the nursing home care of patients. The 1950 amendments to the 1935 Social Security Act provided federal matching funds for medical services in nursing homes, although they excluded matching funds to state and county mental hospitals. Since the federal government supplied matching funds to nursing homes and not to state hospitals, the inevitable effect of this was to divert admissions to mental hospitals in favor of nursing homes. The mental hospital's loss became the nursing home's gain. This happened because mental patients do not disappear as a result of administrative decisions. What happened then was that some nursing homes started to look like minimental hospitals.

Several measures were taken to counteract this trend. Thus it was stipulated that if over one half of the patients in a nursing home were mentally ill, then the home should be recategorized as an Institution for Mental Disease otherwise known as an IMD. It was additionally stipulated that IMDs could not be supported by Medicaid. Obviously there are not many IMDs around. As a result of this policy, mentally ill patients were discouraged from admission to nursing homes. This policy created a backlog of eligible applicants for residential care facilities. This pattern of migration from state hospitals to nursing homes to residential care facilities is customarily thought of as deinstitutionalization, although some maintain that the patients have really remained institutionalized but the institutions have changed—so that the changes may be regarded as occurring as a consequence of transinstitutionalization rather than deinstitutionalization. Be that as it may, it is obvious that changes in mental health systems have ecological consequences that were not anticipated in the past and that mental patients will continue to exist regardless of the admission policies of institutions. Mental patients, somewhat like energy, cannot be created or destroyed.

However, there are ways in which a mental patient can be accepted into a nursing home. Thus if a patient has a concurrent medical illness, the patient may be eligible for admission. This would include patients who have dementia secondary to Alzheimer's disease or related diseases, patients who are terminally ill or comatose or suffering from severe cardiac or pulmonary illnesses, patients who have degenerative neurological diseases, or patients who are convalescing from a recoverable illness following discharge from a hospital.

Have these measures prevented nursing homes from becoming mini mental hospitals? I don't know. I suspect the results are quite variable. My own personal professional experience is in the treatment of non-geriatric patients of residential care facilities so my experiences with nursing homes are quite limited. The one experience I have had with nursing homes occurred after my mother had been hospitalized at the age of ninety-three with a fractured ankle. Her message to me, which I remember quite clearly was, "Martin, get me out of here. The only people here are old people and crazy people." She was only there for about four hours and I have always wondered how Medicare was billed for her hospitalization there.

Appendix F

A Brief History of Medicare

The following brief history of Medicare is provided on the Internet.[1]

1945   Harry Truman sends a message to Congress asking for legislation establishing a national health insurance plan.

Two decades of debate ensue, with opponents warning of the dangers of "socialized medicine."

By the end of Truman's administration, he had backed off from a plan for universal coverage, but administrators in the Social Security system and others had begun to focus on the idea of a program aimed at insuring Social Security beneficiaries.

1965   Medicare and its companion program Medicaid (which insures indigent recipients) are signed into law by President Lyndon Johnson as part of his "Great Society."

Ex-president Truman is the first to enroll in Medicare.

Medicare Part B premium is $3 per month.

1972   Disabled persons under age 65 and those with end-stage renal disease become eligible for coverage.

Services expand to include some chiropractic services, speech therapy, and physical therapy.

Payments to HMOs are authorized.

Supplemental Security Income (SSI) program is established for the elderly and disabled poor. SSI recipients are automatically eligible for Medicaid.

1982   Hospice benefits are added on a temporary basis.

1983   Change from "reasonable cost" to prospective payment system based on diagnosis-related groups for hospital inpatient services begins.

Most federal civilian employees become covered.

1984   Remaining federal employees, including President, members of Congress, and federal judiciary become covered.

1986   Hospice benefits become permanent.

1988   Major overhaul of Medicare benefits is enacted, aimed at providing coverage for catastrophic illness and prescription drugs.

Coverage is added for routine mammography.

1989   Catastrophic coverage and prescription drug coverage are repealed.

Coverage is added for Pap smears.

1992   Physician services payments are based on fee schedule.

1997   Medicare+Choice is enacted under the Balanced Budget Act. Some provisions prove to be so financially restrictive when regulations are unveiled that Congress is forced to revisit the issue in 1999.

1999   Congress "refines" Medicare+Choice and relaxes some Medicare funding restrictions under the Balanced Budget Refinement Act of 1999.

2000   Medicare+Choice Final Rule takes effect.

Prospective payment systems for outpatient services and home health agencies take effect.

Appendix G

The Twenty-Five Warning Signs
of Poor Documentation

The following is a quotation from the *Medicare Bulletin for Northern California* regarding progress note policy:[1]

Today as never before various caregivers depend on the accuracy of your documentation to provide appropriate treatment. Many of these health care providers will never meet you but will judge your professionalism by your chart entries or case summaries. Excellent documentation can distinguish you from others providing the same services and can result in professional referrals. Although you learn the fundamentals of good documentation in school, the passage of time and busy schedules may have caused you to become a bit lax. Here are 25 warning signs of poor documentation.

1. Records that are illegible.
2. Entries that are not dated and timed.
3. Obliterated entries.
4. Entries are not signed or assigned or countersigned without having been read first.
5. Entries for care not performed by the writer.
6. Insufficient information regarding prescriptions.
7. No date noted for followup.
8. No note regarding consent discussion.
9. Notes written more than 24 hours after care was provided.
10. Failure to document noncompliance.
11. No documentation of telephone calls.
12. No documentation of care provided to other physicians' patients.
13. No documentation of patient education offered or provided.
14. Charting only the abnormal.
15. Records kept in pencil.
16. Lots of blank spaces on the page.

17. Use of subjective rather than objective language.
18. No note regarding the patient is taking medications prescribed by another provider.
19. Critical remarks about other providers.
20. Egotistical remarks.
21. Test results that have no indication of physician review and/or patient notification.
22. Pages in the record that do not have the patient's name and identifying number on them.
23. Use of homegrown or unapproved abbreviations.
24. Records that make the patient sound sicker than he or she is.
25. Medication allergies or adverse reactions buried in the record rather than conspicuously evident.

Notes

Preface

1. CPT (2004). *Physicians' Current Procedural Terminology.* American Medical Association, Chicago, IL, p. 57. CPT © 2004 American Medical Association. All Rights Reserved.
2. Fleishman M (2002). Issues in psychopharmacosocioeconomics. *Psychiatric Services,* 53: 1532-1534.

Introduction

1. Rosenstein M, Milazzo-Sayre L, and Manderscheid R (1989). The care of persons with schizophrenia: A statistical profile. *Schizophrenia Bulletin,* 15: 45-58.
2. Lamb HR and Goertzel V (1977). The long-term patient in the era of community treatment. *Archives of General Psychiatry,* 34: 679-682.
3. VanPutten T and Spar JE (1979). The board-and-care home: Does it deserve a bad press? *Hospital and Community Psychiatry,* 30: 461-464.
4. Fleishman M (1985). Board-and-Care homes, 1984: Return of the house call. *Psychiatric Annals,* 15: 654-665; Fleishman M (1989). The role of the psychiatrist in board-and-care homes. *Hospital and Community Psychiatry,* 40: 415-418; Fleishman M (1990). Board-and-care psychiatry and the treatment of the seriously mentally ill. In Cohen NL (Ed.), *Psychiatry takes to the streets* (pp. 256-272). New York: Guilford; Fleishman M (1997). The changing role of the psychiatrist in board-and-care homes. *Psychiatric Services,* 48: 510-513.
5. Suppes T, Calabrese JR, Mitchell PB, Pazzaglia PJ, Potter WZ, Zarina DA (1995). Algorithms for the treatment of bipolar manic-depressive illness. *Psychopharmacological Bulletin* 32:469-474.
6. Sullivan MA (2002). CMHS drug cost update. *Bay Area Psychopharmacology Newsletter,* March, p. 4.
7. Mukherjee S, Decina P, Bocola V, Saraceni F, Scapicchio PL (1996). Diabetes mellitus in schizophrenic patients. *Comprehensive Psychiatry,* 37: 68-73.
8. Buse JB (2002). Metabolic side effects of antipsychotics: Focus on hyperglycemia and diabetes. *Journal of Clinical Psychiatry,* 63 (Supplement 4): 37-41.
9. Rubin RJ, Altman WN, and Mendelson DM (1994). Health care expenditures for people with diabetes mellitus, 1992. *Journal of Clinical Endocrinology and Metabolism,* 78: 809A-809F.
10. Grinfeld JG (1997). Mental health targeted as Medicare, Medicaid expenditures grow. *Psychiatric Times,* 14: 58.

420   THE CASEBOOK OF A RESIDENTIAL CARE PSYCHIATRIST

11. Sullivan AM and Cohen NL (1990). The home visit and the chronically men-tally ill: Board-and-care psychiatry and the treatment of the seriously mentally ill. In Cohen NL (Ed.), *Psychiatry takes to the streets* (pp. 42-60). New York: Guilford.
12. Goldman HH (1984). Epidemiology. In Talbot JA (Ed.), *The Chronic Mental Patient—Five Years Later* (pp. 15-31). Orlando, FL: Grune and Stratton.
13. Bachrach LL (1976). *Deinstitutionalization: An analytical review and socio-logical perspective.* Rockville, MD: National Institute of Mental Health.
14. Goldman (1984), Epidemiology, p. 16.
15. Vaccaro JV, Clark GH (Eds.) (1995). *Practicing psychiatry in the community.* Washington, DC: American Psychiatric Press Inc.
16. Csernansky, JG (Ed.) (2002). *Schizophrenia—A New Guide for Clinicians.* New York: Marcel Dekker Inc.
17. Talbott J (Ed.) (2002). *The Yearbook of Psychiatry and Applied Mental Health.* St. Louis, MO: Mosby.
18. VanPutten and Spar (1979). The board-and-care home.

Chapter 2

1. National Association of Residential Care Facilities, *1987 Directory of Resi-dential Care Facilities.* Richmond: NARCF.
2. Oversight hearing on enforcement of the Keys Amendment before the U.S. House of Representatives (1981). *Select Committee on Aging.* Washington, DC: U.S. Government Printing Office, Comm. Pub. No. 97-296, pp. 6 and 11.
3. Levenson-Palmer G., Chief, Administrative Support Bureau, Community Care Licensing Division, California Department of Social Services. Personal Communication.
4. *HCFA—OSCAR (Online Survey Certification and Reporting)* Form 672:F78-F93, September 2000.
5. *Nursing Home Statistical Yearbook* (1999). American Association of Homes and Services for the Aging.
6. Brown DA (2003). Break the cycle. *The Department of Health and Human Services, 50 Years of Service.* Faircount LLC,Tampa/London, p. 109.
7. Rosenheck R (2000). Cost-effectiveness for mentally ill homeless people: The application of research to policy and practice. *American Journal of Psychiatry,* 157: 1563-1570.
8. Kanapaux W (2004). Guilty of mental illness. *Psychiatric Times* 21 (Janu-ary): 1-5.

Chapter 3

1. Fleishman M (1985). Board-and-care homes, 1984: Return of the house call. *Psychiatric Annals,* 15: 654-665.
2. Delay J and Deniker P (1953). Les neuroplegiclues en therapeutique psychiatrique. *Therapie,* 8: 347.
3. Ayd F (1973). The future of pharmacotherapy: New drug delivery systems. *International Drug Therapy Newsletter.*

4. California State Department of Mental Hygiene (1972). A study of successful treatment, Sacramento, California Human Relations Agency.

5. Thomson C (1989). The president's column. *California Psychiatric Newsletter,* 3:1; *Community Psychiatry,* 40: 415-418.

6. Blaustein M (1985). Introduction and overview. *Psychiatric Annals,* 15: 633-638.

Chapter 4

1. Fleishman M (1985). Board-and-care homes, 1984: Return of the house call. *Psychiatric Annals,* 15: 654-665.

Chapter 5

1. Lerner AJ and Loewe F (1956). *My Fair Lady.*

2. Fleishman M (1985). Board-and-care homes, 1984: Return of the house call. *Psychiatric Annals,* 15: 654-665.

Chapter 6

1. Fleishman M (1985). Board-and-care homes, 1984: Return of the house call. *Psychiatric Annals,* 15: 654-665.

Chapter 7

1. American Psychiatric Association (1994). *Diagnostic and Statistical Manual of Mental Disorders,* Fourth Edition (pp. 285-290). Washington, DC: American Psychiatric Association.

2. Jibson MD (2002). Evidence-based pharmacotherapy of schizophrenia. Con. Journal of Psychotic Disorders, 6(4): 3. (Copyright 2002, Lippincott Williams & Wilkins).

3. American Psychiatric Association (1997). Practice guidelines for the treatment of patients with schizophrenia. *American Journal of Psychiatry,* 154(Supplement 4): 1-62.

4. Lehman AF, Steinwachs DM, and the Coinvestigators of the PORT Project (1998). Translating research into practice: The Schizophrenia Patient Outcomes Research Team (PORT) treatment recommendations. *Schizophrenia Bulletin,* 24: 1-10.

5. Expert consensus guideline series: Treatment of schizophrenia (1996). *Journal of Clinical Psychiatry,* 57(Supplement 12B): 1-58.

6. Chiles JA, Miller AL, Chrismon ML, Rush AJ, Krasnof AS, Shon SS (1999). The Texas Medication Algorithm Project (TMAP): Schizophrenia algorithms. *Journal of Clinical Psychiatry,* 60: 649-657.

7. Porter C (1934). *Anything goes.* Warner Brothers. Inc. All rights reserved. Used by permission.

8. Personal communication, Richard A Shadoan, MD, Director of the 1979 Residential Care Committee, Northern California Psychiatric Society.

9. Tohen MD and Grundy B (1999). Management of acute mania. *Journal of Clinical Psychiatry,* 60(Supplement 5): 31-34.

10. Personal communication, Jeanne Kwong, Health Educator, Community Behavioral Mental Health Services, San Francisco Department of Mental Health.

11. Personal communication, Ed Nasrah, PharmD, and Steve Protzel, PharmD.

12. Bateson G (1972). *Steps to an Ecology of Mind.* New York: Ballantine.

13. Lidz RW and Lidz T (1949). The family environment of schizophrenic patients. *American Journal Psychiatry,* 106: 332-345.

14. Fromm-Reichmann F (1948). Notes on the development of treatment of schizophrenia by psychoanalytic psychotherapy. *Psychiatry,* 11: 263-273.

Chapter 8

1. Donlon PT and Blacker KH (1976). Clinical recognition of early schizophrenia decompensation. *Diseases of the Nervous System,* 36: 323-330.

2. Fleishman M (1985). Board-and-care homes 1984: Return of the house call. *Psychiatric Annals,* 15: 654-660.

3. Ibid.

4. Ibid.

5. Kingsbury SJ, Yi D, Simpson GM (2001). Psychopharmacology: Rational and irrational polypharmacy. *Psychiatric Services,* 52:1033-1036.

6. Rittmansberger H, Meise U, Schauflinger K, et al. (1999). Polypharmacy in psychiatric treatment: Patterns of psychiatric drug use in Austrian psychiatric clinics. *European Psychiatry,* 14: 33-40.

7. Ito C, Kubuta Y, and Sato M (1999). A prospective survey on drug choice for prescriptions for admitted patients with schizophrenia. *Psychiatry and Clinical Neurosciences,* 53: 835-840.

8. Tapp A, Wood AE, Secrest L, Erdmann J, Cubberly L, Kilzien N (2003). Combination antipsychotic therapy in clinical practice. *Psychiatric Services,* 54: 55-59.

9. Young JL, Zonana HV, and Shepler L (1986). Medication noncompliance in schizophrenia: Codification and update. *Bulletin of the American Acacdemy of Psychiatry and Law,* 14: 105-122; Perkins DO (2003). Predictors of noncompliance in patients with schizophrenia. *Journal of Clinical Psychiatry,* 63: 1121-1127.

10. Task force for compliance. Noncompliance with medications: An economic tragedy with important implications for health care reform (1993). *Task Force for Compliance.* Baltimore, MD; Rand CS, Wise RA, Nides M, et al. (1992). Metered-dose inhaled adherence in a clinical trial. *American Revue of Respiratory Disease,* 146: 1559-1564.

Chapter 9

1.VanPutten T and Spar JE (1979). The board-and-care home: Does it deserve bad press? *Hospital and Community Psychiatry,* 30: 461-464.

2. Gerber RA (1981). Psychotropic medicines in long-term-care facilities. *San Francisco Medicine,* August. Medical care guidelines for psychiatric patients in residential care homes (1979) as approved by the *Northern California Psychiatric Society,* March, p. 19.

3. Suppes T, Calabrese JR, Mitchell PB, Pazzaglia CJ, Potter WZ, Zarina DA (1995). Algorithms for the treatment of bipolar manic-depressive illness. *Psychopharmacological Bulletin,* 32: 469-474; Chiles JA, Miller AL, Crismon ML, Rush AJ, Krasnof AS, Shon SS (1999). The Texas Medication Algorithm Project: Development and implementation of the schizophrenic algorithm. *Psychiatric Services,* 50: 69-74.

4. CPT Assistant (1992). *Authoritative Coding Information.* Chicago, IL: The American Medical Association.

Chapter 10

1. Sullivan AM and Cohen NL (1990). The home visit and the chronically mentally ill: Board-and-care psychiatry and the treatment of the seriously mentally ill. In Cohen NL (Ed.), *Psychiatry takes to the streets* (pp. 42-60). New York: Guilford.

2. Mares A and McGuire J (2000). Reducing psychiatric hospitalization among mentally ill veterans living in board-and-care homes. *Psychiatric Services,* 51(7): 914-921.

3. Bachrach LL (1981). Continuity of care for the chronic mental patients: A conceptual analysis. *American Journal of Psychiatry,* 138: 1449-1456.

4. Torrey EF (1986). Continuous treatment teams in the care of the chronic mentally ill. *Hospital and Community Psychiatry,* 37: 1243-1247.

5. Van der Kolk BA and Goldberg LH (1983). Aftercare of schizophrenic patients: Pharamacotherapy and consistency of therapists. *Hospital and Community Psychiatry,* 34: 343-348.

6. Test MA (1979). Continuity of care in community treatment. *New Directions for Mental Health Services,* 2: 15-23.

7. Torrey (1986). Continuous treatment teams, p. 1244.

8. Ibid, pp. 1246-1247.

9. Sharfstein SS (2001). The case for caring coercion. *Psychiatric Review— Sheppard Pratt Health System,* 3(1) (April).

10. Linking mentally ill offenders to community care (2001). *Analysis of the 2000-2001 budget bill, Legislative Analysts Office.*

11. Ibid.

Chapter 12

1. Fleishman M (2001). Medication management, medical necessity, and residential care. *Psychiatric Times,* 18: 6-9.

2. Lamb HR and Goertzel V (1977). The long-term patient in the era of community treatment. *Archives of General Psychiatry,* 34: 679-682.

3. VanPutten T and Spar JE (1979). The board-and-care home: Does it deserve bad press? *Hospital and Community Psychiatry,* 30: 461-464.

4. Fleishman M (1985). Board-and-care homes, 1984: Return of the house call. *Psychiatric Annals,* 15: 654-665; Fleishman M (1989). The role of the psychiatrist in board-and-care homes. *Hospital and Community Psychiatry,* 40: 415-418; Fleishman M (1990). Board-and-care psychiatry and the treatment of the seriously mentally ill. In Cohen NL (Ed.), *Psychiatry takes to the streets* (pp. 256-272). New York: Guilford; Fleishman M (1997). The changing role of the psychiatrist in board-and-care homes. *Psychiatric Services,* 48: 510-513.

5. Suppes T, Calabrese JR, Mitchell PB, Pazzaglia PJ, Potter WZ, Zarina DA (1995). Algorithms for the treatment of bipolar manic-depressive illness. *Psychopharmacological Bulletin,* 32: 469-474.

6. Meghrigian AG (1997). Detecting health care fraud and abuse—Memorandum for the California Medical Association, February.

7. Health care fraud and abuse data collection program: Reporting of final adverse actions. Office of the Inspector General (OIG), HHS Final Rule. *Federal Register* 1999 October 26;54(206):57740-57764.

8. Hanley KK (1998). Definitions of "Screening" and "Medical Necessity," preliminary report to the AMA House of Delegates. Interim Meeting. CMS Report 13-1-98.

9. Fleishman (2000). Economic grand rounds: The management of medication management. *Psychiatric Services,* April 51(4): 457-459.

10. California Medical Association (2001). *2001 California Physicians Legal Handbook.* San Francisco: California Medical Association. Published with permission of and by arrangement with the California Medical Association.

11. California Medical Association (2003). *2003 California Physicians Legal Handbook.* San Francisco: California Medical Association. Published with permission of and by arrangement with the California Medical Association.

12. Doctors irked by states' tactics on Medicaid fraud (2001). *American Medical Association News,* February 19, Vol. 44, p. 1. Copyrighted 2001, American Medical Association.

13. Fleishman M (2001). A psychiatric odyssey. 1997. *Psychiatric Times,* 14 (November): 28-30; Fleishman M (1998). The odyssey continues: The Medicare scissors of 1998. *Psychiatric Times,* 15(July): 54-55; Fleishman M (2001). A psychiatric odyssey—Part III: The Medicare audit (1998); *Psychiatric Times,* 15(October):59-60; Fleishman M (2001). A psychiatric odyssey—Part IV: More secrets of the Medicare audit (1999). *Psychiatric Times,* 16 (January):8-9; Fleishman M (2001). A psychiatric odyssey—Part V: The four little words that killed fee-for-service medicine (1999). *Psychiatric Times,* 16 (April): 31-32; Fleishman M (2001). A psychiatric odyssey—Part VI: Whistleblowers and this crapshoot called medicine (1999). *Psychiatric Times,* 16(June): 17-18; Fleishman M (2001). A psychiatric odyssey—Part VII: Medi-Cal enters the arena of psychiatric audits (1999). *Psychiatric Times,* 16(October): 22-23; Fleishman M (2001). A psychiatric odyssey—Part VIII: Adversarial linguistics and the lexicographer's wars (1999). *Psychiatric Times,* 16(December): 54-56.

14. Grinfeld JG (1997). Mental health targeted as Medicare, Medicaid expenditures grow. *Psychiatric Times,* 14: 58.

Chapter 13

1. Glaser D (2000). Understanding and surviving Medicare audits. *Minnesota Medicine,* 12: 29-31.

Chapter 14

1. *Medicare Bulletin for Northern California,* 96-4, National Heritage Insurance Company.
2. Glaser D (2000). Understanding and surviving Medicare audits. *Minnesota Medicine,* 12: 29-31.
3. Vanderpool D (2001). The privacy rule—how to handle the HIPAA hype. *Psychiatric Practice and Managed Care,* March/April, pp. 6-12.
4. VanPutten T and Spar JE (1979). The board-and-care home: Does it deserve a bad press? *Hospital and Community Psychiatry,* 30: 461-464.

Chapter 15

1. Fleishman M (1985). Board-and-care homes, 1984: Return of the house call. *Psychiatric Annals,* 15: 654-665.
2. Fleishman M (1989). The role of the psychiatrist in board-and-care homes. *Hospital and Community Psychiatry,* 40: 415-418.
3. CPT (2004). *Physicians' Procedural Code Terminology.* American Medical Association, Chicago, IL, p. 269. CPT © 2004 American Medical Association. All Rights Reserved.
4. Levy CJ (2002). Broken homes: A final destination for mentally ill, death, and misery. *The New York Times,* April 28 Section 1, p. 1.
5. Goffman E (1961). *Asylums: Essays on the social situation of mental patients and other inmates.* Garden City, NY: Doubleday, p. XIII.
6. McEvoy JP, Scheifler PL, and Frances A (Eds.) (1999). *The Expert Consensus Guideline Series: The Treatment of Schizophrenia.* Memphis, TN: Physicians Postgraduate Press.

Chapter 16

1. Gutheil TG (1999). Liability issues and liability prevention in suicide. In Jacobs DH (Ed.), *The Harvard Medical School guide to suicide assessment and intervention* (pp. 561-578). San Francisco: Jossey-Bass.
2. Pokorny AD (1983). Prediction of suicide in psychiatric patients: Report of a prospective study. *Archives of General Psychiatry,* 40(30): 249-257.
3. Fenton WS (2000). Depression, suicide, and suicide prevention in schizophrenia. *Suicide—Life-Threatening Behavior,* 30(1): 34-39.
4. Collaborative Working Group on Clinical Trial Evaluations (1998). Atypical antipsychotics for the treatment of depression in schizophrenia and affective disorders. *Journal of Clinical Psychiatry,* 59(Supplement 12): 41-45.

5. Knowlton L (2001). Decreasing suicide in schizophrenia. *Psychiatric Times,* 18: 20-21.

6. Buckley PF (1999). The role of typical and atypical antipsychotic medication in the management of agitation and depression. *Journal of Clinical Psychiatry,* 60(Supplement 10): 52-60.

Chapter 17

1. Shen F, Spencer R (2003). Risperdal Consta: A long-acting injectable atypical antipsychotic. *The Bay Area Psychopharmacology Newsletter,* Vol. 6, Issue 4, pp. 5-6.

2. Glazer WM, Kane JM (1992). Depot neuroleptic therapy: An underutilized treatment option. *Journal of Clinical Psychiatry,* 53(12): 426-433.

3. Ereshevsky L, Mascarenas CA (2003). Comparison of the effectiveness of different routes of antipsychotic administration pharmacokinetics and pharmacodynamics. *Journal of Clinical Psychiatry,* 64(Supplement 16):18-23.

4. Belanger-Annable MC (1985). Long-acting neuroleptics: The technique of intramuscular injection. *The Canadian Nurse,* September, 81(8): 41-43.

5. Curson DA, Barnes TR, Bamber RW, Platt SD, Hirsch SR, Duffy JC (1985). Long-term depot maintenance of chronic schizophrenic outpatients: The seven-year follow-up of the Medical Research Council—fluphenazine/placebo trial. *British Journal of Psychiatry,* 146: 469-474.

6. Hay J (1995). Complications at site of injection of depot neuroleptics. *British Medical Journal,* August 12 (7007): 311-421.

Chapter 18

1. Mowrer OH (1961). *The crisis in psychiatry and religion.* Princeton, NJ: D. Van Nostrand Company, Inc., p. 72.

Chapter 19

1. Porter C (1928). "Let's Do It." From *Paris.* Warner Brothers, Inc. All rights reserved. Used by permission.

Chapter 20

1. Ayd FJ Jr. (1970). The impact of biological psychiatry. In FJ Ayd Jr, B Blackwell (Eds.), *Discoveries in biological psychiatry* (pp. 230-243). Baltimore, MD: Ayd Medical Communications.

2. Roethlisberger F and Dickson W (1939). *Management and the worker: An account of a research program conducted by the Western Electric Company, Chicago.* Cambridge: Harvard University Press.

Chapter 21

1. Fleishman M (2003). Psychopharmacosocioeconomics and the global burden of disease. *Psychiatric Services,* 54: 142-144.

Chapter 22

1. Fleishman M (2002). Issues in psychopharmacosocioeconomics. *Psychiatric Services,* 53: 1532-1534.
2. Wyatt RJ, Henter I, Leary MC, and Taylor E (1995). An economic evaluation of schizophrenia—1991. *Social Psychiatry and Psychiatric Epidemiology,* 30(5): 196-205.
3. The Lewin Group (2000). *Access and utilization of new antidepressant and antipsychotic medications.* Falls Church, VA: Office of Health Policy, Office of the Assistant Secretary for Planning and Evaluation, and The National Institute for Mental Health, Department of Health and Human Services.
4. Ibid.
5. Aboud L (2004). Should family doctors treat serious medical illness? *The Wall Street Journal.* CCXLIII, No. 58, p. A1.
6. DiMasi JA, Hansen RW, Grabowski HG (2003). The price of innovation: New estimates of drug development costs. *Journal of Health Economics,* March, 22(2): 151-185.

Chapter 23

1. Medical Economics Staff (2001). *Drug Topics: 2001 Red Book.* Montvale, NJ: Medical Economics Company.

Chapter 24

1. CPT (2004). *Physicians' Current Procedural Terminology.* American Medical Association, Chicago, IL, p. 24. CPT © 2004 American Medical Association. All Rights Reserved.
2. Ibid.
3. Medicare Bulletin (1996). 96-4, National Heritage Insurance Co., Marysville, CA, p. 35.
4. Ibid.
5. King MS, Lipsky MS, Sharp L (2002). Expert agreement in Current Procedural Terminology evaluation and management coding. *Archives of Internal Medicine,* February 11, 162 (3): 316: 320.

Chapter 25

1. Hogarty CD, Goldberg SC, and the Collaborative Study Group (1973). Drug and sociotherapy in the aftercare of schizophrenic patients. *Archives of General Psychiatry,* 28: 54-64.

2. Lacro PJ, Dunn LB, Dolder CR, Leckband SG, Jest DV (2002). Prevalence of and risk factors for medication nonadherence in patients with schizophrenia: A comprehensive review of the recent literature. *Journal of Clinical Psychiatry,* 63(10): 892-909.

3. Weiden PJ, Olfson M (1995). Cost of relapse in schizophrenia. *Schizophrenia Bulletin,* 21: 419-429.

4. Wing JK (1977). The management of schizophrenia in the community. In Usdin G (Ed.), *Psychiatric Medicine* (p. 427). New York: Brunner/Mazel.

5. Vaughn CE and Leff J (1976). The influence of family and social factors on the course of psychiatric illness. *British Journal of Psychiatry,* 129: 125.

Chapter 26

1. Watson JD and Crick FHC (1953). *Nature,* 171: 737-738.

2. Khayyám O (n.d.). *The Rubaiyat,* st. 71.

Chapter 27

1. Fleishman M (1985). Board-and-care homes, 1984: Return of the house call. *Psychiatric Annals,* 15: 654-665; Fleishman M (1989). The role of the psychiatrist in board-and-care homes. *Hospital and Community Psychiatry,* 40: 415-418; Fleishman M (1990). Board-and-care psychiatry and the treatment of the seriously mentally ill. In Cohen NL (Ed.), *Psychiatry takes to the streets* (pp. 256-272). New York: Guilford; Fleishman M (1997). The changing role of the psychiatrist in board-and-care homes. *Psychiatric Services,* 48: 510-513.

2. Suppes T, Calabrese JR, Mitchell PB, Pazzaglia PJ, Potter WZ, Zarina DA (1995). Algorithms for the treatment of bipolar manic-depressive illness. *Psychopharmacological Bulletin,* 32: 469-474; Chiles JA, Miller AL, Crismon ML, Rush AJ, Krasnof AS, Shon SS (1999). The Texas Medication Algorithm Project: Development and implementation of the schizophrenic algorithm. *Psychiatric Services,* 50: 69-74.

3. McCoy JL and Conley RW (1990). Surveying board-and-care homes: Issues and data collection problems. *Gerontology,* 30(2): 147-153.

4. Gary Levenson-Palmer, California Department of Social Services Community Care Licensing Division, Administrative Support and Program Automation Bureau.

5. HCFA—OSCAR (Online Survey Certification and Reporting) Form 672:F78-F93, September 2000.

6. Hanley KK (1998). Definitions of "Screening" and "Medical Necessity": Preliminary report to the AMA House of Delegates. Interim Meeting. CMS Report 13-1-98.

7. Fleishman (1985). Board-and-care homes, 1984.

8. McEvoy JP, Scheifler PL, Frances A (Eds.) (1999). *The Expert Consensus Guideline Series: The Treatment of Schizophrenia.* Memphis, TN: Physicians Postgraduate Press.

9. Chiles JA, Miller AL, Crismon ML, Rush AJ, Krasnof AS, Shon SS (1999). The Texas Medication Algorithm Project: Development and implementation of the schizophrenic algorithm. *Psychiatric Services,* 50: 69-74.

10. The American Bar Association Commission on Legal Problems of the Elderly and Commission on the Mentally Disabled (1982). *A Model Act Regulating Board-and-Care Homes Guidelines for States.* October.

11. Board-and-care: Insufficient assurances that residents' needs are identified and met (1989). General Accounting Office, Washington, DC. February.

Appendix B

1. Long PW: Internet Mental Health <www.mentalhealth.com> copyright © 1995-1996. Drug list reprinted by permission.

Appendix C

1. Meyer JM (2002). A retrospective comparison of weight, lipid, and glucose changes between risperidone- and olanzapine-treated inpatients: Metabolic outcomes after one year. *Journal of Clinical Psychiatry,* 63(5):425-433. Copyright 2002, Physicians Postgraduate Press. Reprinted by permission.

Appendix E

1. Gurevich T, Cunningham JA (2000). Appropriate use of psychotropic drugs in nursing homes. *American Family Physician,* March 1, 61(5): 1437-1446.

Appendix F

1. Tucker Sutherland (Ed.). <www.SeniorJournal.com>.

Appendix G

1. *Medicare Bulletin for Northern California.* 96-4, November 1996, p. 35.

Index

Page numbers followed by the letter "t" indicate tables.

Printed in the United States
by Baker & Taylor Publisher Services